This book is due for return on or before the last date shown below.

AN OBSTETRICS AND GYNAECOLOGY VADE-MECUM

AN OBSTETRICS AND GYNAECOLOGY VADE-MECUM

Edited by

David K James MA MD FRCOG DCH
Professor of Fetomaternal Medicine, School of Human Development, Faculty of Medicine and Health Sciences, University of Nottingham, Queen's Medical Centre, Nottingham, UK

Ian R Johnson BSc DM FRCOG
Professor of Obstetrics and Gynaecology and Head, School of Human Development, Faculty of Medicine and Health Sciences, University of Nottingham, Queen's Medical Centre, Nottingham, UK

and

Alec McEwan MRCOG
Clinical Research Fellow, University Department of Obstetrics and Gynaecology, City Hospital, Nottingham, UK

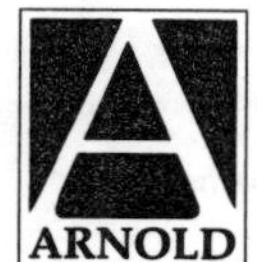

A member of the Hodder Headline Group
LONDON
Co-published in the United States of America by
Oxford University Press Inc., New York

First published in Great Britain in 2000 by
Arnold, a member of the Hodder Headline Group,
338 Euston Road, London NW1 3BH

http://www.arnoldpublishers.com

Co-published in the United States of America by
Oxford University Press Inc.,
198 Madison Avenue, New York, NY10016
Oxford is a registered trademark of Oxford University Press

Arnold International Students' Edition Published 2000
Arnold International Students' Editions are low-priced, un-abridged
editions of important textbooks. They are only for sale in developing countries.

Whilst the advice and information in this book are believed to be true and accurate at the date of going to press, neither the authors nor the publisher can accept any legal responsibility or liability for any errors or omissions that may be made. In particular (but without limiting the generality of the preceding disclaimer) every effort has been made to check drug dosages; however it is still possible that errors have been missed. Furthermore, dosage schedules are constantly being revised and new side-effects recognized. For these reasons the reader is strongly urged to consult the drug companies' printed instructions before administering any of the drugs recommended in this book.

British Library Cataloguing in Publication Data
A catalogue record for this book is available from the British Library

Library of Congress Cataloging-in-Publication Data
A catalog record for this book is available from the Library of Congress

ISBN 0 340 69274 X
ISBN 0 340 76202 0 (ISE)

1 2 3 4 5 6 7 8 9 10

Commissioning Editor: Joanna Koster
Production Editor: James Rabson
Production Controller: Iain McWilliams
Cover design: Terry Griffiths

Typeset in 9/11pt New Baskerville by
Phoenix Photosetting, Chatham, Kent
Printed and bound in India by Ajanta Offset & Packagings Ltd.

CONTENTS

SECTION 2: GYNAECOLOGY

SECTION 3: APPENDICES

CONTRIBUTORS

Philip Baker
Professor, Department of Obstetrics and Gynaecology, City Hospital, Nottingham, NG5 1PB, UK

David K James
Professor of Fetomaternal Medicine, School of Human Development, Faculty of Medicine and Health Sciences, Queen's Medical Centre, Nottingham NG7 2UH, UK

Ian R Johnson
Professor of Obstetrics and Gynaecology and Head, School of Human Development, Faculty of Medicine and Health Sciences, Queen's Medical Centre, Nottingham NG7 2UH

David Liu
Consultant Obstetrician and Gynaecologist, Department of Obstetrics and Gynaecology, City Hospital, Nottingham, NG5 1PB, UK

Alec McEwan
Clinical Research Fellow, University Department of Obstetrics and Gynaecology, City Hospital, Nottingham, NG5 1PB, UK

Marion Macpherson
Consultant Obstetrician and Gynaecologist, C Floor, East Block, Queen's Medical Centre, Nottingham, NG7 2UH, UK

Martin Powell
Consultant Obstetrician and Gynaecologist, C Floor East Block, Queen's Medical Centre, Nottingham, NG7 2UH, UK

Ian Stuart
Consultant Obstetrician and Gynaecologist, Diana, Princess of Wales Hospital, Grimsby DN33 2BA, UK

Ian Symonds
Lecturer, Department of Obstetrics and Gynaecology, Derby City General Hospital, Derby DE22 3NE, UK

Wim van Wijngaarden
Consultant Obstetrician and Gynaecologist, Divisie Verloskunde en Gynaecologie, Academisch Medisch Centrum, Meibergdreet 9, Postbus 22660, 1100 Amsterdam

PREFACE

On the first day of your new post in obstetrics and gynaecology you will probably undergo an induction process. It is likely to involve discussions on health and safety at work, fire drills, study leave applications and perhaps a refresher course in CPR. There will be time allocated for a rapid tour of the department, explanation of the rota and assignment to consultant teams. You may be fortunate enough to be shown a video on 'suturing an episiotomy' and you should have a session devoted to neonatal resuscitation. It may then be a number of days or even weeks before you have any formal teaching on how to actually do the job. Although the situation is improving all the time, education is mostly confined to one session a week. If you are lucky you will be on call with a registrar who is willing to teach you the basics (even if his or her long-term motive is to be called out of bed as little as possible). However, even the best of our seniors forget what it means to know very little and will often assume too much knowledge on your part or make apparent jumps in their reasoning or logic thus confusing you further. Over a 6-month period you are likely to glean small treasures of information from a variety of sources which often cannot be found in standard textbooks. The aim of this manual is to set out the problems facing a new SHO in obstetrics and gynaecology and to take them through the diagnostic and therapeutic steps which they will be expected to follow by their seniors. Rather than having chapters on 'endometriosis', 'placenta praevia' or 'cervical intraepithelial neoplasia' we have incorporated the information into chapters such as 'pelvic pain', 'bleeding in late pregnancy' and 'the abnormal smear". We have done our best to collect as many helpful hints as possible. No apology is given for this simplistic problem-solving approach; we are all aware how inadequately medical school prepares us for work.

Starting obstetrics, and to some extent gynaecology, can come as a confidence blow. You may recently have come from a post where you regularly managed general medical emergencies on your own and with great competence. However, the basic skills you require no longer involve a stethoscope and an ECG. Instead vaginal examinations and CTGs will become your methods of assessment. You may feel incompetent, underutilized and undervalued in your first few weeks, like an on-looking medical student again. Even the essential skills such as blood letting and cannula insertion will usually be done by the midwives. Suturing of perineal tears was once the domain of the junior doctor on the labour ward. Even this now (fortunately) will be done by most midwives unless it is a really difficult tear. However, a major objective of these positions for the GP trainees and new 'career' gynaecologists should be education as well as service.

Therefore, in your first few weeks demand tutoring on CTGs and insist that seniors check your vaginal findings with you. You will not be expected to work in isolation on the labour ward. Difficult deliveries, severe CTG problems, twins, breeches, acute abdomens and other emergencies **must** all be supervised by the registrar. If you are taking on too much responsibility or are being inadequately supported by your second on call, the senior midwife in charge is likely to do something to intervene even if you do not. You will work side by side with the registrar more than in any other specialty. If you are called to a problem it is more than likely that he or she will need to review the patient as well. The aim of this manual is not to allow you to work independently, but to enable you to present the problems clearly to your seniors having already done the basics. Senior midwives can also be extremely helpful and will often gently guide you towards the correct decision. However, if you do not consult your registrar you are ultimately responsible and, as with doctors, there are good midwives and bad.

To live up to its title, a Vade-Mecum must have charts and tables. There are many of these to be found in obstetrics and gynaecology, but few are used frequently by an SHO. In the appendices are those which are most commonly used.

It has been suggested recently that the time for SHOs in obstetrics is almost up and that the ever increasing role of midwives is removing the need for junior doctors on the labour ward and in antenatal clinics. It is difficult to see how this could occur unless we are to introduce would-be obstetricians directly into registrar posts. Similarly, a whole generation of GPs will be created who feel uneasy at managing the simpler problems of pregnancy. Within a few weeks of starting your new role we suspect that you will find yourself a vital part of the team. We hope this manual will help a little during this time and continue to be a useful source of reference whilst you are caring for women and their problems.

David K James
Ian R Johnson
Alec McEwan

SECTION I: OBSTETRICS

SECTION 1: OBSTETRICS

obstetrics

CONTENTS

1

DIAGNOSING PREGNANCY

SYMPTOMS AND SIGNS

AMENORRHOEA

Most pregnant women will have missed a period. It is assumed in dating the pregnancy that ovulation occurs 14 days after the onset of the last period. As this is not always reliable, establishing the cycle pattern is important, especially to identify those women with long cycles and possibly later ovulation. It is helpful to remember that in longer cycles the luteal phase nevertheless only lasts 14 days and it is the follicular phase which varies in length. Therefore a woman with a 5-week cycle is likely to ovulate around day 21. Hence her actual due date will be a week later than the one calculated from her last menstrual period (LMP) using a standard obstetric wheel.

PREGNANCY SYMPTOMS

Subtle sensation of 'feeling pregnant'. Classical pregnancy symptoms are:

- nausea and vomiting (morning sickness)
- breast tenderness
- frequency of micturition
- cravings for certain kinds of food (pica)
- tiredness.

Later in pregnancy, fetal movements are usually felt in nulliparous women from 20 weeks and in multiparous women from 18 weeks.

PREGNANCY SIGNS

- breast enlargement
- pigmentaton of the nipples
- Montgomery's tubercles

- an enlarged soft uterus on bimanual examination
- a mass arising from the pelvis after 12 weeks
- palpable fetal parts and a heart beat audible with a Pinard's stethoscope or Doppler ultrasound later in pregnancy.

Central body temperature

The central body temperature will continue to be elevated by 0.3–0.5°C after fertilization for longer than 7 days after ovulation as a result of sustained progesterone secretion by the corpus luteum. (The central body temperature should be measured rectally and performed at the same time in the morning before rising.)

PREGNANCY TESTS

BIOCHEMICAL TESTS

HCG (human chorionic gonadotrophin) is produced by the trophoblast and consists of two subunits. The alpha subunit of HCG is structurally very similar to that of luteinizing hormone (LH), follicle-stimulating hormone (FSH) and thyroid-stimulating hormone (TSH) and may cause cross reactions when HCG levels are measured. The beta subunit however is different. All current biochemical tests are based on the reaction of antibodies to the beta subunit of HCG in either urine or blood. The beta HCG concentration in urine increases from 5 to 50 IU/L in the first week after implantation (which occurs 5–7 days after ovulation) and is around 100 IU/L on the first day of the missed period. The presently commercially available urine HCG test kits are able to detect HCG concentrations as low as 25 IU/L and therefore may be able to confirm pregnancy even before a period is missed. A number of these early positive results may become negative, as up to 50% of these very early pregnancies may not be viable and regress spontaneously. Very early and weak positive results should be re-tested. Testing is best performed on early morning urine specimens.

Serum beta HCG is usually measured quantitatively. Levels of >15 IU/L beta HCG are indicative of pregnancy and in a normal intrauterine pregnancy it approximately doubles every 36 to 48 hours during most of the first trimester.

ULTRASOUND SCAN

An intrauterine gestation sac is visible at 4–5 weeks' gestation by vaginal scan and at 6–7 weeks by abdominal scan. A fetal heart beat can be seen with a vaginal scan from 5–6 weeks and with an abdominal scan as from 6–7 weeks. An intrauterine pregnancy is normally seen using a transvaginal scan at serum beta HCG levels over 1500 IU/L.

2

THE ANTENATAL CLINIC

AIMS OF ANTENATAL CARE

Antenatal care is primarily aimed at ensuring the well-being of the mother and fetus during pregnancy. For the majority of women at low risk of an adverse outcome to themselves and their baby this will entail the following:

- the provision of education, advice and support
- the treatment of minor ailments (e.g. heartburn, constipation)
- the implementation of a clinical and laboratory screening programme to confirm they remain at low risk.

For the minority of women who are at risk of an adverse outcome, antenatal care will **also** be aimed at addressing these risks and implementing strategies to prevent, ameliorate or treat adverse outcomes.

PRECONCEPTION/PRE-PREGNANCY VISIT

Before conception, women should be offered counselling regarding a number of issues:

- Diet, smoking and alcohol intake.
- The effect of pregnancy on medical disorders they may have.
- The effect of medical disorders and their treatments on the pregnancy.
- Secure rubella immunity.
- Investigate any familial (genetic) disease(s).
- Preconception folic acid supplementation (400 micrograms daily) should be discussed and offered to all.
- Women with a history of neural tube defects, haemolytic anaemia, diabetes and those taking anti-convulsant medication should be prescribed 5 mg of folic acid per day.

- Psychological support is offered in particular to those who had problems in previous pregnancies.
- Moderate non-aerobic exercises should be encouraged, moderate and more severe aerobic exercises discouraged.
- Specific work hazards should be addressed and certain leave arrangements may have to be made to avoid exposure to contaminated environments before conception (e.g. anaesthetists, operating theatre personnel, workers in the pottery, glass, laundry and dry cleaning industry). Exposure to visual display unit (VDU) screens is not associated with any significant complications.
- Consider previous obstetric difficulties the risks of recurrence and how any future pregnancies would be managed.

BOOKING VISIT

The booking visit at the general practitioner or the specialist clinic has the main purpose of confirming the pregnancy and identifying any factors which may have an adverse effect on the fetus or mother, i.e., the identification of high-risk pregnancies. This is usually between 6 and 14 weeks. The professional providing this initial assessment varies with local practice but most women are seen by the general practitioner first followed by the community midwife.

Problems arising during pregnancy may lead to re-categorization from low- to high-risk groups and additional management is instituted where appropriate. Certain risk factors should prompt referral to other disciplines such as cardiology in cases of cardiac murmurs, haematology in cases of thrombocytopenia or a history of thromboembolic disease or to psychiatry in cases with a history of postnatal illness.

The local policy for fetal abnormality screening should be discussed and prenatal diagnosis offered where indicated. The anticipated antenatal progress and management as well as labour and the probable mode of delivery are discussed.

All issues mentioned under 'the preconception visit' should be reinforced, especially smoking and diet, and, if not discussed before, issues such as iron supplementation, dental health, parentcraft classes and maternity benefits should be raised.

At the booking visit a decision is made regarding the form of antenatal care, i.e. whether low-risk GP/community midwife-based, high-risk obstetric specialist care, or shared care between these two. Any problems arising during pregnancy may alter the form of antenatal care.

RISK ASSESSMENT

Risk of an adverse maternal or fetal outcome is identified by history taking, physical examination and specific investigations. It should start at the pre-pregnancy visit, but is formally performed at the booking visit and updated throughout pregnancy, labour and puerperium. Not all risk factors carry the same significance and alterations to planned management should be individualized.

Risk factors possibly requiring additional monitoring and/or interventions in pregnancy are given below (this list is not exhaustive).

HISTORY

- **Present pregnancy:** Uncertain last normal menstrual period, prolonged cycle. History of recent contraception, pill use. Multiple pregnancy, bleeding in pregnancy, intrauterine contraceptive device (IUCD) *in situ*.
- **General:** Extremes of reproductive age (<18 years and >35 years), certain ethnic groups (e.g. haemoglobinopathies, hepatitis B, human immunodeficiency virus [HIV]), poor social circumstances, diet (vegetarian, vegan).
- **Obstetric:** Problems in previous pregnancies and deliveries, cervical cerclage, anaemia, pre-eclampsia, intrauterine growth restriction (IUGR), gestational diabetes, stillbirths, congenital abnormalities, premature labour, previous excessive birth weight, operative deliveries, postpartum haemorrhage (PPH), postnatal depression.
- **Gynaecological:** Fibroids, infertility treatment, polycystic ovarian syndrome, cervical smear test results, cone biopsy of the cervix, prolapse surgery.
- **Past medical history:** Thrombo-embolic disease, cardiovascular disease (e.g. congenital heart problems, valvular diseases, arrhythmias, cardiomyopathies), hypertension, respiratory disorders, diabetes, epilepsy, autoimmune disorders, previous surgery, orthopaedic problems (e.g., prolapsed disc, spinal and pelvic fractures), neurological problems, drug related disorders, allergies, blood transfusion.
- **Family history:** Inherited disease, diabetes, mother and/or sisters with pre-eclampsia.

PHYSICAL EXAMINATION

- Height <152 cm, weight >85 kg or <50 kg, elevated blood pressure, cardiac murmurs, abdominal masses and scars, pelvic examination on indication (e.g. if bleeding, discharge, smear overdue).

INVESTIGATIONS

- **At booking:** Full blood count, Hb electrophoresis for haemoglobinopathies (thalassaemia, sickle cell) if relevant, blood group, rhesus factor and antibody screen, serology for rubella, syphilis, hepatitis B, (HIV if indicated and after counselling), urine analysis (glucose, protein, blood, ketones) and culture. Cervical smear only if at high risk or if unlikely to return postnatally.
- **Diabetes:** Practices vary with respect to screening for gestational diabetes. Often glucose tolerance is tested later in pregnancy, usually around 28 weeks, in women who are at risk of developing an abnormal glucose tolerance or diabetes during pregnancy such as:
  - women with a first degree relative with insulin dependent diabetes mellitus
  - women with a previous unexplained stillbirth
  - women who have had a baby weighing >4 kg at birth
  - women with previous gestational diabetes.

More recently random blood glucose levels have been taken from **all** women at booking and repeated at 28 weeks (*see* p. 14.)

It may also be indicated in specific circumstances occurring during pregnancy, e.g. polyhydramnios, persistent glycosuria.

ULTRASOUND SCAN INVESTIGATIONS

Routine ultrasound screening varies according to availability and local practice. The aims are:

- accurate dating of the pregnancy
- early detection of multiple pregnancies and their chorionicity
- screening for fetal abnormality (see below).

Most centres provide at least one scan during pregnancy and combine dating with detailed fetal anomaly scanning, usually between 18 and 20 weeks. Twelve-weeks scans followed by scans at 20 weeks will allow for more accurate dating and better fetal anomaly screening. Dating scans are important as inaccuracies due to poor recollection of the last menstrual period (LMP) and varying cycle length occur in at least 30% of cases. Because biological divergence occurs after 20 weeks, dating scans should be performed by this gestation. Most units adhere to the 'scan dates' if these differ by more than 7 days from the LMP dates.

SCREENING FOR FETAL ABNORMALITIES

There are a number of different options but their availability varies between units:

- First trimester scanning for increased nuchal translucency (for chromosomal abnormalities).
- Biochemical serum screening in the second trimester (16–19 weeks) for Down's syndrome and neural tube defects (including spina bifida and anencephaly).
- Detailed scanning for structural anomalies (18–20 weeks).
- Invasive testing (chorionic villous sampling or amniocentesis) for certain single gene, metabolic and chromosomal abnormalities.

FOLLOW-UP CLINICS

At each antenatal visit (GP, midwife or hospital) screening for risk factors is continued. This is achieved by history, physical examination and investigations. Support, advice and education are provided at each visit. Attendance to antenatal classes is encouraged.

FREQUENCY OF VISITS

- **Low risk:** A minimum of 5 visits are recommended by the RCOG: 12, 20, 28–32, 36 weeks and term with additional visits for screening purposes which do not require a full examination unless indicated. In practice women are seen more frequently.
- **High risk:** This will depend on the nature of the problem.

AT EACH VISIT

History

- General well-being: Problems at a physical, psychological and social level are discussed and support, advice and/or treatment is given (e.g. varicose veins – thromboembolic disease (TED) stockings).
- The first fetal movements ('quickening') are usually not felt before 20 weeks by nulliparous women and before 18 weeks by

multiparous women, but thereafter enquiry should be made that the mother is feeling movements (see below).

Physical examination

- **General examination:** Blood pressure, mucous membranes (?anaemia), oedema. In some units weight is not routinely recorded during follow-up visits because of its poor clinical value. However, rapid weight gain may be an indicator of inappropriate water retention and oedema accompanying pre-eclampsia.
- **Abdominal examination:**
  - **Fundal height** (Fig 2.1): This may also be measured using a tape measure (number side down) from the fundus to the upper border of the symphysis pubis. This is of more value if the same person performs the examination at each visit. From 24–36 weeks, the fundal height in centimeters approximates to the gestational age in weeks (+/- 2 weeks). However, trends are as important as absolute values.
  - **Liquor volume:** Often unreliable unless there is a gross increase or decrease.

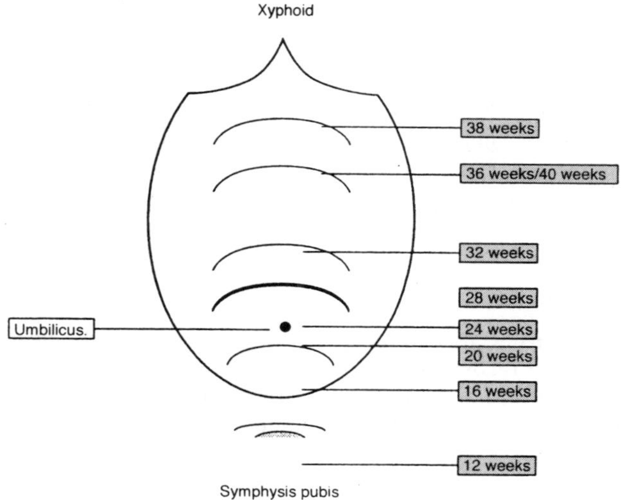

Figure 2.1 Fundal height measurements.

- **Lie:** Longitudinal, transverse or oblique. An abnormal lie in the third trimester may be an indication of placental, uterine, fetal or intra-abdominal abnormalities (e.g. placenta praevia, fibroids, hydrocephalus, ovarian mass).
- **Presentation:** Cephalic or breech. From 36 weeks a breech presentation is increasingly unlikely to turn spontaneously.
- **Engagement:** This is expressed as proportion of the head which can be felt abdominally in fifths. '5/5' means that the whole fetal head can be felt abdominally whereas 0/5 means that none of the head can be felt. Descent of the fetal head into the pelvis commonly occurs in nulliparous women by 36 weeks and may not occur in multiparous women until during labour.
- **Fetal movements:** Should be noted if present; absence of fetal movements during a follow-up visit should be investigated (see pp. 141).
- **Fetal heart:** This should be listened for during each visit either by a Pinard's stethoscope or a Doppler ultrasound device. If it cannot be heard, immediate referral for ultrasound investigation is indicated.

INVESTIGATIONS

- Urine analysis
- Full blood count usually twice more after the booking visit
- Rhesus antibodies, if Rhesus negative, at 28 and 36 weeks
- Random blood glucose at 28 weeks (depending on local policy).

With specific indications

Urine cultures, glucose tolerance test (commonly at 28 weeks and sometimes repeated at 34 weeks), red cell antibodies (e.g. previous blood transfusion), ultrasound scans (subject to local practice), chorionic villus sampling or amniocentesis.

RECORDS

These vary from area to area. All pregnant women should carry some form of record which is jointly used by all professionals (GP, midwife and obstetrician). In some cases the patient held records are the only ones used without separate notes being held by the GP or the hospital.

3

NORMAL LABOUR AND DELIVERY

Definition

Progressive shortening and/or dilatation of the cervix accompanied by regular uterine activity after 24 weeks' gestation. May need two vaginal examinations to diagnose with certainty.

A 'show' (shedding of the mucous plug from the cervix accompanied by blood streaks), or rupture of the membranes (artificial or spontaneous) alone do not constitute labour.

STAGES OF LABOUR

The first stage is between the onset of labour and full dilatation of the cervix. The second stage is between full dilatation and delivery and the third stage is between delivery of the neonate and delivery of the placenta. The first stage of labour can be divided into a latent phase (from shortening of the cervix to 3–4 cm dilatation) and an active phase (from 3–4 cm to full dilatation of the cervix). The third stage is delivery of the placenta.

Progress

Normal progress during the active phase of labour is defined as a minimum cervical dilatation of 1 cm per hour. Progress during the latent phase varies depending on the initial state of the cervix and increase in regularity, strength and duration of contractions. Normal progress during the second stage of labour will on average assure delivery within an hour in nulliparous and within half an hour in multiparous women after starting expulsive efforts. During the third stage of labour, expulsion of the placenta is anticipated to occur within 1 hour of delivery.

Normal progress of labour will depend on the efficacy of uterine activity (**P**owers), the adequacy of the birth canal (**P**assage) and the size, lie and presentation of the fetus (**P**assenger).

Blood loss

Up to 500 mL is considered to be normal.

MANAGEMENT

On admission the antenatal notes **must** be available and reviewed.

- Confirm gestational age, parity and any deviations from normality.
- Establish time of onset, frequency and duration of the contractions and state of the membranes (ruptured or not).
- A general examination including blood pressure, temperature and pulse measurements is performed.
- On abdominal examination the fundal height, lie, presentation and engagement of the presenting part is noted.
- On vaginal examination (if not contraindicated) consistency, length and dilatation of the cervix, position, descent of the presenting part and colour of the amniotic fluid, if present, are noted.
- Urine analysis (dipstick), check for recent full blood count (if haemoglobin is low intravenous [iv] access, group and save, or cross-match of blood may be indicated) and Rhesus status.
- A partogram is commenced on which all observations (fetal and maternal), procedures, and the administration of fluids and drugs are recorded.

FIRST STAGE

- No solid food during the active phase of labour, though normal eating and drinking is possible in the latent phase.
- Practices vary with respect to fetal heart rate monitoring in normal labour. An admission cardiotocogram of 20 to 30 minutes is performed in most units and, if normal, is followed by intermittent fetal heart rate monitoring. If this is performed by auscultation then this should be during and for one minute after contractions every 15 minutes.
- Note frequency and strength of contractions every 15 minutes.
- Note colour of the liquor at regular intervals.
- Four-hourly maternal observations; note fluid input, urinary output and urine analysis.
- Two to four-hourly vaginal examinations to assess progress according to local practice.
- Rupture membranes when indicated (e.g. slow progress or to assess colour of liquor with fetal heart rate abnormalities).

- Pain relief: *see* pp. 114.
- Encourage mobilization: it may stimulate progress.
- Try to provide 'one to one' midwifery care.
- Encourage support from partner and/or relatives.

SECOND STAGE

- The active second stage is timed from when the woman first starts to bear down ('push').
- Start pushing when there is an urge to bear down or sooner if indicated (e.g. 'fetal distress').
- Continuous or intermittent fetal heart rate monitoring (during and for one minute after every contraction).
- Allow epidural analgesia to wear off to achieve a bearing down sensation to allow effective pushing, but not so much that pain relief is totally abolished.
- To optimize the efficiency of pushing allow the mother to assume her preferred position (e.g. semi-recumbent, propped up, squatting, kneeling, the left lateral position). Avoid lying flat on her back as it may produce caval compression.
- Review and consider intervention if the active second stage exceeds one hour (nulliparous) or 30 minutes (multiparous), or earlier if there is no progress. The progress made and the presence of maternal or fetal distress should be taken into account.
- Dry and wrap the baby and hand to mother.

THIRD STAGE

Manage third stage actively:

- Syntometrine Intramuscular (im) 1 amp (5 IU syntocinon + 500 micrograms ergometrine) with delivery of anterior shoulder (use only syntocinon 10 IU im if hypertension has complicated the pregnancy or if other maternal cardiac disease exists).
- Controlled cord traction after signs of placental separation with one hand suprapubically holding the fundus back to avoid uterine inversion.
- Check that the placenta and membranes are complete.

POSTPARTUM

- Record all maternal observations (temperature, pulse, blood pressure, respiration rate).
- Check and record blood loss.

- Check vulval and vaginal lacerations and repair if necessary.
- Keep in the delivery room for one to two hours for observation of blood loss and vital signs.
- Keep baby warm and encourage early breast feeding.
- Practices will vary with regard to examination of the newborn that is healthy. Some examine the baby in the delivery room (beware hypothermia); others delay this until a few hours have elapsed.

4

THE NORMAL PUERPERIUM

Definitions

The normal puerperium is the interval between delivery and 6 weeks postpartum. It involves reversal of the changes of pregnancy into a pre-pregnancy state.

FROM PREGNANCY TO PRE-PREGNANCY STATE

- **Uterine involution:** The fundus is palpable 10–12 cm above the pelvis after delivery. In 7 days it is reduced by 50% in size and abdominally impalpable by day 10 to 14. Thus the height of the fundus reduces by approximately 1 cm a day. Involution is aided by oxytocin and may cause more painful contractions ('after pains') in breast feeding mothers. The internal cervical os closes 2–3 weeks after delivery.
- **Placental site and lochia:** Placental site repair requires some 6 weeks. This is accompanied by shedding of the decidua, debris and necrotic material known as lochia. Normal lochia is, on average, red for 3 days, pink for 7 days and gone in 3–6 weeks.
- **Urinary tract:** Increase in the tone of the urinary tract musculature tone accompanies the decrease in progesterone plasma levels. The gestational dilatation of the ureter decreases over 4–8 weeks. Bruising, oedema and perineal injury may result in inability to void particularly during the first 24 hours after delivery. Stress incontinence is not uncommon after delivery, but in most instances will disappear within 6 weeks, particularly with pelvic floor exercises.
- **Reversal of hormonal changes:** Progesterone and oestradiol levels will return to pre-pregnancy levels within 72 hours. It will take oestrone 4 days, oestriol 8–14 days and LH and FSH 3 weeks to establish pre-pregnancy levels. Insulin sensitivity and glucose tolerance may take 8–10 weeks to return to normal although diabetics return to their pre-pregnancy regime immediately after delivery.

- **Breasts:** The inhibitory action on lactation of hormones responsible for breast enlargement during pregnancy (oestrogens and progestagens) ceases shortly after delivery. Lactation is initiated mainly under the influence of prolactin and human placental lactogen (HPL.) This process is accompanied by vascular engorgement which usually occurs 3–5 days after delivery. This can be very uncomfortable and cause a low-grade pyrexia.
- **Haemoglobin:** Increased on day 1 after which it falls to a minimum by day 5 and increases again until day 9 after which it stabilizes. Check haemoglobin (Hb) on day one to avoid an erroneous diagnosis of anaemia.
- **White blood count:** Increases after delivery (granulocytosis) and is reduced to pre-pregnancy levels by day 6.
- **Coagulation:** Hypercoagulability during pregnancy is further increased after delivery of the placenta, is at its highest during the first 2 weeks and reverts to pre-pregnancy state in about 6 weeks. These changes are accompanied by an increase in platelet levels up to the 50th day post partum.
- **Bowel motility:** Constipation is common for 3–4 days after delivery. Return of intestinal smooth muscle tone, reduction in perineal discomfort and adequate hydration will usually establish normality.
- **Ovulation:** A third of all first cycles are anovulatory. In non-lactating women the first ovulation usually occurs in 6–10 weeks. About 40–50% of women will resume sexual activity within 6 weeks after delivery.
- **Weight loss:** Average weight gain during pregnancy is 12.5 kg. Delivery will reduce weight by 6 kg. Ten weeks after delivery there is, on average, a 2.25 kg increase from booking weight. In lactating women this surplus is reduced to 0.7 kg.
- **Psychological state:** About 40–50% of women will experience mild transient anxiety and/or depression ('postnatal blues') within 7 days of delivery. This is not to be confused with the much more serious postpartum depression which usually occurs later and requires psychiatric management. It is triggered by a combination of major emotional and hormonal changes, fatigue and may be influenced by non-anticipated events during delivery (intervention) and difficulties with breast feeding.
- **Striae gravidarum:** These will remain and become pale in 6–9 months.

MANAGEMENT

Management consists of the monitoring of normal changes, detection and treatment of problems, facilitation of infant feeding and provision of emotional support. In the UK this will be the responsibility of midwives in the absence of complications.

- **Day 1:**
  - **Monitoring the first hour after delivery in the labour suite:** Temperature, pulse, respiration (TPR) and blood pressure, fundal height, bladder, vaginal bleeding.
  - **Thereafter:** 6 hourly TPR and blood pressure, fundal height, bladder, vaginal bleeding.
- **Day 2–14:**
  - **Daily observations:** TPR and blood pressure, bladder (first 48 hours), fundal height, breasts, lochiae, calves. Mental state. Feeding.
- **Further:**
  - **Follow up and treatment of specific problems/complications:** Spinal headache/tears/scars/urinary retention (catheter), constipation (laxatives), breast milk expression, etc.
- **Miscellaneous**
  - Give anti-D 500 IU im (or more if Kleihauer test is positive) within 72 hours after delivery in all Rhesus negative women with Rhesus positive babies.
  - Offer rubella vaccination to those women who are not immune.
  - Check the haemoglobin level within the first 24 hours after delivery.
  - Ensure proper rest. Consider sleeping tablets (e.g, Temazepam 10 mg orally at night) when indicated.
- **Advice on**
  - perineal hygiene
  - exercise abdominal muscles
  - pelvic floor exercises
  - contraception (see below).
- **Arrange postnatal clinic/GP visit at 6 weeks.**

POSTNATAL CONTRACEPTION

Over 90% of women who are less than 5 months postpartum, breast feeding every 4 hours and giving less than 150 mL of supplementary feeding will be anovulatory. However, this should not be relied on as the main form of contraception.

METHODS

Barrier methods

- male/female condoms;
- diaphragm: (re)fit 4–6 weeks after childbirth (size may change).

Intrauterine contraceptive device

Insertion at 6 weeks postnatal check (commonest practice); insertion immediately postpartum may be associated with greater rates of expulsion and perforation.

Combined oral contraceptives

Relatively contraindicated in the early puerperium as they inhibit lactation and there are concerns about their procoagulant effects at a time of natural hypercoagulability. Start on day 21 if not breast-feeding.

Progestagen only pill

Favoured postnatal contraceptive. No effect on lactation. Minimal transfer to infant in breast milk. Need to be taken at same time every day routinely.

Parenteral progestagens

Depo Provera (150 mg im) is an effective postnatal contraceptive but it can cause irregular bleeding. It is secreted in the breast milk with uncertain biological significance for the infant. The injections need to be repeated every 12 weeks.

Progestagen implants/rings

Implants: similar benefits and risks as injectable progestagens but the duration of its action is much longer. Irregular bleeding is the most common indication for removal. Rings are not to be used until after 6 weeks postpartum because of the high expulsion rate.

Sterilization

Can be performed at Caesarean section, just after delivery, or later in the puerperium. Pre-pregnancy or early pregnancy counselling is important and preferable to counselling at a later stage. If there is any doubt, the procedure should be delayed until after the puerperium. In general, interval sterilization is to be preferred over puerperal sterilization. There is an increased failure rate (4 in 1000) compared with interval sterilization (2 in 1000). Risks of puerperal sterilization are regret (increased reversal requests later), general anaesthetic related problems and a hypercoagulable state requiring prophylaxis. Immediately postpartum a mini-laparotomy is performed as the size of the uterus will prevent the safe insertion of a laparoscope. The Fallopian tubes are usually ligated either by applying Filshie clips, or by a (modified) Pomeroy's technique during which the tubes are double ligated with catgut and a segment is removed. Virtually all sterilizations are carried out at the time of Caesarean section or as an interval procedure with very few performed through a postpartum minilaparotomy.

5

PLANNED DELIVERY

ELECTIVE CAESAREAN SECTION

INDICATIONS

Most indications are relative, few absolute. Factors include past obstetric history, age, weight and parental wishes. The decision should be made as early in pregnancy as possible.

Absolute indications

- Fetal
  - transverse or oblique lie
- Placental
  - placenta praevia >grade I
- Maternal
  - tumours obstructing vaginal delivery (fibroids, cysts)
- Previous uterine surgery
  - classical Caesarean section
  - full thickness myomectomy
  - previous hysterotomy.

Relative indications

- Fetal
  - IUGR, breech presentation
- Maternal
  - previous Caesarean section
  - serosal myomectomy
  - colporrhaphy
  - successful incontinence surgery
  - cervical cancer
  - maternal request
- Feto-maternal
  - cephalo-pelvic disproportion
  - multiple pregnancy.

PREOPERATIVE PREPARATION

The patient is preferably prepared for the operation, aftercare and recovery well in advance of the procedure. This includes collaboration in particular with anaesthetists in case of any potential anaesthetic problems.

Anaesthetics

Every patient should be seen by an anaesthetist to discuss anaesthetic management.

Consent

The patient must be aware of the nature, extent and potential complications of the operation and the potential impact on future pregnancies. Signed consent must be obtained after full discussion of these. Ideally consent should be obtained by the surgeon performing the operation.

Investigations

- fetal assessment might be undertaken depending on the indication
- full blood count
- group and save, or cross-matched, depending on local practice and specific problems (e.g. cross-match for anaemia, placenta praevia, anticipated difficult surgery)
- other investigations for specific indications, (e.g. clotting screen, ultrasound scan to confirm lie).

Communication

- inform theatres, anaesthetists and paediatricians.

Prepare patient

- nil by mouth 6 hours prior to operation
- shave suprapubic skin on the same day and as close to the operation as possible.

Drugs

n.b. Local regimens vary and some examples are given

- Thrombo-embolic prophylaxis (e.g. heparin 5000 IU subcutaneously (SC) twice a day (bd), dalteparin 2500 IU SC every day (od), TED stockings)
- prophylactic antibiotics (e.g. co-amoxiclav 1.2 g or cefuroxime 750 mg at induction)

- Ranitidine 150 mg the night before and 2 hours preoperatively. Sodium citrate (30 mL) immediately prior to surgery.

OPERATION

Anaesthesia

- epidural or spinal block (or both) is the preferred method
- general anaesthesia: risk of aspiration syndrome is lessened by the use of cricoid pressure before intubation and rapid/'crash' induction of anaesthesia
- avoid caval occlusion – 15 degree wedge under the patient's right side;
- empty bladder – catheter
- clean abdomen – chlorhexidine or iodine and drape.

Skin incision

n.b. Before the skin incision, ensure that all the required staff are present (paediatrician, midwife).

- low transverse or Pfannenstiel – better healing, wound strength and cosmetic results than a midline incision;
- sub-umbilical midline – only used when greater surgical access to the abdomen is required.

Procedure

- rectus sheath
  - open transversely in a Pfannenstiel incision
  - open longitudinally in a sub-umbilical incision
- peritoneum – incise longitudinally
- utero-vesical peritoneal fold – lift from the lower uterine segment and incise transversely
- bladder – push downwards to allow clear access to the lower uterine segment
- lower uterine segment – incise transversely in a slightly curved fashion with the convexity upwards to avoid downward tearing at the edges
- classical Caesarean section – vertical incision in the upper segment of the uterus
- deliver by sliding hand under the head to direct it through the incision followed by fundal pressure; Wrigley's forceps may be used
- oxytocics – iv oxytocin 10 IU is given by the anaesthetist with the delivery of the baby

- empty cavity – remove placenta, swab the uterine cavity and confirm it is empty.

Closure

- the sutures used for closure vary e.g. Polyglactan (Vicryl), polyglycolic (Dexon) sutures or chromic catgut. Only the skin may be closed with non-absorbable sutures, or staples which need to be removed later.
- uterus – two continuous inverting layers of sutures.
- peritoneum – practice varies. More adhesions have been reported with peritoneal closure and many surgeons do not repair either peritoneal layer.
- check ovaries and fallopian tubes.
- clean blood from abdominal cavity and confirm uterus contracted.
- rectus sheath – continuous suture.
- skin – continuous subcuticular or interrupted sutures, or staples.
- Empty the vagina of blood by fundal pressure. Intravaginal 'swabbing' may introduce infection.
- Ensure proper succinct but comprehensive documentation of the procedure. Note the estimated blood loss. Ensure that postoperative pain relief and fluid regimes and appropriate prophylaxis (antibiotics, antithromboembolic) are written up.

COMPLICATIONS

A summary of possible complications of a Caesarean section is given in Table 5.1.

POSTOPERATIVE RECOVERY AND ADVICE

Mobilization from day 1, usually fully mobilized by day three and home on day 4–6 (depending on local practice).

Pain relief options

- im opiates (e.g. pethidine 50–150 mg every 4 to 6 hours usually with an antiemetic).
- Voltarol 75–100 mg daily im or pr in two divided doses. (Voltarol should not be used with renal compromise, or major blood loss because of risk of renal failure). After day 2 oral analgesia is usually adequate
- Paracetamol 0.5 to 1 g every 4 to 6 hours.
- Dihydrocodeine 30 to 60 mg every 4 to 6 hours.

Table 5.1 Complications of a Caesarean Section

Complication	Management
BLEEDING	
Normal loss is up to 600 mL. Significant loss is over 1000 mL and resuscitation and transfusion must be considered.	
Severed vessels (e.g. from the angle of the uterine wound)	Ligate the bleeding vessels and secure haemostatsis.
Uterine atony (especially after prolonged labour and oxytocin)	Options: Massage the uterus, give oxytocics, prostaglandins (e.g. Haemabate), ligate the uterine arteries or iliac arteries, perform a hysterectomy.
Placenta praevia	As for uterine atony.
HAEMATOMA	Conservative management with antibiotics and resuscitation may be sufficient. Progressive enlargement will necessitate evacuation of blood clot and ligation of bleeding vessels.
URINARY TRACT INJURY	
Bladder (often after previous pelvic surgery)	Repair in two layers by experienced surgeon and leave the catheter on full drainage for 5–10 days under antibiotic cover.
Ureter (particularly after sutures of tears at angles)	Reimplantation by a urologist. Ureteric stents may be sufficient if the ureter is kinked.
ANAESTHETIC	
Epidural/spinal	See page 117
General anaesthesia (aspiration syndrome)	Specialized intensive care
GENERAL	
Thromboembolism (emergency Caesarean section carries a 20-fold increase in thromboembolic risk over vaginal delivery)	Full anticoagulation if suspected until diagnosis confirmed or refuted. Have a low threshold for perfusion scanning in cases of possible PE. Organize venogram or Doppler ultrasonography for investigation of DVT.
Pulmonary problems (pnuemonia, atelectasis)	Diagnosis by X-ray. Treat with physio and antibiotics
Ileus	Treat by NBM and iv infusion. Check electrolytes regularly and correct imbalance
Urinary retention	Catheterize and culture urine. Regimes vary. Resistant cases may require a suprapubic catheter or intermittent self-catheterization.
INFECTION	
Urinary tract	Diagnose with urine cultures and treat with antibiotics.
Endometritis (presenting with pain, discharge or secondary PPH)	Treat with co-amoxiclav or a cephalosporin and metronidazole after taking a high vaginal swab and blood cultures.

Wound infection	Take a wound swab and treat with co-amoxiclav/flucloxacillin/cephalosporin. Drain any haematoma or abscess.
Pelvic abscess	Incision and drainage by an experienced surgeon. Take a swab from the abscess cavity and treat with antibiotics (co-amoxiclav/flucloxacillin/cephalosporin and metronidazole).
RETAINED PRODUCTS Should not occur if the uterus is properly explored before closure.	Evacuation by an experienced surgeon (there is a serious risk of uterine perforation). Do not rely simply on ultrasound findings to make the diagnosis. Antibiotics should be commenced prior to the procedure.

- Thrombo-embolism prophylaxis: continue until fully mobilized or longer if moderate to high risk (e.g. previous pulmonary embolism (PE) or deep vein thrombosis (DVT), pre-eclampsia, thrombophilia, infection).

Postoperative

- Check fundus, lochia, wound, bladder, urinary output.
- Pulse rate and blood pressure every 4 hours or more often if indicated.
- **Day 1:**
  - Full blood count. Start haematinics if low Hb and consider blood transfusion if the Hb is below 8 g/dL or if symptomatic (breathless or dizzy).
  - IV infusion: continue until oral fluids are tolerated.
  - Check: fundus, lochia, wound, bowel sounds, bladder palpation, urinary output; pulse rate and blood pressure every 4 hours.
- **Daily checks:**
  - Fundus, lochiae, wound, breasts, bladder, legs (calves), pulse rate, and blood pressure every 12–24 hours, state of mind, lungs if indicated.
  - Sutures or staples are removed on day 4 or 5 (subcuticular absorbable sutures can be left).
  - Breastfeeding should be started as soon as possible; consider breast pump if the baby is in the special care baby unit (SCBU).

Contraception

To be arranged before discharge – *see* ' Postnatal contraception', p. 21.

Future deliveries

The likely mode of future deliveries should be discussed by a senior obstetrician before discharge from hospital (*see* 'Problems at Booking – previous Caesarean section', p. 41).

INDUCTION OF LABOUR

Definition

The intentional initiation of uterine contractions and cervical dilatation from 24 weeks with the aim to deliver the fetus before the spontaneous onset of labour.

Induction of labour is indicated when the benefit of delivery outweighs the benefits of continuing the pregnancy to the baby and/or the mother. These benefits can range from evident medical reasons (e.g. deteriorating maternal renal function in pre-eclampsia or fetal red cell iso-immunization) to more debatable social indications (e.g., prior to husband going on business trip). Many indications are relative and some will depend on obstetricians' attitudes and the gestational age. The number of days which defines prolonged pregnancy as an indication to induce labour is contentious but most obstetricians agree that induction to prevent postmaturity is undertaken 10 to 14 days after the expected date of delivery. Dates preferably confirmed by an early ultrasound will avoid unnecessary inductions for this indication.

Pre-requisites

- longitudinal lie
- no placenta praevia
- no umbilical cord felt on vaginal examination
- no previous classical Caesarean section
- no history of hysterotomy or full thickness myomectomy
- normal fetal heart rate pattern (CTG).

METHODS

These can be divided into medical (prostaglandins and oxytocin) and mechanical methods (amniotomy, 'membrane sweep', hygroscopic tents or dilators). Other medical and mechanical methods exist but are not commonly used. The choice depends on the state of the cervix as determined by the Bishop Score (Table 5.2) and the obstetric history. Amniotomy is the cornerstone of any method of induction.

Table 5.2 Bishop Score

Score	0	1	2	3
Station of presenting part	−3 cm	−2 cm	−1 /0 cm	+1 cm
Cervical dilatation	Closed	1–2 cm	3–4 cm	>4 cm
Length	>4cm	2–4 cm	1–2 cm	<1 cm
Consistency	Firm	Medium	Soft	
Position	Posterior	Mid	Anterior	

Unfavourable: <5; moderately favourable: 5–8; favourable: >8.

BISHOP SCORE

Unfavourable cervix (Bishop Score <5)

Prior to amniotomy, prostaglandin E_2 (PGE_2) is placed in the posterior fornix to 'ripen' the cervix. This may be done by using pessaries, tablets, gels and polymers. Regimens vary locally. More than one application may be required although three will usually be sufficient. The Bishop Score and parity will determine the dose. The interval between applications varies between 4 and 12 hours depending on the time of the day and local practice. PGE_2 insertion may initiate contractions which may or may not progress into labour. The latter is more likely to occur with a favourable cervix and may be the prime objective of PGE_2 insertion. After each insertion it is recommended that the patient stays in bed for up to 1 hour. The fetal heart rate and uterine activity must be monitored before and for at least 1 hour after each PGE_2 insertion.

Once the cervix is dilated, further doses of PGE_2 are withheld and an amniotomy is performed. Oxytocin and prostaglandins are synergistic. If there is no uterine activity, an oxytocin infusion can be commenced. However, if there is some uterine activity, to avoid uterine hypertonus, oxytocin infusion should not be started too soon after the administration of PGE_2 and amniotomy.

One or more hygroscopic dilators can be inserted into the cervix and produce softening and dilatation through expansion by absorbing fluid. Improvement of the Bishop Score takes from 4 to 8 hours after insertion. After removal of the dilators an amniotomy can be performed and oxytocin commenced if required. This approach is not widely used.

Moderately favourable cervix (Bishop Score 5–8)

PGE_2 may be used to 'ripen' the cervix further and/or initiate contractions. Commonly not more than one insertion will be required.

The higher dose preparations should be avoided. Alternatively, an amniotomy and oxytocin infusion can be started. The latter may be delayed for 2 to 4 hours to see if labour commences spontaneously. The option chosen will be determined by local practice and individual situations.

Favourable cervix (Bishop Score >8)

An amniotomy followed by oxytocin infusion (with or without 2–4 hours delay) is the method of choice.

- **Amniotomy:** This is performed during a digital vaginal examination using an amniotomy hook or a Kocher's forceps. Before rupturing the forewaters a forelying umbilical cord should be excluded. The amount and colour of the liquor is noted. Controlled rupture of the membranes means controlling the outflow of liquor through the vagina digitally/manually by keeping the examining hand in place and is done when the presenting part is not engaged. Always check for cord prolapse before concluding the procedure irrespective of the station of the head.
- **'Membrane sweep':** It is common practice when induction is considered with a Bishop Score of 5 or more for the membranes to be 'swept' digitally by the obstetrician as he performs the cervical assessment. This involves a circular separation of the membranes from the internal aspect of the cervix with the index finger. This procedure is usually undertaken away from the labour suite. Fetal heart rate monitoring is usually not undertaken in these cases, but it must be remembered that it is a form of induction of labour (releasing local prostaglandins). Acceptance and use of this practice varies.
- **Oxytocin infusion:** The rate of intravenous oxytocin infusion is titrated against uterine activity. The aim is to achieve regular 3–4 contractions every 10 minutes. Higher frequencies are associated with uterine hypertonus and fetal hypoxaemia. The rate is controlled with electronic drip counters or infusion pumps. Gravity drip sets are potentially dangerous and to be avoided. Overdilution may cause overhydration. Oxytocin (10 IU) in 500 cc 5% dextrose is an adequate concentration. The infusion rate is commenced at 2 to 4 mU/min and is usually doubled every 15 minutes up to 32 to 40 mU/min or until adequate contractions are established. Regimens may vary locally. The infusion is continued for 1 hour after delivery. Continuous fetal heart rate monitoring is mandatory during an oxytocin infusion. Although multiparous patients and those with previous

Caesarean sections may require oxytocin during induction of labour, it is always best to discuss its use with the registrar. Some units use a different protocol in these circumstances.

KEY POINT

When siting a venflon in the labour ward (size 16 G or larger) for any reason, including the induction of labour, blood should be taken for a full blood count and group and saved, which can be stored in the labour ward fridge and sent to the laboratory if subsequently needed in an emergency.

INDUCTION AFTER SPONTANEOUS RUPTURE OF THE MEMBRANES

This can be done by PGE_2 or intravenous oxytocin infusion. The latter can be started with or without prior ripening of the cervix with PGE_2 as described above. Although not widely practised, PGE_2 can also be given orally (regimes vary from a total of 3 doses of 1.5 mg PGE_2 every half hour to 1 hour, to increasing doses of 0.5 mg to 1.5 mg every half hour with four doses in total).

COMPLICATIONS OF INDUCTION OF LABOUR

- **Failed induction:** No dilatation over 3 cm with an appropriate regime and an adequate time allowed. Mostly in nulliparas with a low Bishop Score and unlikely in multiparous women. This diagnosis should only be made by a senior obstetrician because of the need for alternative management (usually delivery by Caesarean section).
- **Hyponatraemia:** Due to the antidiuretic hormone activity of oxytocin. Prolonged infusions with high doses of oxytocin and diluted solutions may cause fluid retention, pulmonary oedema, electrolyte imbalance, coma and death (these should be exceptionally rare).
- **Fetal distress:** More common with fetal indications for induction (e.g. intrauterine growth retardation). Can also be a result of hyperstimulation – may require iv bolus of a tocolytic (see below). Possible fetal hypoxia and the need for fetal pH estimation and/or urgent delivery should be considered.
- **Hyperstimulation:** Stop oxytocin infusion or wash out PGE_2. Consider an iv bolus of ritodrine (5 mg) or another tocolytic (e.g. salbutamol 2.5 mg). Immediate delivery by Caesarean section may be the only option.
- **Cord prolapse:** Many occur after amniotomy, in particular with an unengaged presenting part and uncontrolled rapid drainage

of liquor. Immediate delivery by Caesarean section is mandatory if the fetus is alive. If the diagnosis is made during a vaginal examination, the examiner should apply upward pressure to the presenting part until delivery (by another obstetrician). Pressure on the uterine fundus towards the pelvis will bring a high head to the pelvic brim and reduce the risks of cord prolapse occurring at amniotomy.

- **Placental abruption:** This may occur particularly following an uncontrolled amniotomy in polyhydramnios. Sudden reduction in uterine volume may result in the placenta shearing off the uterine wall. Management will depend on blood loss and fetal condition, but an emergency Caesarean section may be necessary.
- **Uterine rupture:** Uterine scars (previous Caesarean section/hysterotomy/myomectomy) and high parity are predisposing factors. Very uncommon in nulliparas.
- **Post-partum haemorrhage:** This is more common following prolonged inductions with high doses of oxytocin, failed inductions and long labours (all due to uterine atony). (See page 121 for discussion of management.)

6

THE HIGH-RISK ASSESSMENT UNIT AND DAY CARE

Pregnancies with an increased risk of an adverse outcome to the mother and/or fetus may need more intensive surveillance than the routine antenatal clinic can provide. However, hospital admission to an antenatal ward may not be necessary.

The high-risk day care unit provides a different environment from the antenatal clinic and allows for more time per patient and investigations to be done without having to resort to admission to the antenatal ward. Such a unit is usually run by a specially dedicated team consisting of a consultant with a feto-maternal medicine background and support staff including obstetricians and midwives. Patients can be seen more frequently and flexibly than normal antenatal clinics would allow.

Women seen at such units vary with local practice but might include the following features:

- Women for prenatal diagnosis (counselling and invasive procedures); women with medical problems who need a multidisciplinary input in their management and cases where there is doubt regarding fetal well-being.
- This unit will also function as a direct referral unit for general practitioners and community midwives when they want a woman to be seen and assessed urgently, but not necessarily admitted.
- All invasive procedures not requiring a general or regional anaesthetic, ranging from chorionic villus sampling and amniocentesis, to fetal blood sampling and fetal surgery (local expertise permitting), can be performed in such units.
- Multidisciplinary management is commonly practised. This may involve, for example, clinical genetics, diabetology, obstetric medicine, cardiology, haematology, paediatric surgery, etc.
- Maternal assessment can be performed with the aid of, where appropriate, automated blood pressure machines and full access to emergency laboratory services. Fetal assessment may include

detailed ultrasound scanning, biophysical profile scoring and umbilical arterial Doppler measurements (see pp 88).

The major advantages of this unit are:

- centralization and concentration of high risk pregnancies
- instigation of protocols for the more common problems
- a major reduction in antenatal bed usage.

7

PERINATAL MEETINGS

Definition

These are multidisciplinary meetings held on a regular basis (usually at least monthly) to discuss recent stillbirths and neonatal deaths. They may cover maternal and/or neonatal morbidity as well (subject to local practice). It is an exercise which is aimed at the education of all staff to prevent recurrence where possible and may create a basis for unit policy decisions.

Participants usually include: obstetricians, midwives, neonatologists/paediatricians, pathologists, general practitioners and specialists from other disciplines when appropriate. Proper preparation is crucial and all the results of the requested investigations have to be available and presented where relevant. All levels of staff should participate in the discussion which is preceded by a presentation of the case by the obstetric, paediatric and pathology staff involved. All those present are bound by patient confidentiality. On many occasions the discussion will aid the clinician in counselling the parents at their postnatal visit and therefore it is essential that these meetings are held before such a counselling session takes place.

Checkpoints

Checkpoints in the preparation for perinatal mortality meetings:

- Those involved in the case, and those presenting, know it is going to be discussed: obstetricians, neonatologists, pathologist, general practitioners, midwives and others on occasion.
- The results of all (laboratory) investigations are available (haematology, biochemistry, serology, bacteriology, genetics, post-mortem, etc.)

The aims for each case discussed are:

- Consensus on the cause of death
- Consensus on the factors leading to death
- Identification of preventable factors

- Assessment of the potential value of alternative management
- Consensus on the management during the next pregnancy
- ? Change in unit policy for similar cases/situations.

Perinatal morbidity meetings cover both current and completed pregnancies. Management is discussed. Potential outcomes are reviewed with undelivered cases and alternative and better management strategies are considered with delivered cases. The use of videos for illustration of fetal problems is to be encouraged.

8

THE OBSTETRIC FLYING SQUAD

The obstetric flying squad was developed and introduced to assist pregnant women suffering serious acute obstetric problems away from the hospital.

The common indications to call out a flying squad are:

- bleeding in pregnancy
- labour problems
- pre-eclampsia
- complication of the third stage.

Assessment for the need of a flying squad is performed by senior obstetric staff. It needs to be emphasized that it takes time to organize a flying squad and in the UK it is quicker to bring the patient to hospital by the ambulance service. The debate is whether it is safer to treat the patient before moving her.

A flying squad team normally consists of an obstetrician, a paediatrician, an anaesthetist (all of at least registrar level), a midwife and paramedics. A standard equipped ambulance is used with extras such as O Rhesus negative blood (at least two units), hand-held Doppler machines for fetal heart rate registration, standard delivery pack, forceps, cord clamps, Syntometrine, anaesthetic drugs, full neonatal resuscitation equipment, various size endotracheal tubes and face masks (adult and neonatal), adrenaline, bicarbonate, naloxone, transport incubator etc. Clearly, removal of this team from their hospital duties has an impact on in-patient care.

Every effort must be made to take the hospital obstetric case notes for the patient.

Senior staff have to be aware at all times that a flying squad has gone out so that the labour ward is still covered by experienced obstetric staff.

Proper documentation from the first phone call requesting home assistance including all relevant names, address and times is mandatory.

In most areas of the UK, the obstetric flying service has been discontinued because:

- It is quicker to bring the patient to hospital for treatment by an emergency ambulance than to bring the treatment to her.
- Usually all that will be undertaken in the patients's house is resuscitation, a skill that all ambulance paramedics should have.
- There is no evidence that treatment at home other than resuscitation is of benefit.
- The removal of medical and midwifery staff from hospital is potentially hazardous.

9

PROBLEMS AT BOOKING

The booking antenatal clinic visit (*see* pp. 8) is essentially a **screening exercise**; the findings obtained by taking a history, examining the woman, and performing routine laboratory tests, are used to identify any problems. Each problem requires a specific **management plan** for the remainder of the pregnancy.

PREVIOUS OBSTETRIC PROBLEMS

The past obstetric history may reveal complications in previous pregnancies which should influence the management plan.

PREVIOUS CAESAREAN SECTION

The criteria on which to base a decision whether to opt for an **elective Caesarean section** or to aim for a **vaginal delivery** are contentious. It is important to take a careful history and it is often helpful to study the previous partogram and operation notes. Factors to consider include:

- The **number** of Caesarean sections that have been performed. The risk of uterine rupture in labour increases with the number of previous Caesarean sections.
- Whether the Caesarean section was a **classical** or a transverse **lower segment** incision in the uterus. The vast majority are lower segment Caesarean sections and the risk of scar rupture or dehiscence is approximately 0.3% following a single lower segment Caesarean section. A previous incision in the upper segment of the uterus is more likely to rupture in labour and is considered a strong indication for elective section.
- Whether the previous Caesarean section was for a 'non-recurrent' **cause**, such as placenta praevia or a breech presentation, or a cause that is more likely to recur, such as delay in labour.
- Whether the Caesarean section was performed at **full cervical dilatation**, and whether any unsuccessful attempts at delivery

using forceps or vacuum extraction were made. Recent studies show that vaginal delivery is achieved in over 50% of these cases next time.

- **The views and expectations of the woman.** She may have suffered a long and painful labour which ended in a Caesarean section – and may view any possible repeat performance with great trepidation.
- **The size of the pelvis.** Unless the pelvis is grossly distorted (e.g. pelvic fractures after a road traffic accident, or rickets), clinical and radiological pelvimetry measurements are very poor predictors of the success of a trial of vaginal delivery. Unless the woman has previously delivered a baby vaginally, the only way to accurately determine the size of her pelvis is to see whether a trial of vaginal delivery is successful.
- Whether the pregnancy is otherwise uncomplicated. An additional complication, such as a multiple pregnancy, should lower the threshold to perform a repeat Caesarean section electively.

A provisional plan should be made at the booking visit. This plan can be modified later in pregnancy depending on other complications or features such as a breech presentation. In general, if a woman has had two or more Caesarean sections, or has had her previous Caesarean section at full cervical dilatation, or has had a classical (upper segment) Caesarean section, she is likely to have an elective Caesarean section in the 39th week of pregnancy. Otherwise, the plan would usually be to aim for a vaginal delivery. The majority of women (70–80%) will successfully deliver vaginally after a Caesarean section, even when a previous presumed diagnosis of 'cephalopelvic disproportion' has been made (although success rates are a little lower in this group). The plan for such a labour is discussed with the patient, addressing each of her concerns and anxieties with care and sensitivity. Scar dehiscence and uterine rupture occur rarely (about 1 in 300 trial-of-scars) but carry significant risks of serious fetal and maternal morbidity and mortality. Additional points which need to be considered are how long she should labour before the trial is deemed to be unsuccessful, and whether induction of labour or augmentation of labour with oxytocics, should be permitted (opinions vary).

PREVIOUS HYPERTENSION IN PREGNANCY

An increased risk of pregnancy induced hypertension (PIH) is usually based on a previous obstetric history, although a history of PIH in a first degree relative (mother or sister) increases the risk by 3 to 4-fold.

PIH is defined as two successive blood pressure recordings equal to or greater than 140/90 mmHg, at least 6 hours apart, in a previously normotensive woman, after the 20th week of pregnancy (alternative definitions incorporate rises in blood pressure, typically of 30/15 mmHg). The condition is common, affecting up to 10% of first pregnancies. Mild to moderate PIH in the absence of proteinuria is not associated with increased maternal or perinatal mortality. Thus if a previous pregnancy was complicated by non-proteinuric PIH, you can reassure your patient that a recurrence is unlikely to cause her or the baby any problems.

In contrast, pregnancy-induced hypertension with significant proteinuria (>0.3 g/24 hour urine collection) – termed **pre-eclampsia** – is associated with markedly elevated maternal and perinatal morbidity and mortality. It is wise to check the previous obstetric casenotes to determine whether any previous PIH was proteinuric/non-proteinuric. If the patient's previous pregnancy was complicated by pre-eclampsia:

- Advise the patient that there is a **10% recurrence** rate, although in successive pregnancies pre-eclampsia tends to be less severe and present at progressively later gestations.
- Check that previous pregnancies were not complicated by **intrauterine growth restriction** (IUGR, see below). Pre-eclampsia and IUGR share a common pathogenesis and often coexist.
- Low-dose aspirin **prophylaxis** (75 mg once daily) has not been found to be effective in preventing recurrent pre-eclampsia, although it may be of some benefit in severe, early onset disease.
- If the previous pregnancy was complicated by severe, early onset pre-eclampsia, perform a screen for **autoimmune disease** and **thrombophilia** (*see* page 54) as the incidence of underlying thrombotic tendencies is increased in such patients, and may warrant anticoagulant therapy.
- Alert the community midwife and general practitioner to the possibility of recurrent disease. The patient should be referred back to the hospital if **hypertension** or **persistent proteinuria** or other suspicious features occur (e.g. small for dates uterus, reduced fetal activity).

PREVIOUS INTRAUTERINE GROWTH RESTRICTION

Previous intrauterine growth restriction (IUGR) is commonly defined as a birthweight for gestational age that is below the 10th centile, and is associated with up to ten-fold increase in perinatal mortality. The birthweight and gestational age at delivery of previous infants should be checked. Ideally, use birthweight-for-gestational age charts that have been compiled for the local population. The use of models which correct for parameters such as maternal size, ethnic origin and parity and fetal sex, enable a closer correlation with perinatal morbidity and mortality.

The risk of IUGR is increased 5 to 10-fold if the previous pregnancy was complicated by IUGR compared with a previous normal pregnancy. If the previous pregnancy was complicated by IUGR, plan to review the patient in the third trimester, and plan serial ultrasound estimations of fetal growth and umbilical artery Doppler recordings if IUGR is suspected.

PREVIOUS PRETERM BIRTH

Preterm birth is defined as birth occurring before 37 weeks of completed gestation and such prematurity remains the leading cause of neonatal morbidity and mortality. Babies born prematurely fall into one of two groups. In the first group, labour begins spontaneously or as a result of prelabour premature rupture of membranes. In the second group, a major complication occurs (such as pre-eclampsia or a placental abruption), and the pregnancy is electively ended in the interests of either mother or baby. Attempts to reduce the significant perinatal loss of prematurity must address both of these groups; this section relates to the first group.

A variety of scoring systems have been devised, with the aim of prospectively identifying pregnancies at increased risk of preterm labour. Several associations with preterm labour are recognized – including poor socioeconomic status, smoking, young age and primiparity. However, the scoring systems have had only limited success, and the best predictors are probably a previous history of premature labour or mid-trimester loss, or the presence of a multiple pregnancy. If the risk of preterm birth is increased:

- **Educate** the patient to recognize to the signs and symptoms of preterm labour. The perception of contractions, cramp-like pains, low backache and a 'show' may all prove to be significant, and warrant a careful cervical assessment in order that the advantages of tocolytic and corticosteroid therapy may be obtained.
- If cervical incompetence is suspected on the basis of a previous painless mid-trimester miscarriage, or known traumatic damage

to the cervix, **cervical cerclage** (ideally as a planned procedure) may be performed at 12–14 weeks.

- If an infective aetiology is suspected from a previous preterm labour, cervical microbiological swabs should be taken serially from 20–24 weeks. **Prophylactic antibiotic** therapy can then be targeted to any infective agent identified. Randomized trials of prophylactic antibiotic therapy in the absence of positive swab results have not shown any benefit. Bacterial vaginosis increases the risk of preterm labour or rupture of membranes 2 to 3-fold. Treatment with topical clindamycin or oral metronidazole has been demonstrated to reduce the risks of preterm labour in women who have had such an event previously.
- Other strategies, such as prophylactic administration of tocolytics or corticosteroids are of unproven value.

PREVIOUS ABRUPTION

The incidence of placental abruption, a condition associated with perinatal mortality rates of up to 50% and a maternal mortality rate of 1%, is approximately 1%. Although the incidence is much higher if previous pregnancies have been complicated by a placental abruption (5–15% after one episode, 25% after two), there is little that can be done to prevent such a recurrence. Advise the patient to **stop smoking** (as doing so has been shown to decrease the chance of an abruption), but folic acid supplementation has not been found to be of benefit. Consider checking antiphospholipid antibodies in these patients as the antiphospholipid syndrome (APS) may present with abruption (*see* page 135).

PREVIOUS POSTPARTUM HAEMORRHAGE

The incidence of postpartum haemorrhage, still a major contributor to maternal mortality and morbidity, is 5%. Primary postpartum haemorrhage is defined as the loss of greater than 500 mL of blood in the first 24 hours following delivery. A history of previous primary postpartum haemorrhage is associated with an increased risk of recurrent haemorrhage. Explain the need for preventative measures which include:

- Delivery in **hospital**.
- Serum should be **grouped and saved,** and a **full blood count** should be checked for the delivery.

- Patients who were transfused previously are at risk of having abnormal red cell antibodies – ensure that the blood bank is informed of this when samples are sent.
- The third stage of labour should be managed actively with an oxytocic agent given prophylactically (this is routine in most centres for all women).

PREVIOUS RHESUS ISOIMMUNIZATION

Once a Rhesus negative woman has developed antibodies, she requires careful supervision in a specialized centre. Whilst the magnitude of fetal and neonatal disease may remain unchanged from one pregnancy to another, it more commonly worsens in severity, as evidenced by perinatal mortality rates of about 2% if no previous baby has been affected, rising to approximately 35% when there has been a previous death due to Rhesus disease. When counselling and planning the management of a woman whose previous pregnancy has been complicated by Rhesus disease consider the following:

- **The antibody quantification** (in IU/mL), which is of value in predicting the risk of severe fetal disease in the first sensitised pregnancy, is of limited use when a previous pregnancy has been affected, having a poor correlation with the degree of fetal haemolysis. However, an antibody titre of <5 IU/mL is not usually associated with anything other than mild disease.
- **Serial ultrasound** scans: Findings which may precede the development of hydrops and be predictive of fetal anaemia include: increased amniotic fluid volume, liver size, placental thickness, bowel echogenicity and cardiac diameter and indicate the need for invasive tests.
- **Invasive tests:** To give adequate warning of severe haemolysis in women with a titre ⩾5 IU/mL, invasive tests (amniocentesis or fetal blood sampling) will need to be performed about 10 weeks before the gestation of the earliest previous intrauterine death, earliest birth of a fatally or severely affected baby (cord haemoglobin <10 g/dL), or of the earliest fetal transfusion in a previous pregnancy. Without a history of very severe disease, the first invasive test is usually performed at about 28–30 weeks.

  The severity of the disease is determined either indirectly by the optical density difference (OD) of amniotic fluid at 450 nm (a measure of the excess yellow pigment, i.e. bilirubin) which requires an **amniocentesis** or directly by the fetal haemoglobin which requires **fetal blood sampling** from the umbilical cord.

The latter test carries greater risk of miscarriage, preterm labour and fetal distress but allows a fetal blood transfusion to be performed at the same time. In general, the treatment options for affected fetuses are delivery at term with mild disease, maternal steroid therapy and elective preterm delivery for moderate disease and intrauterine fetal blood transfusion for severe disease. When delivery is planned close liaison with the paediatricians is advisable. Crossmatch of a unit of blood (against mother's blood) may be necessary in anticipation of an urgent neonatal blood transfusion.

- **Obtain the paternal genotype:** Knowledge that the baby may be Rhesus negative (i.e. if the father is heterozygous Rhesus positive) may be helpful – for example, if the amniotic fluid analysis suggests a less serious prognosis than does the previous history. A fetal blood sample will enable the fetal blood group to be determined directly.
- **Anti-D prophylaxis** is of no value once a woman is sensitized.
- **Inform the paediatricians of the forthcoming potential problem:** Haemolytic disease of the newborn (HDN) causes anaemia and hyperbilirubinaemia and treatment involves phototherapy and occasionally exchange transfusion.

OTHER RED CELL ANTIBODIES

All women will have their blood screened for abnormal red cell antibodies. This is particularly important in women who have previously undergone blood transfusion. There are many different kinds of antibodies (with anti-Rhesus D being the best known) and their ability to cause HDN varies greatly. If an unusual antibody is detected contact the blood bank for advice as they will know the potential of that antibody to cause problems, based on past experience. Anti-Kell antibodies for example, can cause severe fetal anaemia and HDN and intrauterine transfusion may become necessary.

PREVIOUS POOR OUTCOME

A previous pregnancy may have ended tragically in a stillbirth, a second trimester loss, or a disabled child. This event may have been linked to another pregnancy complication, such as a placental abruption or a fetal anomaly; if so, management should be directed at prevention (or early detection) of this complication. However, the pregnancy loss may have been otherwise unexplained. Management should include a sympathetic review of the previous pregnancy. When considering the appropriate management, account must be taken of the **psychological** trauma that the couple will be experiencing, and might include:

- Increased antenatal clinic attendance, especially in the third trimester.
- Serial third trimester ultrasound scans, for umbilical artery Doppler recordings, growth and biophysical profile.
- Elective induction of labour, prior to the gestation at which the previous pregnancy loss occurred.
- Previous intrapartum stillbirth or birth injury/asphyxia may prompt the offer of elective Caesarean section.

MEDICAL PROBLEMS

The patient's history, and the examination findings, may reveal medical conditions which should alter management. Remember that medical conditions influence the pregnancy and the pregnancy affects the medical conditions.

MEDICATION IN PREGNANCY (see also pp. 330)

The majority of pregnant women take some medication in pregnancy. This includes medication taken prior to knowledge of pregnancy, prescribed medication, and medication taken without medical advice. Drugs known to have adverse effects on the fetus, and increase the risk of abnormality above the 2–3% observed in the general population, include:

- Hormones: androgens, danazol, stilboestrol
- Warfarin
- Anticonvulsants
- Antibiotics: tetracycline, aminoglycosides, sulphonamides
- Alkylating agents: cyclophosphamide
- Retinoids
- Lithium.

If there is a history of inadvertent exposure to medication in pregnancy:

- Get accurate details of the exposure: dose, gestation, route.
- Obtain as comprehensive and informed risk assessment data as possible. This may involve drug formularies and consulting the hospital drug information service.

If there is a history of continuing medication or about to start medication:

- Obtain as informed risk assessment data as possible, and ensure that the benefits outweigh the risks of medication.
- If possible, try to:
  - avoid the first trimester
  - use drugs which have been extensively used in pregnancy
  - use the minimum dose.
- Consider a detailed anomaly scan at about 20 weeks if a known association exists between the drug and structural abnormalities.
- If the drug has potential effects on the neonate inform the paediatricians in writing of the case with the expected due date (EDD). They should respond with advice for the immediate post-delivery period. Mark this clearly in the maternal records so that the problem is highlighted when the patient attends in labour.

CHRONIC HYPERTENSION

Chronic hypertension is defined as a persistently elevated blood pressure of ≥140/90 mmHg, **before 20 weeks' gestation**. Diagnosis may be difficult in patients who present for the first time after the first trimester, due to the physiological decrease in blood pressure which occurs in mid-pregnancy. Depending on the population studied, the incidence is about 1–2% of pregnant women. Essential hypertension accounts for 90% of cases; other causes include renal disease (glomerulonephritis, nephropathy), diabetes with vascular involvement, thyrotoxicosis, phaeochromocytoma and collagen vascular disease (e.g. systemic lupus erythematosis, scleroderma).

The two most important pregnancy complications are superimposed **pre-eclampsia** (5 to 10-fold increased incidence) and **placental abruption** (5-fold increased incidence). Other risks include an exacerbation of hypertension, renal failure and a cerebrovascular accident. Perinatal mortality is related to the severity of the hypertension.

At the booking visit it is helpful to divide patients with chronic hypertension into two groups:

- **Low risk:**
  - Blood pressure < 160/100
  - Essential hypertension
  - Maternal age < 40

- **High risk (any of the following):**
  - Blood pressure > 160/100
  - Secondary hypertension
  - Maternal age > 40.

Take a careful past medical history (specifically enquiring about cardiac, thyroid, and renal disease, diabetes, and the outcome of any previous pregnancies) from all chronic hypertensive women. Similarly, perform baseline investigations: serum urea, creatinine and electrolytes, urinanalysis and culture, and 24-hour urine collection for protein and creatinine clearance, in all hypertensive patients.

A reasonable management plan for **low risk patients** would be:

- Discontinuation of any antihypertensive medication. This may necessitate review one week and two weeks after discontinuation, but it will be necessary to restart antihypertensive therapy in only a minority of women. If medication is restarted, suitable and safe choices include: methyldopa, labetolol, and nifedepine (never prescribe angiotensin-converting enzyme inhibitors or diuretics – *see* pp. 330).
- Monthly review with ultrasound scans for fetal growth and umbilical artery Doppler recordings if there are concerns about the clinical assessment of fetal size and placental function.
- If there are no complications, and medication has not been necessary, induction of labour before 41+ weeks is not indicated.

A reasonable management plan for **high risk patients** would be:

- Additional investigations at the booking visit: a chest X-ray, and electrocardiogram (especially if there is a long history of hypertension) and antinuclear antibodies (to exclude systemic lupus erythematosis).
- Very close monitoring and surveillance with frequent antenatal clinic visits and joint management by obstetricians and physicians (this may include periods of hospitalization).
- Serial ultrasound scans for fetal growth, umbilical artery Doppler recordings and biophysical profile testing.
- A careful consideration of the timing and mode of delivery – dependent on maternal and fetal well-being, and the presence of any complications.

EPILEPSY

Although epilepsy is the most common neurological disorder in pregnancy, the incidence is less than 1%. In general, if the epilepsy is well controlled, patients have few problems in pregnancy, but seizures increase if the epilepsy is poorly controlled. All anticonvulsant medications are associated with **congenital anomalies** (*see* p. 330), and overall the risk of fetal anomaly is increased 2 to 3-fold compared with the general population. Maternal **seizures** may result in fetal hypoxia and thus perinatal loss or handicap. Management includes:

- Stressing that the risk of seizures are more hazardous to the baby than anticonvulsant medication.
- Stressing the importance of periconceptual and continuing folic acid during pregnancy.
- Opt for **single therapy** medication if possible.
- Offer a detailed mid-trimester ultrasound scan to exclude fetal abnormality.
- The metabolism of antiepileptic medications is affected in a number of ways during pregnancy and routine measurements of drug levels are not usually performed. If fits occur however, check drug levels and adjust the dose to achieve the minimum of the therapeutic range.
- Plan to give the neonate vitamin K at delivery.

DIABETES

About 0.5% of women will have been diagnosed as having diabetes before they become pregnant. Diabetes may result in serious pregnancy complications. There is a 2-fold increase in congenital anomalies. The most common abnormalities are of the central nervous system, but cardiovascular, renal tract and gastrointestinal anomalies can also occur. Sacral agenesis is a very rare – but almost pathognomic – finding in infants of diabetic mothers. Problems which may occur later in pregnancy include: pre-eclampsia, polyhydramnios, premature labour, intrauterine growth restriction, macrosomia (leading to prolonged labour and a danger of shoulder dystocia), and infections. In addition, the neonate is more likely to suffer from respiratory distress syndrome and hypoglycaemia. These complications are more likely, and more severe, when there is poor control of the diabetes. Moreover, progression of any diabetic nephropathy and retinopathy is more likely when control is poor. Optimally, obstetric management should be in conjunction with a nurse specializing in diabetes and a physician–diabetologist.

- Good care of the diabetic patient starts before pregnancy. The main aim is to improve glucose control to reduce the risk of congenital abnormalities. It is also good practice to stress the importance of periconceptual folic acid supplementation in this group of patients.

- Assessment of **glucose** levels, aiming for tight control. Home glucose monitoring using a reflectance meter is the norm. Blood glucose measurements should be performed before each meal, and 2 hours after meals. Aim for fasting glucose levels of 4.0–6.0 mmol/L and 2 hour post-prandial levels up to 7.5 mmol/L. Fructosamine or glycosylated haemoglobin levels give a guide to control over the preceding weeks. The normal ranges for pregnancy vary with different laboratories.
- Treatment of diabetes. The **diet** of patients is important and will often be advised by a dietician. Usually he/she will suggest a program of three meals and several snacks. The aim is to limit periods of hyper and hypoglycaemia. The diet should be about 50% carbohydrate (preferably high fibre), 20–30% protein and 20–30% fat (with only a minority of the fat content being polyunsaturated fats). Calorie intake should be about 30 kcal/kg/day for nonobese women, and 25 kcal/kg/day for obese women. The **insulin** requirement of most insulin-dependent women increases in the second half of pregnancy, and many non-insulin-dependent women will require insulin for the first time during their pregnancy. Women on oral hypoglycaemic agents usually change to insulin for better control. To attain tight glycaemic control, most patients will require multiple injections. The 'basal-bolus' regime is used in many centres. This entails a small dose of medium or long-acting insulin in the evening to ensure constant basal insulin levels, and bolus doses of short-acting (soluble) insulin before each meal to mimic physiological patterns of insulin secretion.

  Hospitalization is only necessary if control is particularly poor, or if the patient cannot cope with self-monitoring.
- An 18–20 week detailed ultrasound scan to check for anomalies.
- There should be frequent antenatal clinic visits. In addition to assessing glucose control, regular ophthalmological examinations are performed to assess retinal vascular changes, and serial tests of renal function are carried out.
- Serial ultrasound scans for fetal growth, umbilical artery Doppler recordings and biophysical profiles.
- Unless there are additional complications, delivery at 39 weeks is common practice.
- **Steroids** may be indicated to promote fetal lung maturity if

preterm delivery is anticipated. Be aware that blood sugar control will be seriously disrupted by their administration and a sliding scale is sometimes required with large doses of insulin. **Betasympathomimetics** (e.g. salbutamol and ritodrine) are often used to suppress uterine activity in cases of preterm labour. They will further disturb glucose homeostasis.

THYROID DISEASE

- **Hyperthyroidism:** The incidence of hyperthyroidism is approximately 1:500 in pregnancy; the majority of cases are due to Grave's disease, an autoimmune disorder that is associated with circulating thyroid-stimulating antibodies. The main maternal concern is uncontrolled disease (or a thyroid storm) which has mortality rates of up to 25%. The incidences of preterm labour, intrauterine growth restriction, and stillbirths are all increased, and there is a 10% incidence of neonatal hyperthyroidism (usually transient). Medical therapy, with drugs such as carbimazole and propylthiouracil, are the mainstay of treatment in pregnancy. Management includes:
  - The level of **circulating antibodies** (which cross the placenta and may affect the fetus) is checked in some centres.
  - Monthly **tests of thyroid function**: free T4 (normal range = 10–19 pmol/L) and TSH (normally <0.5 mU/L).
  - Prescribe carbimazole to all symptomatic patients with laboratory abnormalities. Management of patients with laboratory abnormalities alone is debatable unless there are high levels of circulating antibodies, in which case, treatment should aim to maintain laboratory values at the upper limits of normal. Dose requirements often fall in the second half of pregnancy.
  - Serial ultrasound scans for fetal growth, umbilical artery Doppler recordings and biophysical profile. A sustained fetal tachycardia is suspicious of fetal thyrotoxicosis and requires urgent referral to a fetal medicine centre.
  - Unless there are additional complications, delivery at term can be planned.
- **Hypothyroidism:** The incidence of hypothyroidism is approximately 1:1000 in pregnancy – the major causes are idiopathic, iatrogenic and autoimmune. Provide full thyroid replacement during pregnancy, and perform serial thyroid function tests.

PREVIOUS THROMBOEMBOLIC DISEASE

Venous thrombosis and pulmonary embolism combine to form a serious and often fatal complication of pregnancy and the puerperium. When a history of thromboembolic disease is found:

- Perform a **thrombophilia screen** to check for anti-thrombin III, protein S and protein C deficiency, factor V Leiden mutation, abnormal fibrinogen, homocysteinuria, the prothrombin gene, paroxysmal nocturnal haemoglobinuria and antiphospholipid syndrome.
- Divide patients into those at high and low-risk:
  - **Low-risk**
    Negative thrombophilia screen
    No family history of thromboembolism
    Single previous episode.
  - **High-risk** (any of the following)
    Positive thrombophilia screen
    Strong family history of thromboembolism
    Multiple previous episodes.
- Plan treatment accordingly. Involve a consultant haematologist in decision making. Suitable options include:
  - **Low-risk patients:** Subcutaneous heparin from **36 weeks'** gestation and until **6 weeks after delivery**, or replacing the heparin with Warfarin after delivery. Dose regimens vary greatly.
  - **High-risk patients:** Subcutaneous heparin from **early pregnancy until 6 weeks after delivery**. This treatment has risks of bone demineralisation. In the second trimester, some opt for replacement of heparin with warfarin therapy, however, fetal intracerebral bleeding is a risk with this approach. Furthermore, warfarin has to be changed back to heparin at 36 weeks. Once again dose regimens vary greatly.
- All patients using subcutaneous heparin injections should have their platelet counts checked regularly as serious thrombocytopenia can be a side effect.
- If a clotting screen is normal, an epidural is not contraindicated in the presence of prophylactic heparin therapy.
- Neither heparin or warfarin are contraindications for breast feeding mothers.

PSYCHIATRIC CONDITIONS

Postnatal depression complicates 10–15% of pregnancies, whilst puerperal psychosis occurs in about 1:5000 pregnancies. The most important predisposing factor for these conditions is a previous history of psychiatric disease – either related to pregnancy or outside pregnancy and the puerperium. If there is such a history, liaise with the general practitioner and a psychiatrist, so that the appropriate surveillance after delivery is arranged often through a community psychiatric nurse (CPN). Many women with postnatal depression will be successfully treated without the need for medication, however tricyclic antidepressants and oral chlorpromazine are probably safe for the breast feeding mother but lithium, selective serotonin uptake inhibitors (SSRIs) and benzodiazepines are best avoided.

Pregnant women with **pre-existing psychiatric disorders** pose a slightly different problem and must be managed in conjunction with a psychiatrist. A case conference may be necessary to decide whether the woman is well enough to look after the baby on its arrival and a specialized **mother and baby unit** can be crucially important in maximizing the chances of a successful outcome. Although there are no obvious teratogenic effects of neuroleptic and tricyclic medications, high doses may cause anticholinergic and extrapyramidal side effects in the newborn and a plan should be made to reduce the maternal dose to the minimum in the third trimester. Lithium should not be used in pregnancy, being associated with teratogenicity (e.g. cardiac defects) with first trimester use and fetal hypothyroidism if used later.

CARDIAC DISEASE

The incidence of significant cardiac disease in pregnancy is about 1%. Congenital anomalies are the most common cause; the most prevalent disorders are a patent ductus arteriosis, septal defects, and anomalies of the great vessels. Rheumatic heart disease is still a major problem in areas where streptococcal infections are prevalent (for example in poor socioeconomic conditions). If the history and examination findings indicate cardiac disease:

- Carefully **examine** the patient for clubbing, cyanosis, a raised jugular venous pulse, cardiomegaly, cardiac murmurs, hepatomegaly and peripheral oedema.
- Perform the appropriate **investigations** which may include a chest X-ray, an electrocardiogram, an echocardiogram and possible cardiac catheter studies.
- Divide patients on the basis of the **New York Heart Association classification** as shown in Table 9.1.

Table 9.1 New York Heart Association classification

Grade 1: normal exercise tolerance
Grade 2: breathless on moderate exertion (heavy housework)
Grade 3: breathless on less than moderate exertion (light housework)
Grade 4: breathless without significant activity ('at rest')

Women in classes 1 and 2 can be reassured that with the appropriate care, they should tolerate pregnancy well. Classes 3 and 4 account for only 10% of cases, but 85% of maternal mortality.

- **Termination** of pregnancy should be considered if a patient has pulmonary hypertension, Marfan syndrome with aortic involvement, or grade 4 disease of any cause.
- Arrange an 18–20 week detailed fetal ultrasound scan and fetal echocardiogram as the offspring of women with congenital heart disease are at increased risk themselves.
- Plan antenatal clinic visits in conjunction with a cardiologist.
- Early discussion with anaesthetic colleagues is mandatory. Regional anaesthesia is beneficial in some cases and potentially harmful in others.
- Consider **anticoagulation prophylaxis** against thromboembolic disease in patients predisposed to this complication (for example those with pulmonary hypertension or prosthetic heart valves).
- Prescribe **iron and folate** supplementation to prevent the potential aggravation of anaemia.
- Arrange serial ultrasound scans for fetal growth, umbilical artery Doppler recordings and biophysical profiles.
- Plan **antibiotic prophylaxis** against endocarditis for any patients with: prosthetic valves, a previous history of endocarditis, most congentital malformations, acquired valvular problems, hypertrophic cardiomyopathy and mitral valve prolapse with regurgitation. A suitable regimen (for surgery or delivery) is ampicillin (2 g iv/im) and gentamicin (1.5 mg/kg iv/im) before the procedure, followed by amoxycillin 1.5 g 6 hours later.
- **Delivery** may be elective for worsening maternal symptoms. Caution should be exercised to avoid fluid overload. The second stage should be short to limit maternal exhaustion and a planned forceps delivery may be required to avoid the Valsalva manoeuvre used during pushing which can further compromise cardiac function. Some advocate a physiological third stage; certainly no ergometrine should be given. Facilities for cardiopulmonary resuscitation should be readily available.

CHRONIC RENAL DISEASE

The aetiology of chronic renal disease is varied: glomerulonephritis, diabetes, connective tissue disorders (systemic lupus erythematosus, polyarteritis nodosa, scleroderma), polycystic disease. In general (with the exception of the connective tissue disorders), the outcome of the pregnancy is good and there is little deterioration in renal disease. Complications include an increased incidence of pre-eclampsia, preterm delivery and intrauterine growth restriction. If there is a history of renal disease, plan to:

- Perform baseline **tests of renal function**: serum urea, creatinine, uric acid and electrolytes, 24-hour urinary protein and creatinine clearance.
- Review at 2–4 weekly intervals, in conjunction with a physician. Monthly monitoring of renal function and regular screening for **asymptomatic bacteruria** should be arranged.
- Arrange monthly ultrasound measurement of **fetal growth**, umbilical artery Doppler recording and regular assessment of biophysical profile in the third trimester.
- Monitor blood pressure and treat any **hypertension** with oral agents: suitable and safe choices include: methyldopa, labetolol, and nifedepine.
- Proteinuria is common in renal disease and usually increases during pregnancy. It is therefore an unreliable marker of PET in these patients and distinguishing PET from renal complications can be difficult.
- If renal function worsens or hypertension increases:
  - Exclude **reversible** causes: dehydration, infection.
  - Admit and consider **delivery** of the baby.

RESPIRATORY DISEASE

Lung disease is better tolerated in pregnancy than cardiac disease. **Asthma** is by far the most common respiratory illness encountered in the pregnant population. Fortunately pregnancy and asthma have little influence on one another and the asthma is managed as usual. None of the medications used are thought to be harmful and indeed the greatest risk to the fetus occurs with poorly controlled asthma. Women in labour who have had a recent course of oral steroids should be given extra cover with iv hydrocortisone (100 mg 6-hourly).

Tuberculosis is most common in HIV patients and Asian and West Indian immigrants. The diagnosis is most reliably made by culturing sputum or bronchial washings. Ethambutol and isoniazid are safe in pregnancy, but pyridoxine supplements are necessary. Rifampicin is also considered safe but streptomycin and pyrizinamide are best avoided. Patients remain infectious for two weeks after beginning treatment and this is important for the postnatal ward. Neonates born to mothers undergoing treatment should be vaccinated with isoniazid resistant BCG and given isoniazid. There is no contraindication to breastfeeding.

ANAEMIA

Anaemia in pregnancy (<11.0 g/dL) is a common condition (2–20% of women). Anaemia is associated with increased mortality and morbidity of both mother and baby, with increased incidences of maternal infections, cardiac failure, premature labour and intrauterine growth restriction. It is important to diagnose the type of anaemia and treat accordingly. If the haemoglobin concentration obtained at the booking clinic visit shows anaemia:

- Perform a careful clinical assessment. Pertinent features of the history include: diet and medication, gastrointestinal disorders, previous menstrual and reproductive history and any history of blood loss. On examination, check for skin bruising, koilonykia, hepatosplenomegaly, lymph node enlargement, mouth and gum changes and peripheral neuropathy.
- Perform the following investigations:
  - **Blood film:** a hypochromic microcytic picture suggests iron deficiency or beta-thalassaemia.
  - **Sickle screen:** if the mother is of African descent.
  - **Iron studies and haemoglobin electophoresis:** if the anaemia is hypochromic and microcytic.
  - **Reticulocyte count** (raised in blood loss or haemolysis),
  - **serum folate and B_{12}** if the anaemia is normocytic or macrocytic.
- Instigate the appropriate treatment:
  - **Iron deficiency anaemia**: the haemoglobin level should rise by 1 g every 7–10 days with ferrous sulphate 600 mg od or 200 mg tds (simultaneous treatment with folic acid is necessary) Alternative preparations may be necessary if this therapy produces gastrointestinal side effects.
  - **Folate deficiency anaemia**: folic acid 5 mg od (in malabsorption states intramuscular injection is occasionally required).
  - **Haemoglobinopathies**: if there is a significant fetal risk, the option of antenatal diagnosis (chorion villous biopsy or fetal

blood sampling) should be considered. Folic acid supplementation should be instigated. In sickle cell disease, crises should be prevented by avoiding hypoxia, dehydration and infection. Involve a haematologist early in the care of these patients as there are significant fetal and maternal risks. Placental insufficiency is common and maternal blood transfusions may be necessary before delivery to minimize the risks of sickling crises.

THROMBOCYTOPENIA

The lower limit of the platelet count is normally taken as 150×10^9/L. However, in pregnancy, about 8% of women will have a count between 100–150×10^9/L without any pathology. Platelet counts below 100×10^9/L should be investigated. The common causes for such low values include pre-eclampsia, autoimmune thrombocytopenia and drug induced thrombocytopenia (*see* p. 76).

OBESITY

Obesity in pregnancy is associated with hypertension, gestational diabetes, urinary tract infections, fetal macrosomia (leading to dysfunctional labour, shoulder dystocia and birth asphyxia). In view of these complications, if the maternal booking weight is >85 kg, the management plan should include:

- Screening for gestational diabetes at the booking visit and in the third trimester.
- Serial screening for asymptomatic bacteriuria.
- Ultrasound estimation of fetal size in the third trimester.
- Vigilance for hypertension (using the appropriate sphygmanometer cuff size).

It is inadvisable to advocate drastic dietary manipulation in pregnancy.

PRENATAL DIAGNOSTIC TESTING

There is a variety of circumstances in which the fetus is at an increased risk of abnormality and prenatal diagnostic testing may be of benefit.

ADVANCED MATERNAL AGE

The risk of **chromosomal** abnormalities, in particular Down's syndrome (trisomy 21) rises sharply with maternal age (*see* p. 347).

The incidence of chromosomal abnormalities when the maternal age is 35 years is approximately 1:350 at birth; if the maternal age is 40, this figure rises to about 1:100. If the patient's age is over 35, provide careful and non-directive counselling regarding the risks of chromosomal abnormalities and the options available. These options include:

- No action: the patient may not wish to consider screening for fetal abnormality or to contemplate termination of pregnancy, even if an abnormality was found.
- Non-invasive methods of providing a modified risk assessment. Alternative methods of supplementing the information from maternal age alone have been proposed. These include the triple test (maternal serum levels of unconjugated oestriol, alpha-fetoprotein and beta-human chorionic gonadotrophin) usually at about 16 weeks and ultrasound parameters (such as fetal nuchal translucency scanning at the end of the first trimester). Some units offer these screening tests to all women in pregnancy. *See* page 81 for further discussion of these tests.
- Invasive methods of providing a diagnosis. A comparison of the techniques of amniocentesis and chorion villous biopsy is detailed in Table 9.2:

Table 9.2 A comparison of amniocentesis and chorion villous biopsy

Amniocentesis	Chorion villus biopsy
Lower miscarriage rate (about 1%)	Higher miscarriage rate in first trimester (1–4%)
Usually performed later (15–17 weeks)	Performed earlier (after 10 weeks)
Longer time to obtain results (2–3 weeks)	Shorter time to obtain results (2–3 days)
	Risk of placental mosaicism (0.3%)
Uncommon complications:	**Uncommon complications:**
Preterm labour and postural limb deformities	Limb reduction (in first trimester)
Rhesus isoimmunization	Rhesus isoimmunization

PREVIOUS FAMILY OR SIBLING HISTORY OF A FETAL ABNORMALITY

Ideally, the couple will have had detailed genetic counselling preconceptually. If this has not been performed, counselling should be in conjunction with a clinical geneticist.

- Always take a careful **history**. Pertinent features include; a history of all pregnancies including stillbirths and miscarriages, whether consanguinity exists, and a detailed family history.

- Counselling regarding the risks of a recurrence will depend on the type of abnormality:

Chromosomal abnormalities

Many chromosomal abnormalities have been described, however, they generally have a low risk of recurrence. A typical example is Down's syndrome: if a couple have had one child with trisomy 21, their risk of another affected child is low but increased (to 1:200 for a woman under the age of 35, and twice the normal age-specific risk from 35 years upwards). Counselling should include the option of the invasive prenatal tests discussed above.

Autosomal dominant conditions

These are conditions such as myotonic dystrophy, osteogenesis imperfecta, tuberous sclerosis and Huntingdon's disease, in which the disorder is expressed in the heterozygote. The risk to the offspring of an affected heterozygote will be 1:2, although problems of variable penetrance and expression can make the calculation of risk more difficult.

Autosomal recessive conditions

These are conditions such as thalassaemias and other haemoglobinopathies, cystic fibrosis and phenylketonuria, in which the disorder is expressed in homozygotes. The main risk is for siblings of an affected individual, for whom the risk is 1:4. In counselling for recessive disorders, remember that many are amenable to prenatal diagnosis.

X-linked conditions

The majority of these conditions, such as haemophilia A and Duchenne muscular dystrophy, are recessive. Remember that: male-to-male transmission does not occur, unaffected males never transmit the disease, all daughters of an affected male receive the gene, and that female carriers pass the gene to 50% of their sons (affected) and daughters (carriers).

Other organ or system anomalies

There is a large variety of conditions that follow no clear pattern of inheritance. For some conditions, such as congenital heart disease, it is helpful to offer a detailed second trimester ultrasound scan. For other conditions, the accurate calculation of risk in these cases is the province of the clinical geneticist.

SUBSTANCE ABUSE

The incidence of substance abuse is difficult to quantify and varies markedly between different populations.

ALCOHOL

The incidence of alcohol abuse is approximately 1%, and that of fetal alcohol syndrome is about 1:1000. Maternal risks include tremors and seizures in the chronic user, cardiac arrhythmias, liver damage, gastritis, pancreatitis and Wernicke–Korsakoff syndrome (a life-threatening result of B-vitamin depletion). There is an increased risk of **fetal alcohol syndrome**: intrauterine growth restriction, neurological abnormalities and facial abnormalities (microcephaly, micro-ophthalmia and a poorly developed philtrum) if she consumes more than 10 units of alcohol (= 10 glasses of wine or 10 half pints of lager/beer) /day. Fetal growth restriction without the other features of the syndrome is found if the daily consumption is four units or more. If there is a history of significant alcohol intake:

- Educate the patient regarding the dangers of alcohol abuse in pregnancy.
- Prescribe prophylactic vitamin supplementation.
- Arrange a detailed second trimester ultrasound scan for fetal anomalies.
- Perform an electrocardiogram, liver function tests and hepatitis profile.
- Arrange for serial ultrasound scans of fetal growth.
- Consider referral to a specialist detoxification unit.

OPIATES

Many opiate addicts will not attend for antenatal care; about 50% present in labour. The drug of choice amongst addicts is heroin. An acute opiate overdose is a life-threatening complication to the mother, who is also at increased risk of sexually transmitted disease. There is an increased incidence of intrauterine growth restriction, stillbirths, and preterm labour. Neonatal withdrawal syndrome occurs in about 50% of infants exposed to heroin or methadone *in utero.* If there is a history of opiate abuse:

- Screen for gonorrhoea, chlamydia and syphilis and discuss testing for HIV status.
- Arrange a detailed second trimester ultrasound scan, and serial scans of fetal growth.

- Admit to a **drug dependence unit** and withdraw heroin, replacing it with methadone. This reduces the likelihood of street drug use. The options are then to continue with a **maintenance** methadone program (using the lowest acceptable dose in pregnancy) or slowly reduce the methadone in a **detoxification** program.

COCAINE

Cocaine abuse is an increasing problem. Maternal risks include cardiac arrhythmias, myocardial infarction and permanent central nervous system damage. Adverse effects of cocaine on pregnancies include increased incidences of placental abruptions, intrauterine growth restriction, and preterm labour. The principles of management are similar to those for opiate abuse.

TOBACCO SMOKING

Smoking is a major preventable cause of intrauterine growth restriction. Maternal risks are well recognized and include increased coronary heart disease, lung cancer, respiratory infections and peptic ulceration. In addition to intrauterine growth restriction, smoking is associated with an increased incidence of placental abruption, preterm labour and stillbirths. Once you have elicited a history of smoking, you should strongly encourage your patient to reduce (or preferably cease) cigarette smoking. There is good evidence that cessation of smoking in pregnancy reduces fetal and maternal complications.

PROBLEMS SPECIFIC TO THE PREGNANCY

A variety of problems that are specific to the current pregnancy may be identified at the booking visit.

MULTIPLE PREGNANCY

The incidence of multiple pregnancies varies worldwide, but approximate to 1:80 for twin pregnancies in Europe and the USA. The incidence of triplet pregnancies is rising due to assisted conception technologies. The diagnosis of a multiple pregnancy (often made after a booking visit ultrasound scan), carries an increase in maternal and perinatal morbidity and mortality. Maternal complications of twin pregnancies include an increased incidence of pre-eclampsia (the risk is 5-fold greater), preterm labour (the risk is 8-fold greater), anaemia, antepartum haemorrhage (due to increased risks of both placental abruption and placental praevia), and postpartum haemorrhage. The elevated perinatal mortality (increased 10-fold) is also influenced by greater risks of intrauterine growth restriction, congenital anomalies and cord prolapse. Management of a twin pregnancy includes:

- Prescribing prophylactic **iron and folate** supplementation.
- Determination of **chorionicity** at the end of the first trimester by ultrasound. Chorionicity is determined by ultrasound visualization of the implantation site or the dividing membrane: dichorionic pregnancies have a thick dividing membrane and a lambda or v-shaped attachment to the uterine wall; monochorionic pregnancies have a thin dividing membrane and a T-shaped attachment. The importance of chorionicity lies in the fact that monochorionic pregnancies are at much greater risk of the complications of multiple pregnancy especially the twin-twin transfusion syndrome and growth restriction.
- Arrange a detailed second trimester ultrasound scan for fetal **anomalies**.
- Arrange for serial ultrasound scans of fetal **growth**, amniotic fluid volume, umbilical artery Doppler recording and biophysical profile testing.
- Counsel the patient regarding the signs and symptoms of **preterm labour**. If uterine activity is noted, she should attend the hospital promptly.
- Interventions aimed at reducing the incidence of preterm labour have not been found to be successful. These have included cervical cerclage, bed rest in hospital and betamimetic agents.
- The mode of delivery will depend on the presentation of the first twin. In the absence of other complications, a vaginal delivery is usually planned if the first twin is cephalic, irrespective of the lie and presentation of the second. The place of elective induction at 38 weeks' gestation is controversial, with the benefit unproven; nevertheless, it is a common practice.

In general, the complications are greatest in higher order multiple births; for such cases the planned mode of delivery will usually be by Caesarean section.

BLEEDING IN EARLY PREGNANCY

This subject is discussed on pp. 295.

VIRAL INFECTIONS IN PREGNANCY

At the booking visit, the patient may ask about the implications of a viral infection in a previous pregnancy, or give a history of either a viral-like illness or contact with a viral illness.

Rubella

Rubella affects about 1:1000 pregnancies: after an incubation period of 2–3 weeks, a fine rash and lymphadenopathy are typical of rubella. If the infection occurs in the first trimester, fetal abnormalities (deafness, cardiac defects and cataracts) are common. The classical **TORCH (TOxoplasmosis, Rubella, Cytomegalovirus, Herpes) Syndrome** describes intrauterine growth restriction, hepatosplenomegaly, jaundice, petechiae, anaemia, pneumonia and mental retardation and can be seen with all these congenital infections. If rubella is suspected, take blood samples 2–4 weeks apart for determination of antibody levels. A four-fold rise of complement fixing antibodies indicates a recent infection. The diagnosis can also be made by isolating the virus in urine, blood or pharyngeal swabs. Remember that the majority of women will already be rubella immune. If maternal infection in early pregnancy is confirmed, termination should be discussed (confirmation of fetal infection by invasive tests is an option).

Cytomegalovirus

Cytomegalovirus affects 1:500 pregnancies. The disease may present with the classical TORCH syndrome and if maternal infection is confirmed in early pregnancy, termination of pregnancy should again be discussed. Unfortunately the infection can recur in subsequent pregnancies. If a woman is infected with CMV whilst pregnant, there is a 50% chance her fetus will be also. Of those fetuses infected, 5–10% have evidence of this at birth (e.g. thrombocytopenia, hepatosplenomegaly, choroidoretinitis, intracranial calcification) but a further 15% may develop symptoms later in life (e.g. learning difficulties, intellectual impairment). There is also a high risk of abortion and stillbirth.

Herpes simplex

Reassure any patient who gives a history of previous herpes simplex infections. **Recurrent** episodes of infection are very unlikely to cause effects in the fetus (which will have acquired transplacental immunity) and serial viral cultures of asymptomatic women who have had previous infections are no longer recommended with clinical screening being the preferred option. Women with a previous history should attend for an examination as soon as their membranes rupture or when contractions become regular. If lesions are visible, then Caesarean section is offered. If the membranes have been ruptured for more than four hours, any benefit from Caesarean section is lost.

Primary infections with herpes simplex are very different and carry significant risk to the fetus if it is exposed. If infection occurs in the third trimester then adequate transplacental passage of immunoglobulins may not have occurred by delivery at term. Caesarean section is the preferred mode of delivery in these cases.

Parvovirus

Fifth disease, caused by parvovirus B_{19}, is associated with non-immune **hydrops fetalis**. If the infection is diagnosed, symptomatically treat the presenting symptoms of arthralgia and fatigue and screen using ultrasound scans for fetal hydrops. If hydrops develops, a fetal blood transfusion by a fetal medicine team may be necessary.

Human immunodeficiency virus

Most pregnant HIV patients are asymptomatic carriers. Unless symptoms of AIDS are present, the virus *per se* does not have any effect on the pregnancy. Vertical transmission occurs in 20–30% of untreated undiagnosed cases, the virus reaching the offspring through the placenta, via swallowed secretions and through breast milk.

- If HIV infection is suspected, patients need careful counselling, and need to give informed consent before testing.
- Manage at risk women as if they were HIV positive in terms of **infection control** measures with blood and other body products.
- Screen HIV positive women for other sexually transmitted diseases, cytomegalovirus and *Toxoplasma gondii.*
- Helper T-lymphocyte (**CD4+**) counts should be serially monitored. Counts $<500/mm^3$ suggest that the patient should be seen with an HIV specialist. Counts $<200/mm^3$ require antibiotic prophylaxis against *Pneumocystis carinii* pneumonia.
- Treat any overt opportunistic infection.
- Treatment antenatally with zidovudine and delivery by Caesarean section significantly reduce fetal infection rates. Breastfeeding should be discouraged for the same reason.

Varicella/chickenpox

Immunity to chickenpox is not routinely checked for at booking clinic. If a woman is exposed to chickenpox she should have her immunity checked. The **congenital varicella syndrome** includes eye defects, limb hypoplasia, skin lesions and neurological abnormalities. It occurs in only 2% of cases of maternal varicella prior to 20 weeks. If an exposed woman of less than 20 weeks' gestation is not immune, and if the exposure was within the last 7–10 days then VZIG (immunoglobulin) can be given to reduce the risk of fetal infection. A second serum sample should be taken 2–3 weeks later. A documented rise in varicella IgM signifies maternal infection. Varicella pneumonitis is a complication of chickenpox and carries a significant mortality risk for a pregnant patient. Serious consideration should be given to intravenous acyclovir to women developing the infection during pregnancy.

Maternal chickenpox presenting just before or just after delivery carries grave risks to the fetus which will not yet have received transplacental passive immunity from its mother. Neonatal varicella carries a very high risk of serious morbidity and mortality.

A number of other viral infections can be passed from mother to fetus (influenza, viral hepatitis, mumps, measles, chickenpox, Coxsackie B virus, vaccinia virus), but are either less common or the effects on the fetus are less characteristic.

10

OUTPATIENT (ANTEPARTUM) PROBLEMS

MINOR PROBLEMS

During pregnancy there are a number of 'minor disorders' which are either due to the pregnancy (morning sickness) or exacerbated by the pregnancy. Although none of these conditions place the mother's health at serious risk, they can cause both distress and discomfort, and merit sympathy and consideration.

MORNING SICKNESS

Most women suffer nausea in pregnancy and about half will actually vomit. Symptoms are worst in the morning and are aggravated by the smell of food. It most commonly occurs in first pregnancies, and is often marked in multiple and molar pregnancies. In less than 1% of women, severe nausea and vomiting will necessitate hospital admission.

- Advise all pregnant women with nausea and vomiting to have **frequent small meals**.
  Fatty and greasy foods should be avoided.
- Reassure mothers that the condition is **self-limiting** and will not harm her baby.
- In severe cases: (patients cannot tolerate any food, become clinically dehydrated, and have ketone bodies in their urine) – arrange hospital **admission**.
- In patients who need admission, replace intravenous fluid and electrolytes. Check thyroid function and arrange an ultrasound scan to exclude a molar or multiple pregnancy. Exclude a urinary tract infection and other causes of vomiting. Ensure that the patient takes nothing orally until the vomiting ceases, then gradually increase fluid then solid intake.
- **Avoid antiemetic therapy if possible**, especially in the first trimester. If medication is necessary, try meclozine, promethazine or metoclopromide (rectal or im rather than oral).

- Be vigilant for **Wernicke's encephalopathy** (caused by B_1 deficiency): this can be prevented with water soluble vitamin administration.

BACKACHE

Most patients complain of low backache, especially in the third trimester. Alterations in posture (to counteract the gravid uterus) and relaxation of the ligaments, are probably responsible for this. Rarely, the backache may result from herniation of an intervertebral disc.

Advocate rest, warmth and analgesia; often this is sufficient to alleviate symptoms. A maternity corset or referral to a physiotherapist may be helpful. Occasionally, if the pain is debilitating or neurological deficits are present, referral to an orthopaedic surgeon may be necessary.

HEARTBURN

Approximately two thirds of patients complain of epigastric or retrosternal pain, (the incidence is increased in smokers). The condition is commonly seen in the second half of pregnancy, due to the enlarging uterus pressing on the stomach.

Prescribe an **antacid** (such as aluminium hydroxide) to be taken when symptoms occur. Meals should be frequent and small to prevent overdistension of the stomach (and should contain a milky drink). The avoidance of tight clothing and postural measures such as elevating the head of the bed at night, can often be helpful. H_2 anatagonists (e.g. ranitidine) can be considered for severe cases. If the symptoms do not resolve after such simple measures, consider endoscopic or barium studies to exclude significant gastrointestinal pathology.

CONSTIPATION

Alterations in bowel habit are common in pregnancy, and are exacerbated by medication such as iron supplementation. Encourage an increase in dietary **fibre** (bran, green vegetables), and a reduction of sugar intake. If medication is necessary, prescribe a **bulk-forming** laxative (such as ispagula husk).

VARICOSE VEINS AND HAEMORRHOIDS

Varicose veins (haemorrhoids are varicosities of the veins of the anal canal: the inferior haemorrhoidal plexus) are exacerbated in pregnancy due to the increased levels of steroid hormones and the pressure of the gravid uterus on the pelvic veins. A patient may complain of aching, pain and swelling, and complications include thrombosis or haemorrhage.

Management of varicose veins in the leg should include support stockings and rest with elevation of the feet. Treatment in the form of sclerosing injections or surgical excision is rarely necessary and usually avoided in pregnancy.

Management of haemorrhoids is largely preventative; i.e avoidance of constipation and straining in the second stage of labour, which may exacerbate the condition. If the haemorrhoids prolapse, the patient should replace them and apply an ice-pack to reduce swelling. Anusol is safe in pregnancy.

OEDEMA

Oedema occurs in over 80% of pregnancies and is exacerbated by hot weather. Oedema is aggravated by standing, and usually resolves after resting at night. If swelling compresses the median nerve (as it passes through the aponeurotic tunnel at the wrist) **carpal tunnel syndrome** can result. Management should include reassurance, exercise and splinting of the wrist. Diuretics to reduce oedema should only be considered in extreme cases. Surgical incision of the aponeurosis is rarely necessary.

FAINTING

In the first trimester the progesterone-induced vasodilatation may exceed the increase in blood volume, resulting in **postural hypotension** and fainting. The condition is self limiting so reassure the mother and advise caution when changing positions (e.g. lying to erect, sitting to standing). A history of palpitations preceding the faint may warrant cardiological referral.

MUSCLE CRAMPS

About a third of patients complain of muscle cramps, which are worst at night. Although different medications have been advocated (including quinine and calcium lactate), there is no evidence that these drugs are more effective than simply suggesting that the woman stretches the affected muscle and massages it.

HYPERTENSION IN PREGNANCY

Chronic hypertension should be identified at the antenatal booking visit, and the management of this condition is discussed in

'Problems at booking' (page 49). This section concerns the management of **pregnancy-induced hypertension (PIH)**, which is subdivided on the basis of whether significant **proteinuria** is present or not.

PIH is defined as two successive blood pressure recordings equal to or greater than 140/90 mmHg, at least 6 hours apart, in a previously normotensive woman, after the 20th week of pregnancy (alternative, less useful, definitions incorporate rises in blood pressure, typically of 30/15 mmHg above booking values). The condition is common, affecting up to 10% of first pregnancies.

NON-PROTEINURIC PIH

PIH in the absence of proteinuria is not associated with increased maternal or perinatal mortality. Oedema in pregnancy is usually a physiological finding, and the presence of oedema in a patient with non-proteinuric PIH is not associated with a worse outcome. Patients are usually asymptomatic. Check that the woman was normotensive prior to pregnancy or in early pregnancy, i.e. that chronic hypertension is excluded. Management should include:

- **Reassurance.** Non-proteinuric PIH does not merit in-patient admission or induction of labour. Unless the patient's blood pressure rises to levels associated with a risk of cerebrovascular accident (CVA) (usually not below 160/100) when the blood pressure should be treated, antihypertensive therapy is not indicated. Apart from reducing the risk of CVA, antihypertensive therapy does not benefit either mother or baby.
- **Close surveillance.** Provided the blood pressure remains below 160/100 and there is no evidence of pre-eclampsia, the risks are minimal. Check that proteinuria does not develop. Increased surveillance could include frequent antenatal clinic visits, or visiting by the community midwife, and attendance at an antenatal day-case assessment unit. A reasonable plan is to advocate that your patient be referred back to you if:
  - she develops proteinuria (1+ or more) on dipstick testing;
  - her blood pressure measurements are persistently equal to or greater than 160/100 mmHg; or
  - she develops symptoms.

  Investigations that many undertake at the hospital attendances include maternal (urate, liver transaminases, platelets) and fetal (growth and umbilical artery Doppler recording) testing.

PROTEINURIC PIH OR PRE-ECLAMPSIA

Pre-eclampsia is defined as PIH with the addition of significant proteinuria (>300 mg/24 hour urine collection), in the absence of a urinary tract infection. The emergency management of severe or 'fulminating' pre-eclampsia is discussed in 'Antepartum emergencies' (p. 150). The incidence of pre-eclampsia is between 2–4% of first pregnancies, and the recurrence rate is approximately 10% in subsequent pregnancies. Pre-eclampsia rarely occurs in a multiparous woman whose first pregnancy was uncomplicated, unless there has been a change of partner.

First, establish the diagnosis of pre-eclampsia. Any patient who presents with hypertension and proteinuria should be admitted for assessment. Send a mid-stream urine for **microscopy and culture** (to exclude a urinary tract infection) and arrange for the protein content of a **24 hour urinary collection** to be measured. If the level of proteinuria is insignificant (<300 mg in 24 hours), consider managing the patient as an out-patient (see above). Once a diagnosis of pre-eclampsia has been made:

1. Monitor the condition of the mother

- **Symptoms:** Patients with pre-eclampsia are usually **asymptomatic**; if symptoms develop, they may indicate worsening of the condition. The most sinister symptom is epigastric pain which may reflect subcapsular liver haemorrhages and must never be ignored. Other symptoms, such as headaches, breathlessness, drowsiness, and visual disturbances are less specific but may be helpful.
- **Signs:** The most important of these are serial blood pressure recordings (usually every 4 hours) and daily dipstick assessment of proteinuria. Hyperreflexia, clonus and liver tenderness are signs of fulminating pre-eclampsia.
- **Laboratory tests:** These will identify complications of this multi-organ disease and should include:
  - Full blood count – the **platelet** count and haematocrit are particularly pertinent. If the platelet count is abnormal (<100 × 10^9/dL), a clotting screen is indicated.
  - Blood tests of renal function – serum **uric acid** measurement (*see* p. 344 normal values) is often the most sensitive index, and detects tubular damage before abnormalities in urea, electrolytes and creatinine are apparent.
  - **24 hour urine collection** for measurement of protein and creatinine clearance.

- **Liver function tests:** the first parameter to become abnormal is usually an elevation of the transaminases.

A marked deterioration in any of these parameters may indicate a need for emergency treatment and delivery of the baby (*see* 'Antepartum emergencies', page 148)

2. Monitor the condition of the baby

Pre-eclampsia is associated with **intrauterine growth restriction**. Fetal assessment should include fetal heart rate monitoring, ultrasound measurement of fetal growth, umbilical artery Doppler recording and ultrasound assessment of biophysical profile (particularly amniotic fluid estimation). A deterioration of any of these parameters may indicate a need to deliver the baby.

3. Consider therapy

Remember that **all therapeutic modalities are palliative** and that the disease continues to progress until the baby has been delivered. There is little evidence that any of the suggested therapies improves either maternal or perinatal outcome. In particular:

- Bed-rest is of little or no benefit – the reason patients with pre-eclampsia are admitted is to monitor more closely the disease progression, and ensure that there is no rapid deterioration in the patient's condition, not to impose bed rest.
- Once a diagnosis of pre-eclampsia has been made, low dose aspirin is not helpful.
- Antihypertensive therapy can reduce blood pressure and thus some of the maternal risk. However, it will not alter the multisystemic disease process and may mask the clinical signs of hypertension – and thus mask disease progression leading to a false sense of security. Antihypertensive therapy is rarely indicated unless the patient's blood pressure rises to levels at which there is concern about cerebrovascular accidents (i.e. over 160/100 mmHg), in which case emergency management is necessary (*see* 'Antepartum emergencies', p. 148). Indeed the risk of intracerebral haemorrhage is probably not significantly raised until the BP is 180/120. However a policy of antihypertensive therapy at a lower threshold (e.g. 160/100) is prudent. Outside the emergency situation, suitable antihypertensive therapy includes labetolol (start at 200 mg three times a day [tds]), nifedipine SR (start at 10–20 mg twice a day [bd]), methyldopa (start at 250 mg tds) and hydrallazine (start at 25 mg bd). Diuretics are of little value and are potentially harmful.

4. Consider delivery

The timing of delivery in pregnancies complicated by pre-eclampsia can be very difficult. Once the diagnosis of pre-eclampsia is made, delaying delivery can only be for reasons of benefit to the baby (although the later the gestation the greater the chance of a vaginal delivery). Where there is obvious placental involvement with intrauterine growth restriction, delivery before the biophysical parameters become abnormal may lead to the baby suffering problems due to prematurity. On the other hand, delaying the delivery may lead to the mother's condition deteriorating and the chance of an acute on chronic asphyxial injury to the baby increases.

In general **management guidelines** might be:

- If the patient is >37 weeks, arrange delivery. Unless there are other complications or contraindications, aim for a vaginal delivery.
- If the patient is between 34–37 weeks' gestation, bias should be towards delivering the baby, since the complications of prematurity are mild and short-lived generally.
- If the patient is less than 34 weeks' gestation, expectant management with close surveillance is often indicated. As the gestation advances, the threshold for delivery falls. It is in this group of patients that antihypertensive agents may be of value in allowing the pregnancy to reach a stage when delivery of the baby is less preterm. Manage the patient on a day-to-day basis. If premature delivery is contemplated, prescribe **steroids** to enhance fetal surfactant production (there is some evidence that steroid administration also provides a short-term improvement in the maternal condition), and discuss the case with neonatology colleagues.

5. Educate the patient

Explain the nature and complications of pre-eclampsia. It can be extremely frustrating for an asymptomatic patient to remain in hospital, often with no clear idea of how long her in-patient stay will be.

GESTATIONAL DIABETES

The management of previously diagnosed diabetes is dealt with on page 51.

A new diagnosis of diabetes may be made during pregnancy, usually as a result of an abnormal screening test prompted by the history or the findings of polyhydramnios or a large baby (*see* p. 85).

In most cases, the sugar intolerance is lost after delivery. As most of these women are only temporarily diabetic, there is no concern over renal function or retinopathy. The higher glucose levels usually only occur after the first trimester so there is no excess of fetal anomalies. However there is a risk of macrosomia and neonatal problems, and most obstetricians feel there is benefit in stabilising the blood sugar. This may be done, in some cases, using dietary measures (enrol the help of a dietitician) but if preprandial glucose measurements remain >5.5–6.0 mmol/L and/or postprandial >7.5–8.0 mmol/L, it is likely that insulin will be necessary and the woman will need education on how to self administer it and also how to deal with associated problems such as hypoglycaemia.

If control of glucose levels is good, most advocate IOL (induction of labour) between 38 and 40 weeks. Macrosomia and polyhydramnios can complicate plans for delivery and, in extreme cases, a planned caesarean section may be a safer choice. Gestational diabetics using insulin will need a sliding scale in labour, but all insulin will be stopped immediately following delivery.

Careful screening of these women is necessary throughout the rest of their lives as 40–60% will develop diabetes outside of pregnancy, in the long run. The recurrence risks for gestational diabetes in subsequent pregnancies is 40–70%.

BLOOD DISORDERS

ANAEMIA

Anaemia in pregnancy (definition varies; <10.5 g/dL or <11.0 g/dL) may be detected at the booking clinic visit (*see* 'Problems at booking', p. 58). If anaemia develops later in the pregnancy, it is just as important to perform a careful clinical assessment and establish a diagnosis with the aid of appropriate investigations (red cell indices, blood film, haemoglobin, electrophoresis, ferritin, red cell folate and serum B_{12}). It should be remembered that serum B_{12} values normally fall in pregnancy.

Management will depend on the cause of the anaemia:

Iron deficiency anaemia

Remember causes other than simply pregnancy. Gastrointestinal bleeding will be detected by testing stools for occult blood. The haemoglobin level should rise by 1 g every 7–10 days with ferrous sulphate (600 mg od) and concurrent folate (5 mg daily) therapy. Side effects of iron administration are dose-related. Although some women have gastric symptoms, the main complaint is constipation (usually resolved by increased dietary fibre). Slow-release forms are more expensive and only have fewer side effects because much of the iron is not released and is excreted unchanged. The most common reason for a failure of therapy is poor compliance. Management of iron-deficiency in late pregnancy presents a particular challenge; satisfactory response has to be achieved in a limited time. **Options include:**

- Intravenous administration of iron dextran. The initial intravenous infusion should be slow, as anaphylactic reactions can occur. This is very rarely advocated now.
- Intramuscular injections of iron sorbitol citrate – which can be associated with headaches, nausea and vomiting. Such systemic therapy produces no faster rise in Hb than oral therapy.
- Blood transfusion is only given in extreme circumstances.

The use of such systemic measures should be the decision of a senior obstetrician.

Folate deficiency anaemias

Severe megaloblastic anaemia is very uncommon. Treatment initially should be folic acid 5 mg od (in malabsorption states, glutamic acid or intramuscular folic acid injection are occasionally required).

Haemoglobinopathies

There is no specific treatment to correct the abnormal haemoglobins of sickle-cell and sickle cell C disease. Repeated transfusions reduce the likelihood of sickle crises, by maintaining a high proportion of the circulating haemoglobin as HbA and by reducing the stimulus to erythropoesis (and production of more sickle cells). The aim is for a haemoglobin concentration of 10.5–12.5 g/dL with 60% as HbA. Folic acid supplementation should be instigated, but iron administration may cause haemosiderosis, and should only be given if it is certain that the patient is iron deficient. In women with sickle cell disease, crises should be prevented by avoiding hypoxia, dehydration and infection.

Iron therapy should also be avoided in thalassaemias. It is routine to prescribe folic acid, and blood transfusions are sometimes necessary.

THROMBOCYTOPENIA

A low platelet count ($<150 \times 10^9$/L) is not uncommon in pregnancy. First, repeat the sample to ensure that this is not a **spurious** result. Other causes of a low platelet count are listed below:

- Gestational thrombocytopenia
- Pre-eclampsia and hemolysis, elevated liver enzymes and low platelet count (HELLP syndrome)
- Acute fatty liver of pregnancy
- Disseminated intravascular coagulation
- Haemolytic uraemic syndrome
- Thrombotic thrombocytopenic purpura
- Autoimmune idiopathic thrombocytopenia (AITP)
- Infection and HIV
- Drugs
- Connective tissue diseases
- Bone marrow suppression.

The majority of cases can be labelled as **gestational thrombocytopenia** and the platelet count rarely falls below 100×10^9/L. Counts lower than this are more likely to have a specific cause which should be investigated. **Antiplatelet antibodies** may be positive in **AITP**. A reduction in fetal platelet count is possible in this condition but uncommon. Treatment with high dose steroids or iv gammaglobulin is usually considered when the count falls below 50×10^9/L. Below this level bleeding complications become more common. Liaise with the anaesthetists and haematologists as the due date approaches and repeat platelet counts every 2–4 weeks. Do not diagnose gestational thrombocytopenia or AITP without excluding the other possible causes listed.

DETECTION OF RHESUS ANTIBODIES

The management of a patient with a previous history of Rhesus isoimmunization, or in whom antibodies are detected at the booking visit, has been discussed in 'Problems at booking', (p. 46). Rhesus negative women should have antibody screening repeated at regular intervals during the pregnancy (practices vary but typically are at about 28 and 36 weeks). If antibodies are detected:

- Reassure the patient that as this is the first pregnancy in which antibodies have been detected, it is most unlikely that the baby will be severely affected.
- Perform serial measurements of the antibody quantification every 2–4 weeks.
- If the antibody titre rises above 5 IU/mL, referral or discussion with fetal medicine team is indicated (below that value severe fetal haemolysis is unlikely to be found).

- Arrange serial ultrasound scans. Findings which may precede the development of hydrops and be predictive of fetal anaemia include: increases in amniotic fluid volume, liver size, placental thickness, bowel echogenicity and cardiac diameter. Beware; scanning is an insensitive way of detecting early fetal anaemia.
- Warn the paediatricians and inform them when the patient arrives in labour. (Elective delivery is usual when Rhesus antibodies are present in significant amounts.)

ABNORMAL LIVER FUNCTION

There are a variety of causes of jaundice in pregnancy, which may or may not be related to pregnancy. In addition to taking a careful history and examination, check liver function tests, hepatitis viral serology, hepatobiliary tract ultrasound and an auto-antibody screen (for primary biliary cirrhosis). The differential diagnosis should include:

Related to the pregnancy

- **Intrahepatic cholestasis of pregnancy** (obstetric cholestasis). This condition is characterized by widespread and severe pruritis, hyperbilirubinaemia, bilirubinuria and a 10 to 100-fold increase in bile acids. The stillbirth rate is markedly increased (up to 15%), although the mechanism of fetal demise is unclear. Treatment of the pruritis is difficult; options include skin emollients, chlorpheniramine, cholestyramine and ursodeoxycholic acid (try 300 mg mané and 450 mg nocté. n.b. There is no licence for its use in this situation). The most important part of management should be careful fetal surveillance, including ultrasound assessment of growth, umbilical artery Doppler recordings and biophysical profile. Most advocate delivery at 37–38 weeks gestation.
- **Acute fatty liver of pregnancy.** The diagnosis of this rare but serious condition is usually suspected on clinical grounds. Cases present with vomiting in the third trimester, accompanied by malaise and lower abdominal pain, and followed by jaundice with drowsiness and confusion (hepatic encephalopathy). Liver enzymes are usually elevated, and there may be renal failure, hypertension and proteinuria, with a marked elevation in circulating levels of uric acid. In general, management involves resuscitation of the mother and delivery of the baby as soon as the condition is diagnosed.
- **Severe pre-eclampsia** or eclampsia can occasionally result in liver necrosis, either as a result of disseminated intravascular coagulation, or from anoxic damage due to intense vasospasm.

- **Prolonged vomiting** from hyperemesis gravidarum, or other conditions such as a hiatus hernia can cause liver damage.

Unrelated to the pregnancy

- **Viral hepatitis** is the most common cause of jaundice in pregnancy. It may result from use of contaminated needles, or from contact with excretions of infected people or carriers. Symptoms include anorexia and nausea with right upper quadrant pain, followed by jaundice, dark urine and pale stools. Admit any patient with moderate to severe symptoms, to ensure adequate hydration and to check for signs of premature labour. Reassure the patient that if the baby survives the acute maternal illness, there will be no teratogenic effects of congenital anomalies. Inform the paediatricians of such cases as immunization of babies born to hepatitis B positive mothers may be necessary.

  Other causes include medication (such as chlorpromazine), chronic liver disease (although patients with cirrhosis rarely conceive) and gallstones.

SKIN RASHES

Skin problems in pregnancy can either be due to pre-existing skin disorders or can be secondary to changes associated with pregnancy.

- **Pre-existing skin problems** which can be exacerbated in pregnancy include:
  - Psoriasis: Pregnancy may improve, worsen or have no effect on psoriasis. Generalized pustular psoriasis can occur in pregnancy, and is characterized by coalescing pustules with a marked pyrexia. Treat this rare complication with high dose steroids – termination of pregnancy is sometimes necessary.
  - Eczema: usually improves during pregnancy, although breastfeeding mothers may have problems.
- **Specific skin diseases of pregnancy.** There are a number of these, the most common being the 'polymorphic eruption of pregnancy' which presents late in the third trimester and usually begins on the abdomen. The most common appearance is of urticarial papules which resolve after delivery. It can be intensely itchy but is no threat to the pregnancy. Treatment is with soothing lotions (e.g. calamine), 1% hydrocortisone, antihistamines and promethazine. New onset rashes in pregancy which do not fit this description are best reviewed by a dermatologist. Note that cholestasis of pregnancy does <u>not</u> cause a rash.

- **Other skin problems in pregnancy**: including **infections** (such as scabies) and **drug eruptions**.

Once a diagnosis has been made (and a **skin biopsy** may be needed for this), the management options will often be chosen in collaboration with a dermatologist.

ABNORMAL SCREENING RESULTS

The tests commonly offered for screening the fetus for anomalies are;

- Maternal serum alpha-fetoprotein (MSAFP)
- Double/triple test
- Nuchal translucency
- Detailed anomaly scan.

MATERNAL SERUM ALPHA-FETOPROTEIN

The glycoprotein alpha-fetoprotein (AFP) is made in the fetal yolk sac and then in the fetal liver. Fetal AFP enters the amniotic fluid via fetal urination, and then enters the maternal circulation by diffusion across the placenta. Maternal serum AFP levels rise until 30 weeks gestation and then decline. Between 15 and 20 weeks, maternal serum AFP rises by about 15% each week.

Neural tube defects are the second most common congenital abnormalities (after heart anomalies), with a prevalence in the UK of about 3/1000 births. Over 90% of infants with a neural tube defect are born to parents with no family history of the condition. The screening program was developed when it was apparent that almost all open neural tube defects result in abnormally high levels of maternal serum AFP. AFP is usually expressed as multiples of the median: values over 2.3–2.5 times the median are taken as abnormal. There are many causes of a raised maternal serum AFP:

- Wrong gestational age (i.e. more advanced than anticipated)
- Multiple pregnancy
- Fetomaternal haemorrhage
- Fetal death
- Neural tube defects
- Other fetal abnormalities, including:
  - abdominal wall defects
  - congenital nephrosis
  - bowel obstruction
  - renal tract abnormalities
  - sacrococcygeal teratoma

- Placental/umbilical cord tumours
- Maternal liver disease.

If the patient's serum AFP level is raised she should be managed by a senior obstetrician who will:

- Explain the variety of potential causes of this elevation, and that it is not only due to spina bifida.
- Ask whether there has been any **bleeding** in early pregnancy.
- Check the **gestational age**. Ensure that the laboratory received the correct information; the dates from the last menstrual period should be confirmed by ultrasound dating.
- Exclude **multiple pregnancy**, **anencephaly** and **fetal death** by ultrasound scan.
- Arrange a **detailed ultrasound scan.** Fetal anatomy should be thoroughly assessed with particular emphasis on the central nervous system (head and spine), the abdominal wall, bowel, and kidneys.
- Consider an **amniocentesis**. With advances in the resolution of ultrasound scans, this invasive procedure is rarely indicated. Practices vary locally. If, however, there are problems in visualizing fetal anatomy (for whatever reason), this test should be offered. If amniocentesis is performed, in addition to measuring amniotic fluid (AF) AFP, acetylcholinesterase (AChE) should be measured. AChE is present in high concentrations in the fetal cerebrospinal fluid, and should not normally be found in the amniotic fluid. Fetuses with a neural tube defect will have elevated AF-AFP and AChE, whereas abdominal wall defects are associated with a rise in AF-AFP only.
- If serious fetal structural abnormalities are detected, the couple will need careful counselling as to whether they wish to consider terminating the pregnancy.
- If no abnormalities are detected, the fetus remains at risk of **intrauterine growth restriction, pre-eclampsia, placental abruption, preterm delivery** and **perinatal death**.

  Serial monitoring of the maternal condition and third trimester estimations of fetal growth, umbilical artery Doppler recordings and biophysical profile should be planned.

SERUM SCREENING FOR DOWN'S SYNDROME

All women have a risk of having a pregnancy affected by Down's syndrome. This risk increases with maternal age. The only diagnostic test for Down's syndrome is karyotyping by amniocentesis or placental biopsy. As these tests carry risks to the pregnancy serum screening has been developed to guide invasive testing to those pregnancies most at risk. The levels of three pregnancy associated compounds are subtly different in Down's pregnancies when compared with karyotypically normal pregnancies. Maternal serum AFP and unconjugated oestriol levels are a little lower in affected pregnancies and human chorionic gonadotrophin (HCG) levels are a little higher. Although there is a great deal of overlap between the values the risk estimation calculated solely from the maternal age can be adjusted up or down accordingly. If all three compounds are tested for it is known as the triple test. The levels of the compounds are affected by gestation, race, weight and whether the mother is diabetic and these details must be included with the sample. The ideal gestation for testing is 15 to 18 weeks. The result is given as a risk value. Results of 1 in 200 or greater are considered 'high' risk and further discussion is then warranted with the woman as to further testing (usually amniocentesis). If this is the risk value 'cut-off' at which invasive testing is offered and all women took up the offer of the test then the pick-up rate for Down's syndrome would still be only two-thirds. The 'cut-off' value varies between centres. The limitations of this screening test should be made clear to the woman before she choses to have it performed. *See* p. 60 for further discussion of invasive testing.

NUCHAL TRANSLUCENCY SCANNING

This is a newer alternative to serum screening which has a number of potential benefits over the more traditional screening test. It is performed at an earlier gestation (11–13 weeks), screens for all karyotypic anomalies and also helps point out structural abnormalities which might otherwise have been missed (e.g. structural cardiac anomalies). The nuchal fold is an area of skin over the cervical spine of the fetus which varies in thickness. The thicker it is the greater the risk of fetal anomalies. Values associated with the lowest risk to the fetus are <3 mm. By combining the risk with the maternal age related risk a new risk value is obtained which predicts karyotypic anomalies with greater sensitivity than the triple test (about 80%). If the karyotype is normal in the presence of increased nuchal translucency a detailed anatomy scan is warranted to search for structural anomalies. This screening test requires specialized scan training and is not available throughout the country as yet.

FETAL ABNORMALITIES DETECTED BY ULTRASOUND

Protocols differ both in whether all patients should have a detailed ultrasound scan – or just those at particular risk (on the basis of maternal serum AFP, maternal age, family history, etc), and also in the parameters that are included in a detailed ultrasound scan.

With the improved resolution of fetal ultrasound scanning techniques, increasing numbers of fetal abnormalities are detected. These abnormalities range from:

- **Lethal complications:** These include central nervous system problems such as anencephaly, holoprosencephaly and hydrancephaly, and lethal cardiac abnormalities.
- **Potentially non-lethal abnormalities** which require intervention during the pregnancy: examples include fetal hydrops which may benefit from intrauterine transfusion, and fetal arrhythmias which merit medication.
- **Non-progressive abnormalities** which require no intervention during the pregnancy such as renal tract dilatation which will require paediatric follow-up. Identification of other abnormalities, for example gastroschisis, will prompt liaison with paediatric surgeons, ongoing review by the fetal medicine team and delivery in an appropriate tertiary centre.
- **'Markers'** are features which resolve but may be associated with other conditions. Identification of any fetal abnormality, be it an extra digit or dilated renal pelvis, will lead to a careful check of other organs, as the presence of one aberrant finding increases the chance of another. If such an anomaly is demonstrated and especially if there is more than one, consider invasive determination of karyotype, in view of increased risk of chromosome abnormalities. Similarly, findings such as choroid plexus cysts, which resolve spontaneously, should prompt consideration of karyotyping if any other markers of chromosome abnormality are present and/or the mother is at increased risk because of her age.

If an abnormality is found on ultrasound scan:

- Consider any abnormality on an individual basis, with careful counselling of the couple.
- An interdisciplinary approach is helpful. Depending on the anomaly detected, this may involve perinatologists, neonatologists or radiologists. Depending on the local facilities, referral to a tertiary fetal medicine centre may be indicated.

- Inform all members of the health care team: including the general practitioner and the community midwife.

KEY POINT

Ultrasound scanning can never be a perfect test for the detection of fetal anomalies. It is important that those women having detailed scans appreciate that it is only a screening test and cannot be expected to pick up all abnormalities.

ABNORMAL URINARY DIPSTICK MEASUREMENTS

One of the most important interventions of antenatal care is the testing of a maternal urine specimen at every antenatal visit.

Proteinuria

The differential diagnosis of proteinuria on dipstick testing includes:

- Contamination of urine from a vaginal discharge
- Urinary tract infection
- Pre-eclampsia
- Rupture of membranes (liquor contaminates the urine sample)
- Chronic renal disease, (e.g. chronic pyelonephritis).

If proteinuria is detected:

- A mid-stream urine specimen should be sent for microscopy, culture and sensitivity. Bacteria can be cultured from the urine of 5–10% of antenatal patients. The predominant organisms are bowel commensals (*E. coli, Streptococcus faecalis* and *Aerobacter aerogenes*). Prescribe a course of appropriate antibiotics, determined from laboratory culture and sensitivity testing.
- If there is any suggestion of pre-eclampsia, admit the patient for assessment as discussed above (p. 72).
- Perform a sterile speculum examination if there is a possible history of ruptured membranes.
- It there is no infection, and no evidence of pre-eclampsia, and the proteinuria persists, arrange a 24-hour urine collection for protein quantification. If there is significant proteinuria (> 0.3 g/24-hour collection), arrange a renal ultrasound scan and tests of renal function (plasma urea, uric acid, creatinine and electrolytes, urinary creatinine clearance). Depending on the results, referral to a renal physician may be indicated.

Glycosuria and screening for gestational diabetes

Glycosuria is very variable – its appearance follows no definite pattern. With the increased glomerular filtration rate in pregnancy, the capacity of the renal tubular cells to reabsorb substances such as glucose is exceeded. Detection of glycosuria is therefore usually a normal finding due to this lowered renal threshold. It is of more value as a screen for diabetes if the sample is after meals (i.e. non-fasting). If glycosuria persists, a **random blood sugar** test should be arranged. Normal values:

- ≤6.0 mmol/L (if more than two hours since last meal)
- ≤7.0 mmol/L (if within two hours of a meal)

If the random blood sugar is normal, organize a 75 g **oral glucose tolerance test**. Results at two hours:

- <9.0 mmol/L = normal
- 9.0–11.0 mmol/L = impaired glucose tolerance (*see* p. 74)
- >11.0 mmol/L = diabetes in pregnancy (*see* p. 74)

ABNORMAL HIGH VAGINAL SWAB (HVS) RESULT

The management depends on the organism detected:

Group B beta-haemolytic streptococcus

There is great controversy regarding the management of this finding in pregnancy. If a patient has a high risk of adverse fetal/neonatal outcome many obstetricians would treat during pregnancy with oral antibiotics. However, there is no convincing data to support this approach. Alternatively the swab can be repeated at 36 weeks gestation and if it is still positive there is good data to support the use of iv antibiotics in labour in such patients to reduce postnatal maternal and neonatal septic morbidity. The paediatricians should be informed. If it is detected when the membranes have ruptured there should be no delay in delivery.

Candida

Many obstetricians would not treat the woman unless she was symptomatic.

Other organisms

If **anaerobic organisms**, organisms associated with **bacterial vaginosis** or **clue cells** on microscopy are found, then the woman is at increased risk of preterm labour or membrane rupture. Treatment with metronidazole (and steroids for fetal lung maturity) should be considered although there is no good evidence that this will reduce the risk of these events happening except in the group of women who have had these events occur in a previous pregnancy.

ABNORMAL MID-STREAM URINE (MSU) RESULT

Known urinary pathogens (*E. coli, Streptococcus faecalis, Pseudomonas*) should be treated. However, the use of antibiotics with other organisms is more controversal. The finding of group B beta-haemolytic *Streptococcus* should be managed as discussed under abnormal HVS results (above).

ABNORMAL UTERINE SIZE (AND FETAL SURVEILLANCE)

The uterus may be clinically smaller than expected (small-for-dates; SFD) or larger (large-for-dates; LFD).

Small-for-dates

There are a number of causes of 'small-for-dates':

- Incorrect dates
- Oligohydramnios
  - reduced production of liquor
  - rupture of membranes
- Intrauterine growth retardation (IUGR).

Establish the correct gestation (if possible) and exclude rupture of membranes through history and sterile speculum examination. IUGR is usually suspected clinically and confirmed by serial ultrasound scanning.

Clinical examination is probably the most practical method of screening for IUGR. However, its sensitivity and specificity for detecting a small fetus may be no better than 50%. After 20 weeks' gestation, the symphysis–fundal height should approximate to the gestational age ± 2 cm. If the symphysis–fundal height measurement is too low:

- Check that the dates from the last menstrual period are consistent with ultrasound scan dating in the first half of pregnancy.
- Arrange for **ultrasound** measurement of the head circumference (less sensitive to biological variation than the biparietal diameter), the abdominal circumference, and the liquor volume. Although IUGR may be suspected after a single scan demon-

strates abnormally low measurements (for example, below the 5th centile for gestational age), it can only be diagnosed with conviction after serial scans. An abnormal umbilical artery Doppler recording and/or reduced amniotic fluid volume and/or maternal pre-eclampsia in addition to the finding of a small fetus makes the diagnosis of IUGR more likely (see below).

The aetiology and management of IUGR depends on the gestation at diagnosis and the pattern of IUGR.

Late onset ('asymmetrical') IUGR

The usual cause of IUGR identified in the last trimester is uteroplacental dysfunction, and the pattern of IUGR is characteristically 'asymmetrical', in that the abdominal circumference is reduced to a greater degree than the head circumference.

With suspected or confirmed IUGR the next step is to assess fetal health to distinguish between the normal-but-small fetus and the starved or hypoxaemic small fetus. The options include:

Amniotic fluid volume (AFV)

Definitions for abnormal liquor volumes vary. Some measure the maximum vertical pool depth and define oligohydramnios as a deepest pool of less than 2 cm (and polyhydramnios as a pool depth greater than 8 cm). However, a maximum pool depth between 2 and 3cm may be described as 'subjectively reduced' and may prompt closer observation. Others use the 'amniotic fluid index' (AFI) which is the added total of pool depths from each quadrant. The normal range is 8 to 18 cm, but this may overdiagnose oligohydramnios at term.

Biophysical score (BPS)

This is derived from:

- **A fetal heart rate trace/CTG**
- **Estimation of liquor volume**
- **Fetal tone:** More than one flexor/extensor movement in 30 minutes
- **Fetal movements:** More than three separate body or limb movements in 30 minutes (no fetal movements also scores 0 for fetal tone)
- **Fetal breathing:** more than one episode lasting 30 seconds or more in 30 minutes.

Each parameter is given a score of 0 (if abnormal) or 2 (if normal) for a total score out of 10. All variables together are more predictive than one taken alone. A score of <8 can only be given if the recording period is 40 minutes or more. A score of 8 is considered normal provided the liquor volume is satisfactory. A score of 6 should prompt a repeat measurement within 24 hours. A persistent score of 6 indicates prompt delivery as do lower scores. The predictive value of the test is unproven below 26 weeks or where there is known rupture of membranes. The false negative rate is 0.6/1000 compared to 3/1000 for CTG alone.

Umbilical artery Doppler recording (UAD)

Waveforms of blood flow within the umbilical arteries can be recorded using either pulsed or continuous Doppler ultrasound (Fig. 10.1). Analysis of the waveform can demonstrate one of the following features.

- **Normal:** The placenta is a low resistance organ and thus blood flows through it easily with not only high systolic frequencies (S) but also positive flow even in diastole (D).
- **Abnormal:** Many fetal and placental pathologies are characterized by an increase in the placental resistance manifested as either:
  - **reduced diastolic flow:** There is still diastolic flow but it is reduced so that the ratio of systolic (S) to diastolic (D) flow is increased above the normal range. The S:D ratio is the simplest way of expressing this relationship mathematically. Others are the pulsatility index and the resistance index.
  - **absent end diastolic flow (AEDF):** This is a more extreme state of the same process. It is possible for the diastolic flow to be intermittently absent.
  - **reversed end diastolic flow (RDF):** This is the most severe form of abnormality. The resistance within the placental vessels is so great that blood flow through the umbilical arteries is reversed during diastole.

All these abnormal patterns of UAD flow are associated with an increased risk of adverse outcome in the baby including fetal death, neonatal death, birth asphyxia and neonatal problems such as necrotising enterocolitis. Whilst the UAD can be regarded as a chronic measure of feto-placental function, RDF is associated with the high risk of imminent fetal death. Of all the assessments of the fetus described in this section, use of UAD is the only one which has been proved to significantly improve fetal outcome in randomized controlled trials.

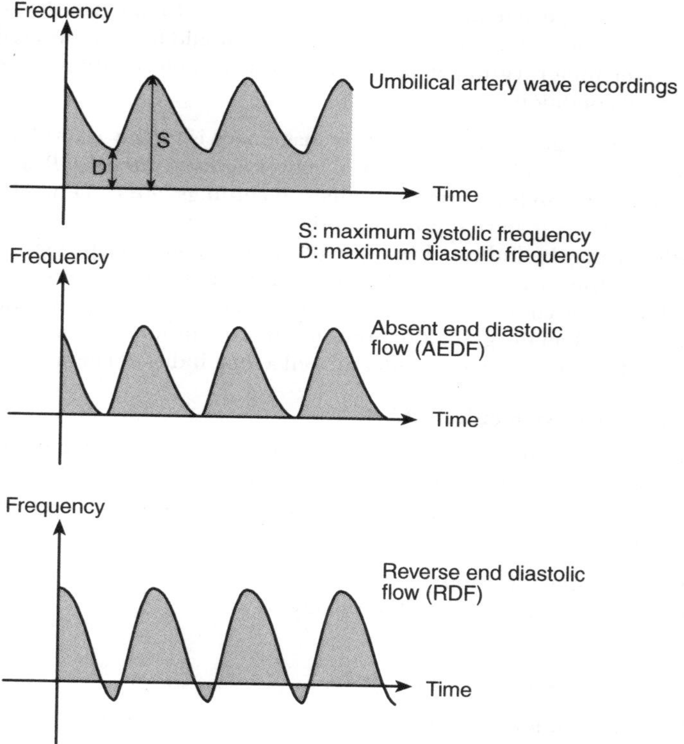

Figure 10.1 Umbilical artery Doppler wave recordings.

Management

In general, the management of a pregnancy complicated by late-onset IUGR might be as follows:

- If the gestation is > 36 weeks; deliver the baby.
- If the tests of fetal well-being indicate acute/active fetal compromise (abnormal CTG or BPS): deliver the baby urgently.
- If there is no evidence of fetal compromise, and the gestation is <36 weeks, monitor the baby carefully. Assessment of liquor volume, biophysical profile and umbilical artery Doppler recordings

can be repeated, and ultrasound estimation of fetal growth can be repeated at 2-week intervals. Steroids should be administered in the preterm group in anticipation of acute deterioration in the fetal condition.

These are generalizations and management is usually individualized. For example, some centres deliver fetuses with IUGR and abnormal umbilical artery Doppler recordings after 33 weeks. Furthermore, maternal pre-eclampsia may coexist (see above) and delivery may be indicated because of her condition (*see* p. 148). A senior obstetrician should decide on the mode of delivery (i.e. induction of labour (IOL) or elective Caesarean section) and this will depend on the gestation, previous obstetric history and the state of the fetus which may not tolerate well a long induced labour.

Early onset (symmetrical) IUGR

If IUGR is identified before the last trimester, or the pattern of IUGR is 'symmetrical' (in that both the abdominal circumference and the head circumference are reduced), the differential diagnosis includes:

- Congenital infection
- Chromosome or other abnormality
- Uteroplacental insufficiency.

Thus assessment should include:

- A **detailed ultrasound scan** to exclude a fetal anomaly (even if a 'routine' anomaly scan was 'normal').
- Consider **karyotyping** (preferably by fetal blood sampling or placental biopsy to obtain a rapid result) if the IUGR is severe. About 20% of such cases will have a chromosomal abnormality. Diagnosis of a structural fetal anomaly or a chromosome abnormality incompatible with life will mean that extensive fetal monitoring and a Caesarean section for fetal indications need not be undertaken.
- Consider **fetal blood sampling** to identify any viral infection and assess fetal acid-base status. The use of cordocentesis in this situation is controversial – in 20% of such cases a fetal bradycardia will result, with fetal death in a proportion, and the test should not be performed outside a tertiary referral centre (if at all). A maternal screening for recent TORCH infection should be performed.
- Tests of **fetal well-being**. If the detailed ultrasound scan and fetal

karyotyping are normal, perform careful assessment of fetal well-being (amniotic fluid volume, biophysical profile, umbilical artery Doppler studies).
- Administer **steroids** to accelerate fetal lung maturation, in case early delivery is necessary.
- Discuss the case with the neonatologists.

EXCESSIVE UTERINE SIZE (LARGE-FOR-DATES)

The differential diagnosis on finding a symphysis–fundal height >3 cm greater than the gestational age in weeks (in the second half of pregnancy) includes:

- Wrong clinical measurement
- Gestational age underestimated
- Excessive maternal size contributing to the measurement
- Multiple pregnancy
- Polyhydramnios
- Normal large-for-gestational age infant
- Macrosomic infant.

The initial assessment includes:

- Checking the gestational age, i.e. that the dates from the last menstrual period are consistent with ultrasound scan dating in the first half of pregnancy.
- Arrange an ultrasound scan to measure head circumference, abdominal circumference and liquor volume.

The subsequent management depends on the diagnosis.

Polyhydramnios

Polyhydramnios is defined as a deepest vertical pool >8 cm or an amniotic fluid index >95th centile for gestational age. Maternal complications include abdominal discomfort, increased risk of post-partum haemorrhage and Caesarean section due to cord prolapse, unstable lie and placental abruption. These factors contribute to perinatal mortality rates of up to 20%. However, the major contributors are increased preterm labour rates and an association with congenital abnormalities. Causes include:

- Maternal diabetes mellitus
- Fetal obstruction through the gastrointestinal tract (e.g. duodenal atresia)
- Impaired swallowing (e.g. trisomy 21, anencephaly)

- Fetal hydrops
- Congenital infection
- Isoimmunization
- Fetal polyuria (e.g. twin–twin transfusion).

Management should be decided by a senior obstetrician and should include:

- A careful maternal history. Pertinent features include a history of diabetes or Rhesus isoimmunization.
- A detailed ultrasound scan to check for fetal anomalies.
- Screening for gestational diabetes and maternal TORCH infections.
- Fetal karyotyping (amniocentesis, placental biopsy, fetal blood sampling) should be considered.
- Therapeutic options include: (i) Indomethacin 50–200 mg/day until 35 weeks' gestation. Fetal risks include premature closure of the ductus arteriosus, cerebral vasoconstriction, diminished renal function; (ii) serial amniocentesis, although risks of the procedure include premature labour, chorioamnionitis and placental abruption.
- Warn all women (irrespective of diagnosis) of risks of preterm labour and/or prelabour membrane rupture necessitating prompt self-referral to hospital.

Excessive fetal size

Excessive growth predisposes the baby to shoulder dystocia, traumatic birth injury and asphyxia. If, after finding a symphysis–fundal height in excess of that compatible with the gestation, the ultrasound measurements of fetal size are above the 90th centile for gestational age, the appropriate mode of delivery has to be reviewed by a senior obstetrician.

The morbidity of infants with birthweights >4.5 kg (4.0 kg in pregnancies complicated by diabetes) is significantly increased. The accuracy of ultrasound estimation of fetal weight is ±10%. The options are:

- Elective Caesarean section: practices vary, but many units have a limit of estimated fetal weight above which this mode of delivery is advised (e.g. 4.5 kg for non-macrosomic fetuses and 4.0 kg for macrosomic fetuses).
- Aim for vaginal delivery: for fetuses with an estimated weight below a certain threshold. If this option is chosen, additional practical guidelines include:

- a critical review of the progress in labour and opting for Caesarean section if poor progress occurs
- avoiding a traumatic vaginal delivery if at all possible
- having an experienced obstetrician present for delivery to anticipate and respond to shoulder dystocia.

There is no good evidence that induction of labour reduces the risks of fetal damage or increases the chances of a vaginal delivery.

REDUCED FETAL MOVEMENTS

This topic is discussed on p. 141.

ABNORMAL PRESENTATION

BREECH PRESENTATION

The incidence of breech presentation at term is approximately 3%, and at 29–32 weeks is approximately 14%. The management of breech presentation at term is one of the most controversial aspects of obstetric practice; in particular, the place of the vaginal breech delivery has been questioned. Perinatal and neonatal morbidity and mortality rates are higher after vaginal breech deliveries than vaginal cephalic deliveries. However, breech presentations are associated with increased incidences of prematurity, congenital anomalies, IUGR and either polyhydramnios or oligohydramnios. The only valid comparison is between breech-presenting babies that were delivered by Caesarean section compared with those that after careful selection, were delivered vaginally. In such comparisons, no short or long-term differences in perinatal or fetal outcome have been found.

The management with a breech presentation at term is the responsibility of a senior obstetrician and should include:

- Explaining the findings, and the need for careful assessment to the couple.
- Arranging an ultrasound scan to:
  - Confirm the presentation
  - Determine the type of breech: extended ('frank', with the fetal legs extended at the knee), flexed ('complete', with the fetal legs flexed at the knee) or footling ('incomplete', with one fetal leg extended and the other flexed).

- Exclude hyperextension of the neck (the 'star-gazing' fetus): which can cause spinal cord and brain injuries at vaginal delivery.
- Estimate liquor volume and placental site.
- Estimate fetal weight.

- Consider performing **external cephalic version** (ECV). Current evidence indicates that ECV performed at term and particularly with tocolysis is a safe procedure for carefully selected women. In such patients, it seems likely that benefits outweigh the risks (of premature labour, fetomaternal haemorrhage, cord accidents). Absolute contraindications are: multiple pregnancy, antepartum haemorrhage, placenta praevia (or any other need for an elective Caesarean section), ruptured membranes or any significant fetal abnormality. Relative contraindications include a previous Caesarean section, IUGR, and Rhesus isoimmunization.

  The tocolytic employed is usually a small intravenous dose of ritodrine (0.2 mg/min) or terbutaline (0.5 micrograms/min). A variety of techniques are described – these involve disengagement of the breech by abdominal pressure, encouraging the baby to somersault into a cephalic presentation, and maintaining the position of the baby for a few minutes.
- If ECV is not performed, or is unsuccessful, the next step is to determine the planned mode of delivery. The criteria listed in Table 10.1 are commonly used.

Table 10.1 Criteria for determining mode of delivery

Favourable for vaginal delivery	Unfavourable for vaginal delivery
Previous vaginal delivery of a normal sized infant	Nulliparity
	Other indication for elective Caesarean section
Estimated fetal weight: <3.8 kg (limit varies)	Estimated fetal weight ≥3.8 kg
Extended breech presentation	Footling breech presentation
	Hyperextended neck
Normal liquor volume	Oligohydramnios/polyhydramnios
Maternal desire for vaginal delivery	Maternal desire for Caesarean section
	IUGR
	Previous Caesarean section
	Grossly contracted pelvis on clinical examination

Most authorities have recommended the abandonment of X-ray pelvimetry measurement of pelvic diameters; it does not appear to be a helpful determinant of the success of attempted vaginal delivery. Clinical pelvimetry is probably only useful if the maternal pelvis is grossly contracted (e.g. after road traffic accident, rickets).

- If a decision is taken to attempt a vaginal delivery, educate the patient regarding the planned management of her labour (*see* p. 105)

UNSTABLE/TRANSVERSE LIE

A lie is described as unstable when the lie and presentation repeatedly change after 36 weeks. The incidence of an unstable lie is <1%, and of a transverse lie in labour is <0.5%. Predisposing factors include:

- Multiparity
- Polyhydramnios
- Multiple pregnancy
- Placenta praevia
- Pelvic tumours
- Fetal anomaly (e.g. hydrocephalus)
- Uterine anomaly
- Fetal macrosomia
- Contracted maternal pelvis.

If the fetal lie is transverse at the time of labour, there are risks of cord prolapse and a compound presentation (with associated risks of fetal death and uterine rupture).

If the abdominal examination identifies an unstable or a transverse lie, the management should be decided by a senior obstetrician and may include:

- A vaginal examination to exclude a pelvic tumour or a grossly contracted pelvis. **n.b.. Do not do this if there is any suggestion of placenta praevia, including antepartum haemorrhage of uncertain origin.**
- Arrange an ultrasound scan to exclude significant fetal anomalies, pelvic tumours and placenta praevia.
- Admit from 37 weeks (the gestation threshold chosen varies). This enables daily observation of fetal lie and presentation, and immediate clinical assistance if membranes rupture or labour begins. If the fetal lie stabilizes as longitudinal for 24–48 hours, the mother can be discharged to await the onset of labour.
- If the unstable/transverse lie persists, there are three options:
  - External cephalic version (ECV) as above, then await spontaneous labour.
  - ECV followed by induction of labour.
  - Elective Caesarean section. (Correct the lie to longitudinal at laparotomy and perform a lower segment incision, rather than a classical incision.)

FAILURE OF ENGAGEMENT

The presenting part commonly only engages in labour, especially if the mother is multiparous. If the presenting part is cephalic and free, and the patient is nulliparous and at term, it is reasonable to:

- Ask your patient to stand, and see if the fetal head enters the pelvis on gentle downward and backward pressure.
- If it does not, many would either perform a vaginal examination to exclude a pelvic tumour or a grossly contracted pelvis **(n.b. do not do this is there is any suggestion of placenta praevia)**, or arrange an ultrasound scan to exclude significant fetal anomalies, pelvic tumours and placenta praevia.
- If no problems are identified, reassure the woman and await spontaneous labour, but stress the need for her to attend early in her labour or immediately her membranes rupture (due to the increased risk of cord prolapse).

Irrespective of which approach is used, the progress in that labour will need to be critically reviewed (cervical dilatation and descent of head) (*see* p. 98).

PROLONGED PREGNANCY

'Prolonged pregnancy', 'postdate pregnancy', 'post-term' and 'postmaturity' are all terms which have been used to describe a pregnancy which has gone beyond 42 weeks. The incidence varies between 3% and 10%, depending on whether the dates are based on the last menstrual period, or have been corrected following an ultrasound scan.

Women become anxious as they go past their expected date of delivery. It is important at the booking visit to establish an accurate gestational age, and warn patients that they should expect to deliver between 37–42 weeks' gestation.

Any patient who has not delivered at 41 weeks should be reviewed in the antenatal clinic, when management should include:

- Checking that there are no risk factors which have been missed. For example, if the patient had previously had an antepartum haemorrhage, a stillbirth or has essential hypertension and is taking antihypertensive therapy, she should really have been delivered at 40 weeks. Likewise, on examination, ensure that there is no clinical suspicion of IUGR. Arrange prompt induction of labour for any such patient.

- If there are no risk factors then there are two options:
  - Arrange induction of labour at 41–42 weeks' gestation.
  - Manage conservatively. If fetal assessment is normal (ideally: weekly ultrasound measurement of umbilical artery Doppler recording, biophysical profile; as a minimum: weekly estimation of liquor volume and fetal heart tracing), induction of labour can be deferred until 43 weeks after which a significant deterioration in perinatal outcome has been reported.

The woman's wishes must be taken into account; however, the evidence from a metanalysis of published randomized trials suggest that the first option (induction of labour at 40 weeks +10–14 days) has a lower incidence of maternal and fetal/neonatal complications. Increased perinatal mortality rates with post-mature pregnancies are caused by an increase in unexplained intrauterine death, fetal distress during labour, traumatic and asphyxial injuries and meconium aspiration.

11

PROBLEMS DURING LABOUR

POOR PROGRESS IN THE FIRST STAGE OF LABOUR

Definition

Poor progress in first stage is said to occur when the plot of recorded progress in the active phase of labour is two or more hours to the right of an action line approximating to 1cm cervical dilatation per hour. Prolonged labour is somewhat arbitrarily defined as labour lasting more than 24 hours in a primigravida or more than 16 hours in a multigravida.

Causes

- Inadequate uterine activity – 'the powers'
- Malpresentation or malposition – 'the passenger'
- True cephalopelvic disproportion and other physical obstructions – 'the passages'.

MANAGEMENT

1. Decide whether the patient is in active labour or not

Labour is defined as the onset of regular painful uterine contractions resulting in cervical change and/or descent of the presenting part into the pelvis. It may be difficult to distinguish the uterine contractions that occur towards the end of pregnancy from true labour. The presence of a show (the passage of a mucous plug sometimes mixed with a small amount of blood) may precede labour by several days and is not a reliable sign. Similarly, rupture of the membranes precedes the onset of regular contractions in up to 15% of women. The active phase of labour is usually said to have begun once the cervix is more than 3 cm dilated, although this may be a normal finding in multiparous patients from 37 weeks. Where the cervix is less than 4 cm dilated it may be necessary to carry out more than one vaginal examination to assess change in the cervix before confirming a diagnosis of labour. Poor progress cannot be diagnosed until labour is established. Unless there is another reason for induction of labour (and provided the fetal heart rate pattern is normal) women who are contracting but not in established labour should be allowed to mobilize or rest at home or on the antenatal ward until either the uterine activity subsides or they progress to established labour.

2. Determine the presentation and position

Palpate the uterus abdominally between contractions and feel for the long axis of the fetus and the position of the fetal head. Carry out a vaginal examination and note the **position** (relation of the presenting part to the maternal pelvis) and **station** (i.e. how far above or below the ischial spines) of the presenting part. If in doubt about the lie or presenting part ask a more senior member of staff to examine the patient or arrange an ultrasound scan on delivery suite. Oblique and transverse lies are not compatible with vaginal delivery and will need to be delivered by Caesarean section. Delay in progress in a breech presentation in the presence of adequate uterine activity (see below) would generally be regarded as an indication for Caesarean section. Even where uterine activity appears suboptimal, the use of syntocinon in breech presentations should be discussed with the consultant on-call. Occipito-posterior and occipito-transverse positions or face presentation may be associated with delay in progress but may be deliverable vaginally with judicious use of syntocinon.

3. Look for evidence of obstruction

In cephalopelvic disproportion the relative diameter of the presenting part or the absolute smallest diameter is greater than the bony pelvis. True disproportion resulting from contraction of the bony pelvis is rare in the UK (<3%) and the commonest causes are the relative disproportions produced by malpositions and large babies. Those at risk include patients with a history of pelvic injury, abnormal gait or short stature, primiparous women where the head is more than three-fifths palpable above the pelvic brim at 39 weeks and multiparous women with a history of difficult operative delivery. Examination findings of a pubic arch of less than 90 degrees or being able to feel the sacral promontory per vaginam are suggestive of a narrow pelvis, but the best guide is descent of the presenting part in labour. This should be assessed by abdominal palpation as well as vaginally as the presence of caput may give a false impression of descent. Signs of obstruction in labour include failure of the presenting part to descend, a prolonged latent phase, secondary arrest, the presence of moulding (overlapping of the fetal skull bones) and an abnormal fetal heart rate pattern.

KEY POINT

A diagnosis of obstructed labour, especially in a multiparous patient, is an obstetric emergency because of the risk of uterine rupture and is an indication for delivery by Caesarean section.

4. Correct any inadequate uterine activity

Having excluded presentations incompatible with vaginal delivery and obstruction, assess the uterine activity. Palpation is a reasonable indicator of frequency, but a poor measure of duration and strength of contractions. External tochography may be difficult in obese or restless patients and gives no real information of intrauterine pressure. It is most useful as a record of contraction frequency and in the interpretation of changes in the fetal heart rate. Intrauterine pressure catheters are not widely used but should be considered if available where external monitoring is difficult or if using syntocinon in patients who have had a previous Caesarean section. If uterine activity appears inadequate (contractions less frequent than 4 in 10 minutes or of short duration on external monitoring) start an infusion of syntocinon and increase according to the local protocol until either the maximum recommended dose is attained or there are 4–5 strong sustained uterine contractions every 10 minutes. Reassess the cervix after 4 hours of adequate uterine activity for primigravidae who are less than 8 cm dilated, otherwise after 2 hours and if there is no evidence of progress consider delivery by Caesarean section.

KEY POINTS

- ***Multiparous patients should be assessed by an experienced obstetrician before starting syntocinon.***
- ***The use of syntocinon in patients who have had a previous Caesarean section, or with breech presentations should be discussed with a consultant.***
- ***If obstruction is suspected, ask a more senior person to examine the patient before using or continuing syntocinon.***

POOR PROGRESS IN THE SECOND STAGE OF LABOUR

Definition

This is somewhat arbitrarily defined as an active second stage of more than 40 minutes in multigravid patients or more than 1 hour in a primigravid patient. Active pushing is often delayed an hour after full dilatation is reached in the presence of an epidural or if there is no desire to push. However, there should still be evidence of progress after 1 hour. Concern regarding progress may be expressed in patients where uterine activity is thought to be inadequate prior to these time limits.

Causes

- Inadequate uterine activity
- Maternal exhaustion
- Obstruction
- Malposition.

ASSESSMENT

- Examine the abdomen for the number of fifths of the head palpable, the size of the fetus and the position of the fetal back.
- Perform a vaginal examination to confirm full dilatation, determine the station of the presenting part, position and any evidence of caput or overlapping of the skull bones (moulding). Where there is marked oedema or an occipito-posterior position abdominal and bimanual examination gives a more reliable guide to descent of the presenting part.
- Assess the strength and regularity of the uterine contractions and review the progress during the first stage.
- Review the CTG (see below).

MANAGEMENT (FOR CEPHALIC PRESENTATION)

Ensure that the bladder is empty.

- **If the cervix is found not to be fully dilated**: manage as per first stage. If there is evidence of fetal compromise or obstruction arrange for examination in theatre and proceed to Caesarean section. Otherwise review overall progress and reassess after an appropriate interval (depending on the actual dilatation, but usually 1 hour with augmentation if uterine activity appears inadequate). This is a potentially dangerous situation and should be discussed with a senior obstetrician. The fetal heart should be monitored continuously and if there is any doubt about the condition of the baby a fetal scalp pH performed before allowing labour to continue. **It may be necessary to arrange an epidural to prevent involuntary pushing against the incompletely dilated cervix.**

- **If maternal and fetal condition are satisfactory and there is evidence of progress (e.g. descent of the presenting part):** allow the active phase of the second stage of labour to continue and reassess progress after a further 30 minutes.
- **If uterine activity is poor and there is no evidence of obstruction or fetal compromise consider augmentation with syntocinon:** This would be of most value at the onset of second stage where uterine activity is felt to be poor and would not normally be appropriate where there has already been a prolonged active second stage. The same cautions (multiparous patients, previous Caesarean sections) apply as for the management of secondary arrest in the first stage of labour.
- **Indications for abdominal delivery:** Caesarean section may be indicated in second stage presentations that are incompatible with vaginal delivery (such as brow presentations) or where the head remains above the ischial spines or more than one fifth palpable per abdomen or where there is no descent of the presenting part during an attempted vaginal delivery.
- **Other circumstances:** In circumstances other than those above the management of delay in the second stage will normally be by **instrumental delivery**. Details of different methods are outlined in Practical Procedures (p. 171). The instrument chosen will depend on whether a rotational delivery is required, the experience of the operator, maternal analgesia and fetal maturity (*see* Table 11.1). Generally vacuum extraction is associated with less maternal trauma and requires less analgesia so should be considered first. Always ensure that there is adequate analgesia (this may mean arranging a spinal block) and that the bladder is empty. Rotational deliveries (i.e. for positions other than occipito-anterior) should be done by or under the supervision of an experienced registrar and consideration be given to carrying out fetal blood sampling first if the fetal heart rate pattern is abnormal.

If instrumental delivery is to be carried out in theatre as a trial by an experienced obstetrician (*see* Table 11.1) the patient should be consented for an emergency Caesarean section and theatre team and anaesthetist contacted. Blood should be sent for urgent group and save and arrangements made for a fetal heart rate monitor to be available in theatre so that continuous FHR recording is maintained until delivery.

Table 11.1 Operative delivery in the second stage

Suitable for experienced SHO	Call Registrar	Trial in theatre by experienced obstetrician	Caesarean
Fully dilated Direct OA Nothing felt PA No moulding Minimal caput Normal 1st stage Head below ischial spines	Any head palpable PA Abnormal CTG Unsure of position/ not OA No movement/descent after one pull	Needs spinal Marked caput or moulding More than 3 hours from 8 cm to fully dilated	Brow >1/5th palpable PA/ above spines PV pH <7.15 Requires rotation but unable to apply forceps or rotate No descent after 3 pulls

OA: occipito-anterior; PA: per abdomen; PV: per vagina; CTG: cardiotocograph.

MALPRESENTATION/MALPOSITION

OCCIPITO-POSTERIOR (OP) POSITION

The commonest of malpositions occurring in 10–15% labours and persistent in 5%. As labour progresses the head is more likely to extend than flex leading to larger transverse diameters with a poor fit onto the cervix and poor uterine activity. It may arise as a result of pelvic shape (android and anthropoid, prominent sacrum) or abnormalities of fetal tone, fetal tumour or a deflexed head at onset of labour (more common with inadequate pre-labour or epidural).

Diagnosis

May be suspected antenatally if the back is difficult to palpate or the umbilicus is lower than the fundus. Failure to progress in labour with a poorly applied cervix and marked backache with contractions are suggestive but diagnosis is usually made by vaginal examination by palpating the anterior fontanelle under the pubic symphysis.

Management

If progress is normal no intervention is required as a proportion of cases undergo spontaneous rotation or deliver OP. For delay in the first stage augment with syntocinon (see above), ensure adequate hydration and analgesia. Changing maternal position may be of help in encouraging spontaneous rotation and relieving pressure on one part of the cervix. If there is failure to progress in the second stage consider:

- **Outlet forceps:** If direct OP with a low station Neville Barnes forceps can be used to deliver the vertex face-to-pubes.The head should descend with the first pull and a large episiotomy should be made.
- **Manual rotation:** (may need to disimpact head with a risk of cord prolapse). An assistant should move the shoulders by pressure on the abdomen and forceps are applied when the head is in the direct occipito anterior/occipito posterior (OA/OP) position.
- **Rotational forceps** (Kiellands/Bartons): somewhat more difficult to perform and associated with greater maternal and fetal trauma in the wrong hands.
- **Vacuum extractor:** associated with less maternal trauma but requires a special (posterior) metal cup for OP positions. Applied correctly increases flexion and allows head rotation.
- **Caesarean section:** If more than one fifth palpable per abdomen or if difficulty anticipated with rotation because of pelvic assessment or fetal size or where fetus already acidotic/hypoxic.

KEY POINT

Serious consideration should be given to performing these deliveries in theatre with anaesthetic backup ready for early recourse to Caesarean section.

FACE PRESENTATION

This occurs in 1:500 deliveries. Diagnosis is by palpating orbit, mouth and nose on vaginal examination. Vaginal delivery is possible if mento(chin)-anterior. Treat delay in first stage with syntocinon as for vertex. Can be delivered by low cavity forceps but vacuum extraction and rotational forceps are contraindicated.

BROW PRESENTATION

This occurs in 1:1500 labours. As the presenting diameter is the occipito-mental (13.5 cm) it is not compatible with vaginal delivery unless the infant is small. Diagnosis is made by being able to feel the supra-orbital ridges and bridge of the nose on vaginal examination. The management is expectant in the first stage (most convert to face or vertex) and delivery by Caesarean section in the second stage or if progress is slow in first stage. A short trial of syntocinon may be considered but uterine rupture is a risk.

BREECH PRESENTATION

This occurs in 3–5% of pregnancies at term but a higher proportion of preterm labours. For **antenatal** examination, assessment and management *see* p. 93.

Undiagnosed breech in labour

Confirm the diagnosis by pelvic examination and determine if the presenting part is a foot ('footling breech'). Ultrasound may be of value in confirming presentation, type of breech and excluding gross fetal abnormalities such as hydrocephalus. Assess cervical dilation and station of the presenting part; exclude any gross pelvic contraction. From the notes determine the current gestation and previous obstetric history. Commence a CTG. The decision to allow vaginal delivery should then be made in conjunction with the obstetric consultant and the patient's wishes. Delivery by Caesarean section is commonly performed when:

- Footling presentation
- Gestation 26–32 weeks
- Abnormal fetal heart rate (FHR) pattern
- Additional fetal risk factors (e.g. IUGR, diabetes)
- Suspected fetal abnormality
- Low-lying placenta
- Previous history of obstructed labour
- Maternal request
- Suspected disproportion (large fetus and/or small pelvis).

Management of breech labour

Progress in the first stage should be as for cephalic presentation. An epidural may be of value to prevent pushing on an incompletely dilated cervix and if an operative delivery is required. Keep the membranes intact if the CTG is normal. The decision to use syntocinon for failure to progress should be made after assessment by an experienced obstetric registrar and discussion with a consultant.

Vaginal delivery of a breech presentation should only be undertaken by or under the supervision of an experienced obstetrician. Once fully dilated allow descent of the presenting part and active second stage as for cephalic presentation. Failure to progress will normally be an indication for Caesarean section. It is a good idea to perform an episiotomy just before the buttocks deliver. Allow spontaneous delivery to the level of the shoulders. When the scapulae are visible deliver the shoulders by flexing the arms at the elbows and deliver the head with either low cavity forceps or the Mauriceau–Smellie–Veit technique as follows. When the nuchal line is visible grasp by ankles and lift so as trunk rests on the right forearm. Insert your right middle finger into mouth and place index and ring fingers on malar bones. With the fingers of the left hand hooked over the shoulders, deliver head by gentle traction downwards then upwards in an arc, the right hand maintaining flexion of the head.

- **If unable to deliver the shoulders:** An experienced obstetrician should be conducting the delivery. He/she is likely to hold the pelvis with thumbs over sacrum, body lifted slightly to cause lateral flexion and rotate clockwise through 180 degrees so that the posterior shoulder comes to lie in front and can be lifted out by placing a finger in the bend of the elbow. The body is then rotated counterclockwise through 180 degrees, keeping the back uppermost and the second shoulder is delivered.
- **Head entrapment:** Again an experienced obstetrician should be conducting the delivery. This occurs at the level of the pelvic inlet or from an incompletely dilated cervix and accounts for 25% of intrapartum deaths in breech deliveries and is most likely where the fetal weight is < 1000 g or more than 3.5 kg. If unable to deliver the head follow these options:
  - flex the head with abdominal pressure and Mauriceau–Smellie–Veit technique
  - turn the head laterally
  - cut cervix at 4 and 8 o'clock if incompletely dilated
  - perform symphysiotomy.

SHOULDER DYSTOCIA

This describes the situation when one or both of the fetal shoulders remain above the pelvic brim despite delivery of the head. Its risks are fetal injury, asphyxia and death.

RISK FACTORS

- Previous shoulder dystocia
- Estimated fetal weight >4.5 kg
- Evidence of macrosomia (i.e. an increased abdominal to head circumference ratio)
- Diabetes

Intrapartum evidence of impending shoulder dystocia includes:

- secondary arrest or slow progress in first stage in multiparous women (although this is not a sensitive indicator)
- descent followed by retraction of the head during second stage (Turtle neck sign)
- chin pulled up against the introitus after delivery of the head.

MANAGEMENT

DON'T PANIC! Ask for the most experienced obstetrician in the hospital and a pediatrician to be called then start working through the following sequence. DO NOT use excessive lateral traction on the head as this seriously risks brachial plexus injury.

- Place the patient in lithotomy or left lateral position with the hips maximally flexed and abducted to increase the diameter of the pelvic outlet (McRobert's manoeuvre).
- Ask an assistant to press suprapubically (not fundally) to displace the anterior shoulder below the symphysis and attempt to deliver the head avoiding excessive lateral traction.
- Extend or make an episiotomy.
- Reach inside the vagina and try to rotate the shoulders to the oblique position with digital rotational pressure on the anterior shoulder.
- If delivery still not possible try to rotate through 180 degrees to deliver the posterior shoulder.
- If unable to rotate try bringing the posterior arm down vaginally to deliver the posterior shoulder.
- Consider symphysiotomy or displacing the head back into the abdomen and delivery by Caesarean section (Zavanelli manoeuvre).
- Fracturing the fetal clavicles is another possibility (reduces the bisacromial diameter) but is difficult and further increases risk of lung and brachial plexus injury.

After delivery take blood for a cord pH. Identify and repair any vaginal lacerations and make a careful note of the manoeuvres used.

ABNORMALITIES OF THE CARDIOTOCOGRAPH

The cardiotocograph (CTG) comprises a (upper) recording of the fetal heart rate (FHR) and a (lower) record of uterine contractions. The fetal heart rate pattern is determined either by external Doppler ultrasound detection of movement of the fetal heart or measurement of the interval between QRS complexes detected by an electrode attached to the presenting part. The frequency and duration (but not strength) of uterine contractions is measured by a pressure transducer placed on the maternal abdominal wall. A horizontal scale/speed of 1 cm per minute is usually used, with a machine generated record of the time. In North America the paper speed is 3 cm/min. Each record must be clearly marked with the patient's name, date and time commenced. Any intervention or point at which the trace is assessed for possible abnormality should be marked on the record and signed. The CTG forms part of the antenatal records and must be stored securely with the notes.

DEFINITIONS

- **Baseline:** The mean FHR in beats per minute (bpm).
- **Variability:** The small deviations from the baseline lasting less than 15 seconds expressed in bpm.
- **Accelerations:** An increase in fetal heart rate of more than 15 bpm lasting for more than 15 seconds.
- **Reactive:** A CTG with accelerations.
- **Decelerations:** A fall in FHR of more than 15 pbm for more than 15 seconds (some use a definition of 20bpm for 30 seconds). These may be early (onset coincides with onset of uterine contractions with the nadir of the deceleration at the peak of the contraction), variable (no fixed relation to contractions and/or varying in depth and duration) or late (FHR begins to fall only after the peak of the contraction).
- **Bradycardia:** A fall in FHR below 100 bpm for more than 3 minutes or less than 80 bpm for more than 2 minutes
- **Uncomplicated:** A FHR pattern with normal variability and no decelerations.
- **Sinusoidal pattern:** A saw tooth pattern comprising 2–5 cycles per minute of 5–15 bpm amplitude.

Always confirm the presence and rate of the fetal heart with a fetal stethoscope or ultrasound scan if there is any doubt about the quality of the CTG recording, as the maternal heart beat may be misidentified as fetal especially where there is a maternal tachycardia.

When interpreting the CTG bear in mind that:

- The fetal heart rate pattern can be affected by maternal temperature, drugs, fetal anaemia, congenital abnormalities and infection as well as hypoxia.
- Interpretation of the CTG needs to be made in the context of the clinical situation. Fetal hypoxia develops more rapidly in pre and

post term labours, infants affected by intrauterine growth retardation or infection and where there is meconium staining of the liquor.

- Isolated abnormalities of the CTG need to be viewed in the context of the rest of the CTG. The presence of accelerations with normal baseline variability is reassuring. Periods of decreased variability may occur normally during fetal sleep periods (though these do not usually last for more than 40 minutes) and after the administration of opiates. The sequence of loss of accelerations, followed by a rise in baseline then reduced variability suggests increasing hypoxia.

Deciding who should be monitored

For spontaneous labour, most units carry out a 20-minute CTG on admission. If the baseline is between 110–150, with a variability of 5–25 bpm, two or more accelerations and no decelerations the fetal heart can be monitored by intermittent auscultation.

Continuous monitoring should be performed where there is an increased risk of intrapartum hypoxia, namely:

- The admission CTG does not fulfil the above
- Labour <37 weeks or more than 41 weeks
- Meconium stained amniotic fluid
- Where prostaglandins or syntocinon are used
- Epidural analgesia
- Intrauterine growth retardation
- Intrauterine infection
- Previous Caesarean section
- Vaginal bleeding or suspected concealed abruption
- Hypertension or diabetes
- Malposition or presentation
- (Second stage of labour).

A CTG should be described as **normal**, **suspicious** or **abnormal** (Table 11.2).

If there are no accelerations in 20 minutes continue and reevaluate after 40 minutes.

With either suspicious or abnormal CTGs, standard 'first-aid' measures include:

- turn mother onto left side
- stop oxytocin infusion (if in use)
- give oxygen by face mask.

Table 11.2 Interpretation of the CTG in the first stage

	Normal	Suspicious	Abnormal
Accelerations	2 in 20 min	None in 40 min	None in 40 min
Baseline	110–150 bpm	150–170 bpm or 100–110 if uncomplicated	>150 bpm with decelerations or variability <5bpm
		Isolated transient bradycardia	Bradycardia >3 minutes or with a suspicious trace
Variability	5–25 bpm	>25 bpm (if no accelerations) or <5 bpm for 40 minutes	<5 bpm for >90 min Sinusoidal pattern with no accelerations
Decelerations	None/early (especially in late first stage)	Variable <60 bpm for <60 s	Variable >60 bpm or >60 s Late

If suspicious continue the CTG if clear liquor and otherwise uncomplicated pregnancy. Carry out amniotomy if possible. Check fetal scalp blood pH if high risk pregnancy, meconium liquor or if FHR trace not normal in 30 minutes.

If abnormal deliver if clinically indicated (cord prolapse, evidence of abruption or uterine rupture, failure to progress despite adequate uterine activity) or if unable to obtain fetal scalp pH. Otherwise perform amniotomy if membranes still intact and obtain **fetal scalp blood sample** (*see* below and p. 177). If pH <7,2 deliver as a matter of urgency. Ask for the obstetric registrar, anaesthetist and theatre team to be called. Stop oxytocics and take blood for group and save and prepare for Caesarean section unless now fully dilated. If pH 7.2–7.25 or base excess >–7, repeat blood sampling after 30 minutes even if the CTG improves.

If the pH remains above 7.2 but is worsening, the decision to deliver or continue will depend on the rate of progress in labour, current dilatation and an assessment of the other risk factors which may reduce the baby's ability to tolerate hypoxia. Remember acidaemia develops more rapidly and is associated with greater neonatal morbidity in preterm infants. Fetal pH may NOT be a reliable guide to the condition of the baby in the presence of infection or fetal anaemia.

SECOND STAGE CTG INTERPRETATION

Second stage CTGs are more difficult to interpret and the definitions of 'normal','suspicious' and 'abnormal' differ slightly from first stage. Variable decelerations are more common and can be observed provided recovery to the baseline is not prolonged, the baseline does not rise and the variability remains adequate (>5 bpm). The baseline may fall to 100–110 bpm without causing too much anxiety provided the other aspects of the CTG are normal.

If the CTG is suspicious observe for change in baseline. In the presence of rising baseline, worsening bradycardia or any abnormal features perform vaginal and abdominal assessment and arrange immediate operative intervention unless delivery imminent.

Sudden deterioration of the CTG

Prolonged bradycardia is a fall in the baseline fetal heart rate below 100 bpm for more than 3 minutes or to less than 80 bpm for 2 minutes. Possible causes include:

- **uterine hypertonus** (e.g. excessive syntocinon)
- **maternal hypotension** (e.g. after siting of epidural)
- **maternal vomiting**
- **intrapartum abruption**
- **uterine rupture or scar dehisence**
- **cord prolapse**
- **fetal vertex stimulation** (e.g. during vaginal examination).

Immediate action

- Alter patient position, stop syntocinon and administer facial oxygen.
- Perform a vaginal examination to exclude cord prolapse and establish cervical dilation.
- Have someone check maternal pulse and blood pressure and ask about/palpate the abdomen for uterine hypertonus.
- Mobilise emergency theatre staff ready for urgent Caesarean section.
- Correct any maternal hypotension with intravenous fluids.
- Try a bolus of ritodrine to reverse uterine hypertonus.

Immediate delivery is indicated if there is evidence of cord prolapse, scar dehiscence or abruption and should be considered where there has been a previously abnormal CTG, thick meconium or IUGR.

If there are no signs of recovery by 6 minutes or the baseline remains below 100 for more than 10 minutes deliver. **There is no role for fetal blood sampling during a persistent bradycardia.**

Action following a recovered bradycardia

This will be determined by the clinical situation and the fetal heart rate pattern before and after the bradycardia. In the presence of clear liquor and a normal term labour with a previously normal CTG observe the FHR over the next 20–30 minutes. If this is normal no further action is required apart from continued monitoring. If the the preceding or following CTG is suspicious or abnormal, or where there are other risk factors obtain fetal blood sample (allowing 5–10 minutes for correction of acidosis) if possible, otherwise deliver.

Generally, the prognosis following an isolated bradycardia is good where baseline variability is maintained throughout the bradycardia, the subsequent trace is normal and where an identifiable (and reversible) cause such as hypotension following an epidural can be identified.

MECONIUM STAINING OF THE AMNIOTIC FLUID

This is a relatively common finding in posterm pregnancies. It may also be associated with any stress or injury to the fetus occurring before or during labour, including acute or chronic hypoxia. The presence of fresh meconium or the passage of meconium during labour are usually thought to be associated with a more acute insult. The presence of meconium is associated with an increase risk of fetal acidaemia with any abnormal fetal heart rate pattern but is not usually considered an indication for fetal blood sampling or delivery if the CTG is normal. A paediatrician should be present at delivery of all infants with meconium-stained liquor to reduce the risk of meconium aspiration.

STILLBIRTH (see also Intrauterine fetal death, p. 143)

Intrapartum fetal death is uncommon, although it may result if a persistently abnormal CTG is not acted on. The causes (*see* Table 11.3) are generally the same as those for antenatal stillbirth as is the management and investigation afterwards with the following important provisos.

- It is more likely to be perceived as avoidable by the parents and staff.

Table 11.3 Causes of intrapartum stillbirth

Cause	Mechanism	Risk factors
Acute hypoxia	Abruption	Pre-eclampsia
	Cord prolapse	Unstable lie
	Uterine rupture	Previous Caesarean section
	Delay delivery second stage	
	– failed instrumental delivery	Malposition
	– shoulder dystocia	Macrosomia
	– trapped head with breech delivery	Breech
Acute on chronic hypoxia	Lack of metabolic reserve to cope with labour	IUGR Pre-eclampsia Preterm APH
Haemorrhage	Vasa praevia	
	Feto-maternal transfusion	Abruption
Unknown	Unknown	Diabetes Obstetric cholestasis Post-term

- Unless there has been a previous diagnosis of a lethal congenital malformation or in cases of extreme prematurity where a decision not to intervene during labour has already been made, there will be little if any time for parents and staff to come to terms with the event before delivery of the baby.
- The baby is more likely to be delivered operatively as a result of preterminal changes in the fetal heart rate pattern and may undergo extensive attempts at resuscitation at delivery.

MANAGEMENT

In most cases the diagnosis is made at the time of delivery. Except as noted above the sudden loss of the fetal heart beat will usually be an indication for immediate delivery (by Caesarean section if not fully dilated). If it can be established that the fetal heart activity has been absent for more than 15 minutes before delivery can be arranged the prognosis is likely to be so poor that allowing labour to continue to vaginal delivery should be considered. If there are no signs of life after 30 minutes of active resuscitation after delivery this should be discontinued, but remember that if at any point a heart beat is detected this will be a neonatal death and not a stillbirth. The decision to discontinue resuscitation would be made by a senior paediatrician.

MATERNAL PROBLEMS

ANALGESIA DURING LABOUR

Non-pharmacological methods

Around 30–40% of women will labour without any formal form of analgesia. Training in coping with pain in antenatal classes using approaches such as breathing exercises will help to achieve this. Hypnotherapy and acupuncture may, in some cases, have good results. Self- controlled transcutaneous electrical nerve stimulation (TENS) with the skin electrodes attached to the back below T10 is commonly found to be of help during the early first stage of labour. Mobilization has been shown to reduce formal analgesia requirements.

Pharmacological methods

- **Simple analgesia:** Paracetamol is usually of benefit when labour is just establishing and may allow for a few more hours without stronger forms of pain relief.
- **Entonox:** This inhalational 50:50 mixture of oxygen and nitrous oxide gives almost immediate pain relief. It is self-administered and this helps avoid overdosage, although it may cause confusion and reduce cooperation. It is eliminated very quickly by the lungs. It is best avoided during the second stage.
- **Opiate analgesia:** This is easy to administer, and has a very low incidence of serious side effects. Should they occur then antagonists are available. It is usually administered intramuscularly in the form of pethidine, diamorphine or sometimes omnopon and will take effect within about 20 minutes. Although diamorphine provides better pain relief than pethidine, the law in England does not allow for its administration by midwives, unlike in Scotland where it is widely used and given by midwives. Opiates may, in acute situations, be given intravenously.

- **Dosage:** Pethidine is commonly given 4–6 hourly in dosages ranging from 50 to 100 mg, although 150 mg may be required on occasion. Diamorphine is given in similar time intervals in a dose ranging from 10 to 20 mg. Simultaneous administration of an anti-emetic is advisable (e.g. prochlorperazine 12.5 mg im or metoclopramide 10 mg im every 8 hours maximally).

- **Side effects:**
  - Inadequate pain relief in up to 40% of women.
  - Nausea and vomiting.
  - Confusion.
  - Delayed gastric emptying.
  - Neonatal respiratory depression. (This can be reversed with naloxone 10 micrograms/kg.)
  - Overdose can lead to respiratory depression in the mother.
  - Opiates may reduce the reactivity of the fetal heart rate pattern and influence CTG interpretation.
- **Contra-indications:**
  - Previous adverse reactions.
  - monoamino oxidase inhibitors.
  - if delivery is anticipated before full benefit will be achieved (over 8 to 9 cm dilatation or within 2 hours).

Nerve blocks

- **Sensory nerve pathways:**
  - **Uterine body:** sympathic – T11, T12, L1, L2 – superior and inferior hypogastric plexus
  - **Cervix and lower uterus:** parasympathetic – S2, S3, S4 – pelvic plexus
  - **Vagina and vulva:** somatic – S2, S3, S4 – pudendal nerve.

1. **Epidural block:**

- **Summary:** This involves the placement of a small catheter in the epidural space allowing the administration of a local anaesthetic, commonly 0.25–0.5% bupivacaine (Marcaine), or sometimes lignocaine, with or without opiates such as fentanyl, diamorphine or morphine, via a bacterial filter, to give pain relief. These drugs work by a direct action on the nerve roots. They can be given in boluses on demand or in a 'mobile' set-up in which there is a continuous infusion. The motor deficit (but not the analgesia) of the anaesthetized area is substantially reduced with this form of administration. In case of 'breakthrough pain' top-up doses can be administered whilst continuing the infusion.
- **Indications:** These are all relative and include:
  - maternal choice.
  - augmentation of labour with oxytocics.
  - persistent occipito-posterior positions.
  - operative deliveries.
  - twin deliveries (to allow manipulation of the second twin if required).

- breech presentation (said to help by (i) reducing an urge to push before full cervical dilatation; (ii) allowing the presenting part to come down; (iii) pain-free application of forceps to the head).
- management of hypertension during labour (it causes peripheral vasodilatation through a sympathetic blockade and so causes a fall in blood pressure).

- **Contraindications:**
  absolute:
  - clotting disorders
  - systemic or local sepsis
  - allergy to local anaesthetics.

  relative:
  - fetal distress
  - haemorrhage
  - hypovolaemia
  - placenta praevia
  - cardiac disease with outflow tract obstruction (e.g. aortic valve stenosis, certain CNS disorders).
- **Procedure:** Verbal consent must be obtained with explanation of complications and side effects. Fluid preloading to avoid hypotension, as a result of vasodilatation, is achieved with 500–1000 mL Hartmann's solution. An epidural catheter is usually sited in the L1–L2 or L2–L3 space to anaesthetize level T10 and below. After a test dose (to check drug is not given intrathecally and the block is not ascending beyond T4) wait 5 minutes and check blood presssure before the full loading dose is given. The level of the block is assessed with ethyl chloride spray. Top-ups are given in divided doses when required. No more than 5 mL should be given at any one time. A midwife needs to be present for at least 20 minutes after each top-up and the blood pressure and pulse are recorded every 5 minutes. The fetal heart rate is recorded continuously.
- **Advantages:** Pain free, lucid and cooperative parturient. The block can usually be quickly adapted to accommodate a Caesarean section.
- **Disadvantages:** Necessity of a dedicated anaesthetic service, immobility of the parturient, common need for catheterization, loss of a bearing down reflex and a slight increase in the instrumental delivery rate. A 'mobile epidural' (bupivacaine plus opiate by continuous infusion and 'escape' top-ups when required) allows for more mobility and maintenance of some of the bearing down reflex enhancing active pushing during the second stage.

- **Complications:**
  - **Fetal bradycardia:** Usually transient. Check blood pressure and correct if hypotensive with fluids or ephedrine. Otherwise manage as other bradycardias (*see* p. 111).
  - **Hypotension:** A particular risk after the first bolus but can also occur after a top-up. Preventable by pre-loading with intravenous fluids. Treatable by increasing iv fluid rate.
  - **Incomplete block:** Missed segment, unilateral block or patchy anaesthesia. Remedies include increasing the dose or re-siting the catheter.
  - **Subdural block:** High block (can be total spinal) with missed segments and persistent pain. The catheter should be removed as further boluses may rupture the arachnoid mater and give an acute total spinal block. The epidural can be re-sited with reduced doses.

Dural tap

This describes breaching the subarachnoid space by the needle or catheter. It may go unrecognized and lead to a 'spinal' headache or total spinal block. A spinal headache is characterized by being worse when sitting upright and being relieved by lying flat. If no headache occurs during labour there is no need for elective instrumental delivery. Consider leaving the catheter in for 24 hours and infuse 1–1.5 L of normal saline intravenously to prevent or treat the headache. If the headache persists consider a blood patch (performed by the anaesthetists).

- **Total spinal:** This is potentially fatal to mother and fetus. It may occur after inadvertent placement of local anaesthetic in the subarachnoid space (i.e. a dural tap; sometimes several hours after siting of epidural), or after spinal anaesthesia. Dyspnoea progresses to apnoea, severe hypotension and unconsciousness. Treat with O_2, ventilation, intubation, iv fluids, iv ephedrine and atropine if bradycardia develops. Prevent by aspiration of catheter prior to administration of anaesthetic and the use of test doses. Suspect intrathecal administration if there occurs a rapid onset of analgesia, severe hypotension, or increasing motor block within 5 minutes of administration.
- **Haematoma:** Pressure on the spinal cord or nerve root(s) may lead to a variety of pains and deficits including paraplegia.
- **Intravenous local anaesthetic:** This may cause light headedness, paraesthesias (lips and fingers), convulsions, cardiac conduction defects and cardiac arrest. Treatment depends on the

severity, but includes avoiding the supine position (15 degree wedge), raising the legs, defibrillation and adrenaline.

2. Spinal block

This describes the intrathecal installation of a local anaesthetic such as 1–2 mL of 0.5% bupivacaine to anaesthetize T10 and below. The mode of action is similar to that of an epidural block. The level of the block can be tailored somewhat by making use of gravity on the 'heavy' anaesthetic compound by positioning the patient in a head-up position. It has an almost instantaneous onset allowing for any form of emergency operative procedure. It is not suitable for procedures longer than one hour unless a spinal catheter is inserted. The contraindications are similar to those for an epidural block.

3. Caudal block

Local anaesthetic (up to 20 mL of 0.5% bupivacaine or 0.5% lignocaine) is injected through the sacro-coccygeal membrane in the sacral hiatus outside the dura mater to block the sacral nerves. Used for instrumental deliveries and perineal repair in the absence of an epidural or spinal block.

4. Pudendal block

The pudendal nerve (S2–4) runs through the foramen infrapiriforme just behind the ischial spine medial to the pudendal artery into the ischiorectal fossa to supply the sensory innervation of the perineum, vulva, clitoris, lower vagina and external urethral meatus. It can be used for a range of vaginal procedures including outlet forceps and ventouse deliveries. The ischial spines are identified on vaginal examination and the tip of a Kobak guarded needle is passed through both the vaginal mucosa and the sacrospinous ligament. Lignocaine (10 mL at 0.5–1%) is injected immediately medial and 1 cm behind the tip of each ischial spine. Vacuum withdrawal of the syringe before injecting is paramount as the pudendal vessels are just lateral from the nerve and may be punctured inadvertently. The nerve block will take about 5 minutes to establish. Additional perineal infiltration for an episiotomy is often required. The maximum total dose allowed is 20 mL 1% lignocaine. The block lasts for about one hour.

5. Perineal infiltration

As the presenting part distends the perineum, the latter is infiltrated in a fanlike fashion with 0.5–1% lignocaine to allow for episiotomies to be placed, sutured and tears to be repaired. Perineal infiltration before rather than after delivery has the advantage that the anaesthetic is more accurately placed where required most. Again, the maximum total dose allowed is 20 mL 1% lignocaine. Analgesia is usually effective within 3 minutes and lasts for about 45 to 90 minutes (*see also* p. 169).

General anaesthesia

With the recognition of safer methods such as spinal and epidural blocks the use of general anaesthesia (GA) has decreased. Although on the decline, it is an associated factor in maternal mortality. Vomiting and inhalation of gastric contents resulting in Mendelson's syndrome is a potentially fatal complication. Premedication with ranitidine and sodium citrate and cricoid pressure lessen the risk. A GA is indicated when regional anaesthesia is contraindicated, or not wished by the mother.

HYPERTENSION

There should be local guidelines/protocols for hypertensive patients in labour. Hypertension may occur for the first time during labour. Exclude proteinuria (if necessary with a catheter specimen of urine). No specific action is necessary if there is no proteinuria and the blood pressure remains below 160/100. Otherwise the patient should be managed as for severe pre-eclampsia as detailed below (*see also* pp. 148–153).

- Take blood for full blood count, electrolytes and clotting screen.
- Start a fluid balance chart and aim to restrict fluid intake to 100 mL/hour.
- If clotting is normal encourage epidural analgesia as this will lower the blood pressure to a degree.
- If the blood pressure remains >160/100 give an iv bolus of 5–10 mg of hydralazine over 10 minutes and commence an intravenous infusion as previously described.
- Consider magnesium sulphate if there are features of hyperreflexia, clonus, epigastric pain, headache, visual disturbance or altered consciousness.
- Avoid a prolonged active second stage.
- Syntometrine should not be used in the third stage since the ergometrine it contains may elevate the blood pressure even further. Syntocinon (5–10 units) im is a suitable alternative.

During labour and after delivery check:

- Clinical condition (reflexes, level of consciousness and chest for evidence of fluid overload) every 4–6 hours.

- BP, urine output hourly.
- serial bloods for platelet count, clotting times, renal and liver function and serum magnesium levels if a magnesium sulphate infusion is in place.
- central venous pressure if oliguric (varies as a practice between units).
- oxygen saturation by pulse oximetry if available.

Avoid fluid overload. After delivery continue high dependency care on labour suite for at least 24 hours after clinical, biochemical and haematological indices have stabilized.

ECLAMPSIA

(*See* pp. 153)

DIABETES

There should be local guidelines/protocols for diabetic patients in labour. In spontaneous or induced labour monitor blood glucose concentrations hourly. The normal subcutaneous insulin is omitted once in established labour and blood glucose controlled using a combination of short acting insulin (usually 1unit/mL in saline) and 5% dextrose according to a sliding scale. The fetal heart rate should be monitored continuously during labour with a lower threshold for fetal blood scalp sampling and delivery in theatre than in non-diabetic pregnancies. Insulin requirements fall dramatically after delivery. Diabetic control should be managed in consultation with the physicians.

SUDDEN COLLAPSE

This includes cardiac or respiratory arrest, sudden loss of consciousness or profound hypotension occurring during labour or after delivery.

Causes (relevant to pregnancy)

- Eclampsia
- Thromboembolism
- Amniotic fluid embolus
- Bleeding (including uterine rupture and inversion and abruption)
- Local anaesthetic toxicity from regional analgesia
- Profound syncope.

Management

- Summon help
- Change position to left lateral if sitting or lying supine
- Ensure the **airway** is clear, check if **breathing** and ventilate if appropriate, check the **circulation** and commence external cardiac compression if there is no output. Administer oxygen. Check for any response to voice. Check pulse blood pressure and fetal heart rate.

- Establish intravenous access and save blood for crossmatching, clotting, full blood count, electrolytes and liver function. Enquire for details of the delivery, drugs given, blood loss and hypertension.
- Further management will depend on the diagnosis (*see* eclampsia, massive haemorrhage pp. 153, 146). Initial treatment for thromboembolus and amniotic fluid embolus is supportive as above.

The first priority is the mother's life and adequate resuscitation takes priority over delivery of the fetus. However, in the event of cardiac arrest if resuscitation has failed to revive the mother within 10 minutes and a fetal heart beat is still present then the baby should be delivered.

PRIMARY POSTPARTUM HAEMORRHAGE

Definition

A vaginal blood loss of more than 500 mL within 24 hours of delivery of the placenta. This incidence is 6–12% of deliveries. The causes are listed in Table 11.4.

Management

- Place a hand on the patient's abdomen and stimulate the uterus to contract by massaging it through the abdominal wall. As you are doing this assess the patient's general condition and ask whether the placenta has been delivered, the mode of delivery and approximate blood loss so far.
- Unless the bleeding stops immediately and the patient shows no sign of haemodynamic compromise summon extra help (an additional midwife, the obstetric registrar, the anesthetist, a porter and the haematology technician on-call).
- Ask the midwife to check pulse and blood pressure. Site a 14 G venflon, two if the bleeding is severe. Take blood for cross-match (minimum four units). If hypotensive give fluids (*see*

Table 11.4 Causes of primary post-partum haemorrhage

Uterine atony (90%)	Prolonged labours Multiple pregnancy, large baby Anesthetic agents Age Multiparity, especially if >4 Tocolysis Operative delivery Previous history Retained placenta/membranes Placenta accreta/percreta Placenta praevia, abruption
Lacerations (7%)	**Uterine rupture** (spontaneous/iatrogenic, scar/non-scar) Risk factors: previous CS, uterine perforation, D&C, MROP, myomectomy, syntocinon use in multips **Cervical** (may extend up to uterine arteries or lower segment) **Vaginal** (episiotomy, laceration, damage from instrumental delivery) **Vulval** (unsecured vessel. Presentation may be delayed with blood tracking to ischiorectal fossa)
Clotting defects (3%)	Pre-eclampsia and HELLP syndrome Abruption Infection Inherited clotting disorders and anticoagulants Massive blood loss

CS: Caesarean section; D&C: dilatation and curettage; MROP: manual removal of placenta.

'Management of major haemorrhage' p. 146–7). If the uterus remains poorly contracted give an additional bolus of syntocinon 10 iu iv or syntometrine 1 ampoule im and follow through the following management options in sequence, until the bleeding ceases. Many of them require the decision to be taken by an experienced obstetrician.

- Commence a syntocinon infusion (40 iu in 500 mLs 5% dextrose over 4 hours).
- Catheterize.
- Examine the vagina and cervix and suture any lacerations.
- If bleeding continues arrange for an examination under anaesthesia to check there are no retained products or uterine, cervical or vaginal lacerations.
- Give carboprost 250 micrograms im or intramyometrially (with repeat doses if necessary).

– Consider laparotomy for uterine rupture, extended cervical lacerations, broad ligament haematomas, direct myometrial injection of the prostaglandin PGF, ligation of internal iliacs, placement of a B-Lynch brace suture and hysterectomy.

RETAINED PLACENTA

Definition

Failure to deliver the placenta within 60 minutes of delivery of the baby.

Risk factors

More common in conditions where the uterus fails to contract properly after delivery (prolonged labour, grandmultiparas), in certain congenital malformations of the uterus and where placentation occurs over a previous uterine scar or invades into the myometrium (placenta accreta).

Management

- **Prevention:** Active management of the third stage with administration of oxytocics at the time of delivery of the fetal shoulders. Given via the intramuscular route, these take 1–2 minutes to stimulate the uterus to contract. Placental separation is indicated by lengthening of the cord, a slight increase in blood loss from the uterus and a rise in the uterine fundus. Keeping the left hand on the abdomen pressing down above the symphysis the placenta is delivered by pulling downwards on the cord.
- **Established retained placenta:** This may be associated with postpartum bleeding. Establish an intravenous line and take blood for cross matching. If the patient is shocked manage as for massive obstetric haemorrhage whilst keeping the uterus as contracted as possible with oxytocics and rubbing the uterus per abdomen. Empty the bladder. If the placenta remains undelivered arrange transfer to theatre for manual removal (*see* 'Practical procedures', p. 179). It is reasonable to leave this for up to an hour if there is no sign of bleeding and spontaneous delivery of the placenta may occur with this extra time. However, beware the rising fundus which may represent a uterus filling with blood.

UTERINE INVERSION

This occurs when the fundus of the uterus is pulled through the cervix, usually as a result of traction on an incompletely separated placenta. The patient can quickly become profoundly shocked and there is often significant bleeding.

Management

- If still attached do not attempt to remove the placenta. It may be possible to push the fundus back up into the uterus manually if the diagnosis is made immediately.
- Commence resuscitation as for massive obstetric haemorrhage and arrange immediate examination under general anaesthetic when uterine relaxation may make further attempts at manual removal successful.
- Using one hand to block the introitus fill the vagina with (warm) saline using hydrostatic pressure to push the fundus back up into the uterus (O'Sullivan's technique).
- Once this has been achieved keep the uterus contracted with a syntocinon infusion and syntometrine and remove the placenta manually.
- Whilst these steps ideally should be undertaken by an experienced obstetrician, delays might make the situation worse and an attempt to push back and re-vert the uterus at the moment it occurs is permissible irrespective of the grade of the operator.
- If these techniques fail then a laparotomy may be necessary. Tenacula or Lanes' tissue forceps may be used to grasp the inverted fundus and correct it (Huntington's technique). If the constriction ring is too tight then it can be incised posteriorly (Haultain technique).

12

ANTEPARTUM EMERGENCIES

ABDOMINAL PAIN

Most women experience one or more episodes of abdominal pain during pregnancy. Many of these resolve spontaneously and a specific diagnosis is never made. Where no pathological cause is found for an episode of abdominal pain there does not appear to be a greater risk of complications in the remainder of the pregnancy.

It is important to be able to distinguish pathological from physiological causes of pain and between those causes that are pregnancy related and more general causes of abdominal pain. Avoiding overintervention and providing reassurance are as important as prompt appropriate treatment where indicated.

CAUSES OF ABDOMINAL PAIN IN PREGNANCY

- **Uterine**
  - labour
  - abruption
  - fibroids
  - polyhydramnios
  - chorioamnionitis
  - rupture.
- **Ovarian**
  - cyst rupture/torsion/haemorrhage
- **Intestinal**
  - constipation
  - appendicitis
  - obstruction
  - peptic ulceration.
- **Hepatic**
  - cholecystitis
  - hepatic distension of pre-eclampsia
  - acute fatty liver of pregnancy.

- **Renal**
  - urinary tract infection and pyelonephritis
  - urinary calculus.
- **Abdominal wall**
  - hernia
  - rectus haematoma
  - varicella zoster
  - symphysis pubis pain.
- **Other**
  - ruptured splenic aneurysm
  - pancreatitis
  - sickle cell crisis
  - ketoacidosis
  - referred pain (MI, PE, pneumonia).

THE KEY STEPS

- ***To determine whether the woman is in labour and if so whether it is uncomplicated.***
- ***If she is not in labour is the pain still uterine and if so is it due to an abruption?***
- ***If the pain is not uterine is the cause pathological and in need of treatment?***
- ***If it is pathological is the treatment likely to be surgical?***

HISTORY

- Re-calculate and check the current gestational age from early ultrasound and last period.
- Has the pregnancy been uncomplicated to date? If not take particular note of previous bleeding, prolonged rupture of membranes, multiple pregnancy, previously noted uterine fibroids or ovarian cysts and hypertension.
- Ask about the pain. Was the onset sudden or gradual? Is it intermittent or continuous? Where is it felt and is it associated with uterine contractions? Ask about associated symptoms, especially vaginal bleeding, nausea or vomiting, and any problems with defaecation or micturition. Labour usually presents as intermittent central or lower abdominal pain of gradual onset lasting 1–2 minutes and associated with uterine contractions. The pain should markedly improve between contractions. There may be a preceding history of passing a blood streaked mucous plug (show). Remember uterine activity occurs throughout pregnancy

and painful Braxton–Hicks contractions may be difficult to distinguish from labour. **Also labour (especially if pre-term) may be triggered by other causes of abdominal pain such as abruption and infection.**

- Enquire about previous obstetric history. Previous abruptions (recurrence risk 6%), pre-term labour and operations resulting in a uterine scar (Caesarean section, myomectomy) may all carry significance for the current pregnancy.
- Ask whether there is any history of abdominal pain or abdominal surgery prior to the current pregnancy.
- Remember that recurrent admissions for abdominal pain may be the presentation of social problems. Tactfully explore this possibility.

KEY POINT

Beware of attributing abdominal pain to labour in a multiparous woman who says it is different from labour pain.

EXAMINATION

- Assess the patient's general condition and check pulse, blood pressure and temperature.
- Look for evidence of previous abdominal surgery. Palpate the abdomen starting away from the area of maximal tenderness. Does the uterine size seem large or small for dates ? Is the uterus soft, hard or contracting ? If the abdomen is tender to palpation determine if this is over the uterus and if not whether there is any associated peritonism. Check for tenderness over the renal angles. Ask the patient to turn onto her left side keeping a hand over the area of tenderness. If the pain shifts to the left it is more likely to be uterine or adnexal (Alder's sign). Listen for bowel sounds and a fetal heartbeat.
- Perform a gentle speculum examination. If there is evidence of ruptured membranes take a swab and estimate cervical dilation. Otherwise carry out a digital examination to determine cervical dilatation and effacement and to feel for any adnexal masses.

INVESTIGATIONS

These will be determined by the examination and history findings.

- A urinalysis is mandatory. Proteinuria may be due to urinary tract infection but may also occur in pre-eclampsia presenting as epigastric pain or with an abruption. Renal colic is unlikely in the absence of haematuria but vaginal bleeding from a show or abruption contaminating the sample occur more commonly. Send urine for culture.

- Where the diagnosis is unclear a **full blood count**, looking for a raised leucocyte count (interpretation of a single value is difficult unless it is markedly raised because of the normal leucocytosis of pregnancy), **serum amylase** and **Kleihauer** (to look for evidence of concealed abruption by the detection of fetal red cells in the maternal circulation) may be of help.
- Ultrasound is of limited value in the diagnosis of abdominal pain. An abruption large enough to be seen on scan is usually evident clinically and occasionally large venous sinuses may be erroneously diagnosed as abruptions. A scan may help in the diagnosis of ovarian tumours, uterine fibroids, polyhydramnios, gallstones and hydronephrosis.

MANAGEMENT

General principles

- Check for a fetal heart beat and commence external monitoring if 26 or more weeks.
- **If the patient is shocked** the most likely diagnosis is massive abruption (see below). If the uterus is soft consider other causes of intra-abdominal bleeding such as ruptured splenic or hepatic aneurysm, uterine rupture, intestinal perforation and septicaemic shock from chorioamnionitis, appendicitis (see below) or pyelonephritis. Site two 14 G canulae, take blood for full blood count, clotting, biochemistry and crossmatch (six units) and summon help.
- If the **patient is stable but unwell** with a pyrexia and tachycardia the most likely diagnoses are **chorioamnionitis** if there is a history of ruptured membranes or uterine tenderness and **pyelonephritis** in the presence of loin tenderness. Otherwise consider **appendicitis** and **cholecystitis** (see below). Take urine, blood and vaginal swabs for culture. Check the white cell count (as stated above however, serial values may be more helpful).
- If the **patient is systemically well** or only mildly tachycardic but distressed by the pain the most likely diagnosis is labour. If there is no evidence of this on abdominal palpation and vaginal examination consider abruption, degeneration of uterine fibroids or ovarian cyst accidents if the pain arises in the genital tract and renal or intestinal colic if not.

The further management of labour, abruption, pre-eclampsia, chorioamnionitis and urinary tract infection are discussed elsewhere.

Appendicitis

This is the most common non-gynaecological condition requiring surgery during pregnancy. Although it is no more common in pregnancy (1–2/1000 pregnancies) mortality is four times higher than the general population due to delays in diagnosis and treatment. Pregnancy displaces the appendix upwards, laterally and away from the anterior abdominal wall and a white cell count of 10–15×10^9/L can be normal. Appendicitis may present with right loin pain and sterile pyuria mimicking pyelonephritis and the temperature remains normal or slightly raised in two thirds of cases. Despite these caveats the commonest presentation remains periumbilical pain shifting to the right iliac fossa. A resting tachycardia, low grade pyrexia and negative urine culture are all suspicious if present but their absence does not exclude the diagnosis. Similarly appendicitis is unlikely where the white cell count is less than 10 and there are no symptoms of nausea or loss of appetite. **The most important step is to think of the diagnosis**. Early surgical referral is essential. Check white cell count, electrolytes and start an intravenous infusion. The morbidity of an 'unnecessary' laparotomy is far lower than that of a perforated appendix so a high index of suspicion with early recourse to surgery is essential. Classically the incision for an appendicectomy in pregnancy is over the point of maximal tenderness.

Cholecystitis

Cholecystectomy is the second commonest non-obstetric operation in pregnancy (1–6/10 000 pregnancies). Half the patients will have had symptoms before pregnancy. Epigastric or right upper quadrant pain radiating to the loin is associated with nausea, vomiting and sometimes jaundice (5% only). Initial management is usually **conservative** with intravenous fluids, sedation, analgesia and antibiotics. Check liver function tests, electrolytes, white cell count and arrange ultrasound examination of the biliary tract. Ask for a surgical opinion. **Surgery** should be considered if there is obstruction of common bile duct, cholangitis, pancreatitis, empyema or failure to respond to medical treatment.

Fibroids

These are the commonest of gynaecological tumours and are found in 0.5–5% of women and are commoner in the Afro-Caribbean population. If not previously diagnosed they may be identified on ultrasound examination or present as a large for dates uterus. They increase in size during pregnancy as a result of hypertrophy and oedema in response to elevated oestrogen levels. Red degeneration occurs as a result of thrombosis in the capsular vessels and venous engorgement presenting as acute abdominal pain and vomiting. The uterus is tender and there may be an associated low grade temperature and raised white cell count. Management is medical with analgesia and bedrest. The pain normally resolves in 4–7 days. Laparotomy is indicated only where there is doubt about the diagnosis to exclude other causes of pain or where there is a pedunculated sub-serous fibroid which has undergone torsion.

Acute fatty liver of pregnancy

A rare condition of unknown aetiology with a maternal and fetal mortality rate possibly as high as 85%. It presents with sudden onset nausea, vomiting, upper abdominal pain and liver tenderness, usually in the third trimester. It may be associated with hypertension, proteinuria, oedema, renal failure and haematemesis. Jaundice is a late development and may be accompanied by disseminated intravascular coagulation (DIC) and hepatic encephalopathy. The diagnosis is confirmed by finding hypoglycaemia, deranged liver function tests, and hyperuricaemia. There may be liver changes detectable with ultrasound or CT, but this is variable. Management essentially involves making the diagnosis and immediate delivery of the baby. Large amounts of dextrose may be necessary to treat the profound hypoglycaemia with supportive care for the other organ systems. Liver transplantation is sometimes needed.

Renal colic

This usually presents in the second half of pregnancy with acute loin pain and superimposed abdominal colic. Microscopic haematuria is usually present. Check a urine sample for infection and consider renal ultrasound or a plain abdominal X-ray (as part of a modified intravenous urogram). Once the diagnosis is confirmed treat with analgesia and antibiotics. If the stone is not passed (50% chance) ask for a urological opinion.

ANTEPARTUM HAEMORRHAGE

Definition

Bleeding from the genital tract prior to labour after the 23rd week of pregnancy.

Incidence

Ten per cent of pregnancies.

CAUSES

- Abruption
- Placenta praevia
- Lower genital tract lesions
  - cervical erosion
  - cervicitis and vaginal infections
  - trauma and foreign bodies
  - genital tract varicosities
  - genital tract tumours (benign/malignant)
- Heavy 'show'
- Unspecified/undetermined
- Other sites, e.g. rectal.

GENERAL PRINCIPLES OF MANAGEMENT

Assess patient's general condition for signs of haemodynamic compromise.

KEY POINT

If the patient is shocked or bleeding heavily call for immediate senior assistance* (see *'Major haemorrhage' p. 146)

Most patients will be cardiovascularly stable and will appear well. Once the patient has been resuscitated, if necessary, use the history, examination and ultrasound findings to establish the likely cause. In practice for most significant bleeds this will mean distinguishing placenta praevia from placental separation or abruption (*see* Table 12.1).

History

- Re-calculate and confirm the current **gestational age.**
- Ask about the duration of bleeding and the estimated amount.
- Were there any **precipitating factors**? Postcoital bleeding is suggestive of local cervical causes or placenta praevia. Bleeding following external trauma to the uterus may be a sign of placental abruption.
- Was the bleeding associated with **abdominal pain** or **uterine contractions**? Classically a placental abruption is painful and often triggers uterine activity. A bleed from a placenta praevia is said to

Table 12.1 Distinguishing features for antepartum hemorrhage

	Abruption	Placenta praevia
Bleeding	Painful	Usually painless
Haemodynamic signs	Often greater than observed loss	Proportionate to observed loss
Uterus	Tender and irritable; may be hard to feel fetal parts	Soft
Fetal position	Normal	Presenting part not engaged, breech transverse and oblique lie more common
Fetal heart rate	Absent or abnormal	Normal

be painless; however, it may occur after contractions begin and can be associated with abruption also. To confuse matters further an abruption can be 'silent'.

- Have there been previous episodes of bleeding in the present pregnancy ?
- Abruption and placenta praevia both have **recurrence risks** and a past history of either condition is significant. Previous Caesarean section is a risk factor for placenta praevia and maternal hypertensive disorders predispose to abruptio placentae.
- Check the notes for any **ultrasound scans** indicating the placental site.
- What was the date of the **last cervical smear?**

Examination

- What is the **general condition** of the patient? Placenta praevia and abruption can both cause shock; however, if the degree of this is out of proportion to the severity of the bleeding a concealed abruption is the more likely diagnosis.
- Check for **uterine tenderness, contractions and increased tone**. If the uterus is tender, is it still possible to feel fetal parts and does it relax between contractions?
- Check for **abnormal lie or presentation** as this may indicate a low lying placenta preventing engagement of the presenting part.
- The presence of **hypertension and proteinuria** may signify pre-eclampsia, a known risk factor for placental abruption.
- **Do not carry out a pelvic examination without first discussing with a senior obstetrician.** A speculum examination is important to exclude lower genital tract causes but should also be deferred until the placental site has been determined by ultrasound scan.

Investigations

- Full blood count.
- Group and save and crossmatch if moderate or heavy bleed (4–8 units). Rhesus negative patients will require immunoprophylaxis with anti-D.
- Clotting screen. Clotting abnormalities are most commonly associated with abruption but will occur in any scenario involving haemorrhage and multiple blood transfusion.
- Kleihauer test. This is performed on all Rhesus negative patients who bleed. It quantifies the amount of fetal blood reaching the maternal circulation at times of possible haemorrhage. Treatment with 500 iu of anti-D is the standard amount given to women who have vaginal bleeding after 20 weeks' gestation. However if the feto-maternal transfusion is large, more will be necessary and this will be indicated by the Kleihauer result. The Kleihauer can also be used in Rhesus positive women to retrospectively show that fetomaternal haemorrhage has occurred.
- Carry out or arrange an ultrasound to establish the placental site. Do not rely on the placental location from an 18–20 week scan. False-negatives are recognized, particularly with posterior placentas. Also, most low lying placentas at 20 weeks will have been pulled clear of the lower segment by the third trimester. Remember that placental abruption can occur in patients with placenta praevias and that measuring the distance between the lower edge of the placenta and the cervical os is less accurate in posterior placental sites.
- Cardiotocography. Any CTG abnormalities in the presence of vaginal bleeding are highly suspicious of abruption and may indicate the need for immediate delivery. However, CTG changes can be a late event in an evolving abruption and so a normal CTG does not exclude an abruption.

PLACENTA PRAEVIA

Definition

Placental implantation in the lower segment

Incidence

An incidence of 0.5% pregnancies at term. Note that 20–30% of women may have a low-lying placental site on scan at 20 weeks, but only 3% of these will be praevia at term.

Risk factors

Multiparous older women, multiple pregnancy, previous Caesarean sections and diabetes.

Classification is by 'grade'

- I: reaching the lower segment, i.e. within 5 cm of the internal os at term (the lower segment is shorter at earlier gestations and is nonexistent until approximately 28 weeks).
- II: reaching the internal os.
- III: eccentrically covering the internal os.
- IV: centrally/symmetrically covering the os.

MANAGEMENT

- If under 37 weeks with no evidence of fetal or maternal compromise, ensure that blood is available and hospitalize for bed rest.
- Give steroids (two doses of 12 mg betamethasone or dexamethasone 12 hours apart) if under 34 weeks (some units use 35 weeks as the limit).
- How long a patient stays in hospital will be determined by the severity and frequency of the antepartum bleeds, the proximity of their home to the hospital, the experiences and preferences of their managing consultant and perhaps the grade of the placenta praevia. Traditionally these women stayed in hospital from 32–34 weeks' gestation until delivery. Recently, there has been a move to manage them at home with the compromise being admission from 36 weeks gestation. The advantage is reduced social disruption and psychological morbidity but this policy risks emergency admission with major antepartum haemorrhage (APH) with possible fetal and maternal morbidity/mortality.
- For asymptomatic grade I and II placenta praevias diagnosed early in the third trimester repeat scanning may be of value as the relationship of the internal os to the placental lower edge may change as the lower segment preferentially develops over the third trimester.
- ***Vaginal delivery*** may be possible with a grade I anterior praevia as the placenta can be displaced anteriorly and superiorly by the fetal head. This is more likely if the head is engaged by 37 weeks. An examination in theatre with the patient awake, but prepared for Caesarean section is carried out after 38 weeks by an experienced obstetrician and if no placenta can be palpated through the vaginal fornices or within 5 cm of the internal os labour is induced by rupture of the membranes.

- *Caesarean section* is indicated for all other types of praevia once the patient reaches 38 weeks or earlier if the patient labours or there is persistent bleeding. There is an increased risk of intrapartum and postpartum bleeding because the lower segment is less able to contract to secure haemostasis at the site of implantation of the placenta. Such operations should be carried out with consultant supervision with six units of blood available. Some consider that regional anaesthesia should only be used after discussion at consultant level as there is a theoretical risk of increased haemorrhage. Anterior placentas may have to be incised to enter the uterine cavity. An infusion of syntocinon (40 units in 500 mL of normal saline over 4 hours) should be commenced following delivery of the infant. A hysterectomy is needed more frequently in this scenario and most believe that all women with a placenta praevia should be consented for this prior to the Casarean section commencing.

PLACENTAL ABRUPTION

Definition

Bleeding into the decidual space causing separation of trophoblast from chorion. The blood subsequently leaks out and is 'revealed' or infuses into the myometrium causing increased tone and reduced placental perfusion with release of thromboplastin.

Incidence

An incidence of 1% of pregnancies.

Risk factors

Increased maternal age, hypertensive disorders (10% of pre-eclamptics, 24% of eclamptics), smoking (two-fold relative risk), collagen vascular diseases, trauma, decompression of polyhydramnios and a history of abruption in a previous pregnancy.

MANAGEMENT

- If there has been a small bleed only, under 38 weeks, with localized tenderness at most, normal fetal heart rate pattern and stable maternal signs then conservative management may be possible. Check full blood count (FBC) and clotting, ensure iv access and watch closely. Keep in hospital until the bleeding has stopped. Hospitalization after that point will vary with clinical circumstances. If under 34 weeks, consider giving the mother dexamethasone. Arrange serial scans for growth and treat the remainder of the pregnancy as high risk.

- **Deliver** if other than above. Any bleeding not attributable to placenta praevia or a 'show' occurring after 37 weeks is an indication for delivery, vaginally if possible, with continuous intrapartum monitoring. In earlier pregnancies the decision may be more difficult especially in concealed abruptions where the diagnosis is based only on abdominal pain. Remember that the longer the delay before delivery the worse the outcome, that premature infants tolerate abruption poorly and a terminal deterioration in the fetal heart rate pattern may occur with relatively minor abnormalities on the preceding CTG. Because abruption will often stimulate uterine activity it may be possible to deliver even preterm pregnancies vaginally although there should be a low threshold for Caesarean section if there is evidence of fetal compromise. Delivery by **Caesarean section** is indicated where there is a persistently abnormal fetal heart rate pattern and delivery is not imminent, or if vaginal delivery is unlikely soon and there is evidence of continued bleeding. During labour and after delivery monitor blood pressure, urine output and check FBC and clotting at regular intervals for signs of disseminated intravascular coagulation. Inform the obstetric consultant, haematologist and anaesthetist of any patient with a significant abruption.

Complications

Complications of abruption include:

- DIC
- PPH (25%; commonest cause of maternal death)
- renal failure
- isoimmunization
- intrauterine fetal death.

PRETERM UTERINE ACTIVITY

Definition

Preterm labour can be defined as regular uterine contractions resulting in cervical effacement/dilatation before 37 completed weeks and after 23 weeks of pregnancy. It can be very difficult to distinguish between preterm uterine activity that will settle spontaneously and that which will result in premature labour.

Incidence

Preterm labour occurs in 5–9% of pregnancies but accounts for 85% of perinatal deaths (excluding lethal malformations). This has remained largely unchanged over recent years.

CAUSES AND RISK FACTORS FOR PRE-TERM LABOUR

Note that the causes of preterm delivery are subtly different from those of preterm labour; for example severe PET may result in preterm delivery by IOL or Caesarean section, but in most cases does not cause preterm labour. (The causes of pre-term labour are unknown in about 30% of cases.)

Maternal

- Age (<15, >35)
- Socioeconomic class
- Smoking
- Race (black > white)
- Weight (<50 kg)
- Illegal drug abuse
- Infection and high pyrexia, e.g. pyelonephritis
- Trauma e.g. road traffic accident
- Uterine anomalies.

Previous history

- Previous preterm labour (35% recurrence)
- Previous cone biopsy (cervical incompetence)
- Vaginal bleeding in the current pregnancy.

Fetal/placental

- Chorioamnionitis (infection) e.g. bacterial vaginosis
- Polyhydramnios (30–40% preterm)
- Multiple pregnancy
- Fetal abnormality
- Pre-term rupture of membranes (30–40%)
- Abruption and bleeding placenta praevia.

History

- Ask about the onset and frequency of pains and any vaginal loss (?show ?liquor ?blood ?infected discharge).
- Check for risk factors and symptoms of infection or abruption (see above)
- Check the current gestation carefully. This is especially important at extremely preterm gestations.

EXAMINATION

- Check routine maternal observations and the fetal heart beat.
- Palpate the uterus and note whether size corresponds to dates. Is there is any tenderness or uterine contractions?
- Try to determine the presentation and whether the presenting part is engaged.
- Carry out a gentle speculum examination and look for any evidence of blood or liquor and any obvious cervical dilatation.Take swabs for culture from the cervix.
- If there is no evidence of ruptured membranes cervical dilation should be assessed by gentle digital examination.

KEY POINT

About 50–86% of contractions will settle on no therapy and it is often not possible to diagnose true preterm labour on the basis of one examination. Although these should be kept to a minimum (especially if the membranes have ruptured) repeat examinations may be necessary to document cervical change.

INVESTIGATIONS

- Take blood for white cell count, CRP and urine for culture. A cervical swab should already have been done during the examination. Perform blood cultures if there is a high pyrexia.
- An ultrasound scan may be necessary to define lie, presentation and placental site.

MANAGEMENT

The risk of true labour developing will be higher if painful uterine contractions are more frequent than every 8 minutes, if the cervix is soft and less than 2 cm long or more than 2 cm dilated or changing its characteristics over 2 hours.

Treatment

- Treat any underlying precipitating factors such as urinary tract infections (UTIs).
- Admit and ensure adequate analgesia, rehydration and rest.
- Give steroids if less than 34 weeks (in some units 36 weeks).
- Ensure that the paediatric staff are aware. The lower gestational limits for care of preterm infants vary between units. Whether there is potential free cot space will vary from day to day also.

- Decide if attempts at labour suppression are warranted. If less than 34 weeks' gestation consider **tocolysis** in order to allow time for steroids to take effect or to allow transfer to a unit with neonatal cots. The most widely used agents are intravenous beta-sympathomimetics (terbutaline, ritodrine, salbutamol) although non-steroidal anti-inflammatory drugs, calcium channel blockers and glyceryl trinitrate (GTN) patches are also under evaluation.
  Contraindications to the use of tocolytics are:
  – Fetal death/lethal malformation
  – Abnormal CTG
  – APH
  – Chorioamnionitis
  – Maternal heart disease.

Diabetes is a relative contraindication to beta sympathomimetics which disturb glucose control (an insulin sliding scale may be necessary). Extra care must also be taken with multiple pregnancies (see below).

Pethidine alone can be an effective intermediate treatment and can be justified for maternal analgesic reasons.

Beta-sympathomimetics should be given in as small a volume of fluid as possible at the minimum dose which stops contractions (see prescribing sections for more information). Before starting treatment exclude any evidence of maternal cardiovascular disease. Monitor maternal pulse (keep below 120) and blood pressure very regularly and auscultate the lungs every 6 hours as there is a risk of pulmonary oedema with this treatment (this contributes to a number of maternal deaths each year and is greater in multiple pregnancies and when steroids have also been administered). Check blood glucose and potassium levels at regular intervals (risk of hyperglycaemia and hypokalemia). Once contractions have stopped gradually reduce the dose of tocolytic.There is no evidence for using oral therapy subsequently.

- If tocolysis is contraindicated or unsuccessful the **mode of delivery** must be decided upon. Aim to deliver vaginally but consider Caesarean section if the presentation is breech between 26 and 32 weeks (800–1500 g), or if there are CTG abnormalities.

KEY POINTS

The use of tocolysis, in utero transfers and the mode of delivery for patients with preterm labour are all consultant level decisions and policies vary from unit to unit. At very preterm gestations (less than 26 weeks) careful

counselling from senior obstetricians and paediatricians is necessary before management is decided. Caesarean sections at these times are difficult and carry risks for future pregnancies. The rates of survival and neurological handicap change dramatically with gestation and over-aggressive attempts to deliver a liveborn infant may not always be justified.

PRETERM (PRE-LABOUR) RUPTURE OF MEMBRANES

Spontaneous rupture of membranes occurs in up to 10% of pregnancies prior to the onset of labour. Many more women notice some watery vaginal discharge which is not liquor. The differential diagnosis includes vaginal discharge and urine. Ask about the amount of fluid lost, its colour and whether the loss occurred after micturition. Check the pulse and temperature and examine the abdomen for any signs of tenderness. Carry out a sterile speculum examination and look for any pooling of fluid, any evidence of cord prolapse and estimate cervical dilation. If there is no obvious liquor seen ask the patient to cough. Take a sample of any fluid for Gram stain and culture. Monitor the fetal heart. If the diagnosis is still unproven but the history is suggestive admit for observation for any further loss.

PRE-LABOUR RUPTURE OF MEMBRANES AT TERM

More than 80% of women will labour spontaneously within 24 hours. If there are any features of infection at initial assessment or if labour does not occur within 24 hours most centres would induce labour with syntocinon if the cervix is effaced and open. If the cervix is long and/or closed a course of oral or vaginal prostaglandins can be used prior to the syntocinon. In the absence of signs of infection some centres will treat conservatively and await the onset of spontaneous labour over several days. Pre-labour rupture of membranes may be associated with an abnormal presentation or poorly applied presenting part and is more likely to be associated with prolonged labour and operative delivery. In all cases vigilance for chorioamnionitis should be maintained until delivery:

- Pyrexia
- Maternal and fetal tachycardia
- Uterine tenderness
- Raised white cell count ($>15 \times 10^9$/L)
- Raised CRP.

PRE-TERM (BEFORE 37 WEEKS) RUPTURE OF MEMBRANES (PTROM)

There is a 30% chance of labour. After 34 weeks this should be allowed to continue if it occurs. Furthermore, many units would wait 24 hours and then induce labour at 34 weeks or more because of the low risks from prematurity at and beyond this gestation. Tocolysis should be used with care if at all below 34 weeks as the onset of uterine activity in these patients may be the first sign of chorioamnionitis. The benefit of steroids in pre-term pregnancies with ROM is unproven though many units will use them. If labour does not occur and there are no signs of infection admit for 4 hourly pulse, temperature and blood pressure, twice weekly white cell counts, CRP measurements and weekly vaginal swabs. (Beware the usual rise in WCC following steroid administration). Treat any proven vaginal infection. The timing and mode of elective delivery should be considered by an experienced obstetrician. The value of routine administration of antibiotics in all cases is under evaluation but is preferred by some units. Deliver if any signs of infection or after 37 weeks (34 weeks in some units). Ensure that the Special Care Baby/Neonatal Unit can accommodate a premature infant with possible sepsis.

DECREASED FETAL MOVEMENTS

Fetal movements are normally felt from about 18 weeks onwards. In some mothers it can be earlier. Perception of movements may be reduced by obesity or an anterior placenta or when the mother is distracted by events or other symptoms. Most women notice a change in the quality of movement towards term and of quantity just prior to labour. Periods of inactivity associated with fetal sleep are normal but these are short-lived and last no more than 40 minutes. Some mothers will report more fetal activity at night than during the day. Absence or significant reduction in movements in a previously active fetus should always be treated seriously as it may be a sign of impending or actual fetal demise. Statistically the fetus is at greater likelihood of death and thus the pregnancy should be managed as one 'at risk'.

MANAGEMENT

Practice varies. Establish whether a fetal heart beat is present. If less than 24 weeks it may be necessary to use a portable Doppler ultrasound but the mother can then normally be reassured without hospital admission. If more than 24 weeks or if a fetal heart cannot be heard patients complaining of reduced movements should be seen in hospital. If fetal heart sounds cannot be heard either by auscultation or using an external CTG **or if there is any doubt about the quality of the CTG recording carry out an ultrasound to look for fetal heart movements.** If the fetal heartbeat is absent on ultrasound have your findings confirmed by a more experienced sonographer and manage as for an intrauterine fetal death (IUFD) as below.

Where the fetal heart rate appears normal next try to establish if there is any evidence of a problem perceiving movements. Are the fetal movements seen, palpated or heard on the CTG felt by the mother? Has the mother had difficulty feeling movements throughout the pregnancy? Recent cessation of movements is a worrying feature.

Unless there is clear evidence of a perceptual problem or the pregnancy is less than 24 weeks any woman admitted complaining of reduced movements requires as full an evaluation as possible of fetal well-being. This should include at least a review of any risk factors, clinical examination and a cardiotocograph (CTG). An ultrasound evaluation of fetal growth and biophysical score (or at least liquor volume) and umbilical artery Doppler is also desirable but can be delayed until the next day if no suitably experienced sonographer or equipment is available on admission provided the CTG and examination are normal. Many units do not perform this ultrasound evaluation of the fetus. However, this is illogical. The antenatal CTG is a poor long-term predictor of fetal death in high risk pregnancies, whilst for example, umbilical artery Doppler recording is a good predictor.

CLINICAL HISTORY AND EXAMINATION

Confirm the current gestation. Ask whether there have been any episodes of vaginal bleeding during the pregnancy after 20 weeks. Was the reduction in movements associated with any pain? Look at the notes and look for recent scans, evidence of growth restriction, pre-eclampsia, or isoimmunization. Ask about the outcome of any previous pregnancies especially previous stillbirth, abruption or growth retardation. Examine for hypertension and test the urine for protein. The symphysial-fundal height in cm should correspond to the gestation in weeks (±2 cm). Does the amount of liquor around the baby appear normal? Is the uterus tender or irritable?

ANTENATAL CARDIOTOCOGRAPHY

Interpretation can be difficult in pre-term pregnancies. In particular, isolated abnormalities need to be evaluated in the context of the rest of the trace and other assessments of fetal well-being. It also should be remembered that the CTG only gives short term (hours) reassurance of fetal health. It is a poor long-term predictor of fetal risk. The antenatal CTG is interpreted in much the same way as a CTG from the first stage of labour (*see* p. 107) and can be described as normal, suspicious or abnormal. However, any form of deceleration is abnormal in a non-contracting patient and should cause significant concern in this setting.

ULTRASOUND

Liquor volume, biophysical profile scores and umbilical artery Doppler waveforms can all be measured and used to ascertain whether this pregnancy is normal or not. Indeed, fetal movements seen on scan are often not felt by the patient and it is valuable to note this. *See* p. 86 (Fetal surveillance) for more information.

MANAGEMENT

Table 12.2 gives the four possible options for management. Opinions vary, especially at very preterm gestations and there is not always good trial evidence to guide the clinician. Exactly how abnormal do antenatal monitoring tests have to be before one considers delivering an infant at 25–26 weeks, for example ? Is the delay of 48 hours for steroid administration harmful or beneficial in this situation ? Clearly management of preterm pregnancies needs to involve a senior high-risk obstetrician and the paediatric team and steroids should be administered to pregnancies of less than 35 weeks' gestation if preterm delivery is a possibility.

INTRAUTERINE FETAL DEATH (IUFD)

Definition

Intrauterine fetal death (IUFD) is fetal death diagnosed after 23 weeks. This term applies even if it is suspected that fetal demise occurred before 24 weeks.

Causes of fetal death

- **Fetal**
  - Congenital malformation/syndrome/karyotypic anomaly

Table 12.2 Possible action for reduced movements in an anatomically normal fetus

Immediate delivery	Persistently suspicious or abnormal CTG Suspicious CTG and abnormal BPS (<8) Reversed end diastolic flow (? all gestations)
Delivery within 24 hours	High risk pregnancy at term Maternal indication (e.g. pre-eclampsia) Reduced AFV (in the absence of ruptured membranes) at 34 or more weeks Persistently abnormal umbilical artery Doppler at 34 or more weeks
Continued fetal monitoring	Preterm high risk pregnancy or suspected IUGR with normal umbilical artery Doppler, BPS and CTG Reduced AFV before 34 weeks Abnormal umbilical artery Doppler record (not reversed flow) before 34 weeks
Normal care	Low-risk pregnancy with normal fetal assessment where movements return to normal

  - Cord accident (compression or knot)
  - Infection (e.g. parvovirus, listeria, CMV, toxoplasmosis)
  - Isoimmunization
  - Fetomaternal haemorrhage
- **Placental**
  - pre-eclampsia
  - anti-phospholipid syndrome
  - abruption
  - chorioamnionitis
- **Maternal**
  - diabetes
  - cholestasis of pregnancy.

Diagnosis

Presentation is usually with absent fetal movements or when a fetal heart is not heard during an antenatal examination. The diagnosis is confirmed by ultrasound examination.

MANAGEMENT

The aims are to deliver the fetus, treat any coexisting maternal illness and initiate investigations to establish a cause whilst providing sympathetic support for the patient and her family.

Immediately after confirmation of the diagnosis inform the senior obstetrician on-call and discuss the findings with the parents. Unless there is a pressing maternal medical indication to do otherwise allow the parents time to ask questions and be alone together or with other members of the family. When they are ready, carry out a full clinical examination in particular checking blood pressure and urinalysis. Document fundal height and look for any evidence of abruption. Carry out a gentle pelvic examination taking swabs for bacterial culture and to establish cervical dilation. Unless there is a maternal indication for admission (such as ante-partum haemorrhage or pre-eclampsia) induction of labour can be according to the parents' wishes.

Investigation for intrauterine death (IUD)

- Full blood count
- Blood glucose/glycosylated Hb
- Liver function tests, uric acid
- Clotting screen
- Blood group/anti-red cell antibodies
- Kleihauer test (before labour induced)
- Serum for toxoplasma, rubella, cytomegalovirus, parvovirus B_{12} testing
- Anti-phospholipid antibody screen
- Blood cultures
- High vaginal swab
- Bacterial cultures from fetus and placenta
- Karyotype
- Post-mortem and examination of placenta.

Delivery should be vaginal if possible using amniotomy and syntocinon and/or prostaglandins. Caesarean section might be indicated for abnormal presentation, some types of uterine scar and occasionally for maternal request. Provided severe PET or abruption has not been the cause, it takes many weeks for a coagulopathy to occur after IUD and most women will be quite safe to go home prior to admission for the delivery. Prior to the delivery discuss with the parents whether they wish to see and hold the baby after it has been delivered. Most couples later will say how valuable it was to have time alone with their child. Tangible mementos such as photographs and foot prints should be taken and stored carefully. Many who decline the offer of seeing the baby at delivery will later ask for the photographs.

- After delivery examine the fetus for any obvious congenital malformations, note the fetal weight and any evidence of maceration.
- Check for cord entanglement or true knots.
- Weigh the placenta and look for evidence of any retroplacental bleeding or abnormalities.
- Take a small piece of fetal skin, a sample of placenta and if possible blood from a cardiac stab from the fetus for karyotyping.
- Discuss sensitively with the parents the value of a limited or full post-mortem examination of the baby. Ideally request for post-mortem should come from a senior obstetrician who is responsible for the patient's care.
- If the offer of a post-mortem is declined take an X-ray. This will occasionally highlight a skeletal dysplasia which has been the underlying cause of the IUD.
- Always send the placenta for histological examination.
- Write out a death certificate.
- Inform the patients GP and community midwife prior to discharge and arrange a follow-up appointment for 6–8 weeks.
- Remember most units have a standard protocol for managing fetal death including a check list of investigations.
- Many units also have a designated midwife or chaplain who acts as grief counsellor and coordinates care of bereaved parents but that does not absolve obstetricians from contributing to the sensitive and sympathetic care needed by the woman.
- A number of support organisations, e.g. SANDS (Support after Neonatal Death or Stillbirth) exist. All couples should be informed of these groups but they do not suit all and bereaved parents should be allowed to contact them independently.

SEVERE OBSTETRIC EMERGENCIES

MAJOR HAEMORRHAGE

Definition

- Blood loss >25% circulating volume
- >1500 mL blood loss
- heavy continuing blood loss (it would be irresponsible to wait until 1500 mL of blood have been passed before implementing prompt management).

Table 12.3 gives details of the clinical features by which the amount of blood loss can be estimated.

Table 12.3 Clinical features of massive blood loss

Volume Lost	Signs	Heart rate	Syst BP	Output	Symptoms
10–15%	Postural hypotension	80–100	Normal	Normal	Dizzy on standing
15–30%	Cold peripheries	100–120	Normal	Oliguric	Thirst, weakness
30–40%	Pallor, cold	120+	70–80	Oliguric	Restless, syncope
40%	Sweaty pale cold	120+ Thready	50	Anuric	Air hunger Collapse

Common causes of major obstetric haemorrhage

- *Antepartum*
  - Placenta praevia
  - Abruption
  - Uterine rupture
  - Difficult haemostasis at Caesarean section.
- *Postpartum*
  - Uterine atony
  - Lower genital tract trauma (perineal, vaginal and cervical lacerations; uterine perforation during curettage for retained products)
  - Retained products of conception
  - Uterine inversion
  - Endometritis.

MANAGEMENT

The aims are:

- to stop blood loss
- to resuscitate the patient and restore/maintain oxygen carrying volume to tissues.

All units should have major obstetric haemorrhage protocols. Everyone working in the obstetric unit should be familiar with these.

See sections on Antepartum haemorrhage and Postpartum haemorrhage for specific measures to stop bleeding and in addition do the following:

- Summon all extra staff especially a senior anaesthetist. Inform blood bank and porters.
- Take 20 mL of blood for crossmatch (at least six units), FBC, clotting studies, renal and liver function tests.

- Administer oxygen by face mask.
- Site two 14 G iv lines.
- Insert a Foley catheter.
- Give a plasma expander (crystalloid or colloid). Beware, however, fluid overloading patients, especially those with severe pre-eclampsia (see below).
- Give blood as soon as possible. Wait for cross-matched blood if the blood pressure improves with fluids and remains stable. Otherwise give ABO compatible blood or even O Rhesus negative blood if the loss is >40%. Use a compression cuff if the volume expansion is needed rapidly and a blood warmer if > 2 units are given. If >40% volume is replaced extra colloid (HAS) should be given.
- Consider central venous pressure (CVP)/Arterial lines.
- Recheck haematology, clotting and biochemistry at regular intervals – the results quickly become 'out-of-date'.
- Give FFP, platelets and cryoprecipitate as appropriate (via consultation with the consultant haematologist who should already have been involved).
- Consider transfer to intensive treatment unit (ITU).

KEY POINT

Involve senior obstetricians, anaesthetists, haematologists and nephrologists early, especially where there is ongoing bleeding or deranged clotting.

SEVERE HYPERTENSION

Definitions

- **Hypertension** is best defined as a BP of greater than 140/90 mmHg on two or more occasions 4 hours apart.
- **Severe hypertension** is a diastolic of 110 or more or a systolic of 170 or more.
- **Pre-eclampsia** (PET) is hypertension with >0.3 g proteinuria/24 hours after 20 weeks' gestation.
- **Pregnancy-induced hypertension** is new onset hypertension arising after 20 weeks' gestation without significant proteinuria. It is associated with a better outcome than pre-eclampsia but may progress onto it.

Severe pre-eclampsia can be defined in a number of ways:

- severe hypertension, especially when resistant to treatment

- heavy proteinuria
- persistent symptoms of epigastric pain, headache, nausea, vomiting or visual disturbance
- hyperreflexia (three beats clonus), papilloedema, epigastric tenderness, cyanosis, pulmonary oedema
- worsening biochemistry (↑ urate, ↑ Cr, ↑ Urea, ↑ aspartate aminotransferase (AST), ↓ Alb)
- abnormal coagulation (↓ platelet, ↑ PTR, ↓ fibrinogen ↑ fibrinogen degradation products (FDP))
- decreasing urinary output
- evidence of fetal compromise (abnormal Dopplers or CTG).

CAUSES OF HYPERTENSION IN PREGNANCY

- Pre-eclampsia
- Non-proteinuric gestational hypertension
- Essential hypertension
- Renal disease
- Phaeochromocytoma
- Connective tissue disease.

The major risks from uncontrolled severe hypertension are cerebrovascular accidents and placental abruption. Pre-eclampsia carries additional risks of eclampsia, pulmonary oedema (often iatrogenic due to fluid overload) and DIC. The risks are particularly great where there is a rapidly evolving clinical picture when failure to recognize the significance of symptoms or to initiate prompt treatment can be fatal.

HISTORY

- From the notes calculate the current gestation, check the blood pressure at booking, check for any history of chronic hypertension or renal disease.
- Pre-eclampsia is five times more common in first pregnancies and 10 times more common where a previous pregnancy was affected.
- There is a definite familial tendency to pre-eclampsia. Is there any family history?
- Ask about headache, visual blurring, epigastric pain and vomiting.
- Enquire about fetal activity.

EXAMINATION

- Does the patient look puffy around the face and eyes?
- Is there any impairment in the level of consciousness?

- Check the blood pressure again yourself with the patient sitting at 45 degrees and using a large cuff if obese. 'Wedge' the patient to provide a 30 degree pelvic tilt. The Korotkoff IV phase (muffling) is often used but phase V (complete disappearance) corresponds more closely with actual intra-arterial pressures.
- Listen to the lung bases for crepitations and note any sacral oedema.
- Examine the uterus for a tenderness and measure fundal height.
- Test for epigastric and right upper quadrant (RUQ) abdominal tenderness.
- Examine for clonus and examine the fundi for papilloedema.

INVESTIGATIONS

- Test urine for proteinuria (if necessary catheterize to obtain a sample).
- Send urine for microscopy and culture.
- Take blood for FBC, liver function tests, electrolytes, clotting studies and group and save.
- Request a full fetal assessment (Umbilical artery Dopplers, biometric measurements, AFV, BPS/CTG).

MANAGEMENT OF SEVERE DISEASE

If the patient has severe hypertension, symptoms or signs suggestive of severe disease or rapidly deteriorating blood test results, involve senior staff, obtain intravenous access and then;

1. Transfer to delivery suite

2. Stabilize the blood pressure

Aim to bring the blood pressure to (140–160)/(90–100). Too rapid a drop in blood pressure may risk intracerebral events and the decline should be gradual. Patients with pre-eclampsia have a lower circulating blood volume and may tolerate a drop in BP poorly. Some advocate volume loading with colloid prior to bringing down the blood pressure. As the risks of cerebral and pulmonary fluid overload are very great any fluid given needs to be done cautiously after discussion with senior colleagues.

Each consultant is likely to have their own preference for the agent used. All maternity units should have guidelines which will include the preferred antihypertensive of that unit. Possible options for control of severe hypertension include:

- **oral methyl dopa 500 mg stat,** followed by 250 mg every 6–8 hours. **Oral nifedipine 10 mg** can be given between doses of methyldopa if control is not adequate. Nifedipine causes headaches which may confuse the clinical picture.
- **oral labetalol, 200 mg** followed by repeat doses every 6–8 hours.
- **intravenous hydralazine 5–10 mg** given over 5 minutes and repeated after 15 minutes if necessary. This takes 10–15 minutes to work and the effect lasts up to 6 hours. Side effects include tachycardia and headache.
- **intravenous labetolol.** Start with a bolus of 20 mg followed by further doses of 40 mg and 80 mg as required, up to a total of 200 mg.

Although oral preparations take somewhat longer to take effect, the response is usually rapid enough such that intravenous drugs can be avoided in most cirumstances.

The blood pressure needs to be maintained at the level stated above. This is done with oral doses as already mentioned, or with continuous infusions of hydralazine (5–40 mg/h) or labetalol (20–160 mg/h) which can be titrated against their response.

3. Fluid management

Aim to restrict fluid intake to 100 mL/h (remember to calculate the fluids used in antihypertensive and syntocinon infusions). Urine volumes of <30 mL/h can be tolerated for a few hours as the risks of acute tubular necrosis are outweighed by those of pulmonary and cerebral oedema. However, central venous pressure measurements (or even pulmonary capillary wedge pressure readings) may be necessary to accurately monitor fluid status. Diuretics should not be used to increase urine output unless there is good evidence of fluid overload. Extra colloid can be used if the central venous pressure is low but 'blind' fluid challenges are to be avoided.

4. Seizure prophylaxis

There is some evidence that eclamptic fits can be prevented by using intravenous magnesium sulphate infusions. This is by no means accepted practice as yet and large randomized controlled trials are underway in this country to determine if the use of magnesium sulphate in severe pre-eclampsia is indeed 'best-practice'. The criteria for its use as a prophylactic agent have not yet been established but see the section on eclampsia for a dosage schedule.

5. Delivery

Delivery of the placenta is the only way of actually treating the underlying pathophysiological processes of pre-eclampsia. The options are induction and Caesarean section. Assess the cervix. If it is favourable induce labour and deliver vaginally. An epidural may be helpful in reducing blood pressure by vasodilating and reducing afferent pain stimulation. It is safer than a spinal or general anaesthetic if Caesarean section is required. A coagulopathy is a contraindication to regional anaesthesia and platelet counts of <100 may limit the options for analgesia. Delivery by Caesarean section is indicated in pre-term pregnancies where the cervix is unfavourable (i.e. a Bishop score of less than 4), where labour can not be established within 24 hours and if maternal or fetal condition deteriorates. Avoid prolonged active second stage and do not use syntometrine in the third stage due to its hypertensive action (syntocinon is fine).

6. Continuous observation and monitoring

Vigilance must be maintained throughout for complications and deterioration in maternal or fetal condition.

- BP and urine output hourly.
- Oxygen saturation by pulse oximetry.
- Central venous pressure if oliguric.
- Serial measurements of platelet count, clotting times, renal and liver function and serum magnesium levels if having magnesium sulphate.
- Maternal clinical condition; level of consciousness, reflexes, basal crepitations, tachycardia (a sign of pulmonary oedema).
- Continuous fetal monitoring should be considered, whether labouring or not. Pre-eclampsia occurs as a result of placental dysfunction and fetal compromise is most likely during labour.

7. After delivery

Continue intensive treatment on labour suite for at least 24 hours after clinical, biochemical and haematological indices have stabilised. Antihypertensive medications may be necessary for a number of weeks postpartum. Advise at least a 5-day hospital stay after the delivery. Pre-eclampsia may deteriorate in the first week and continued monitoring is necessary.

8. Follow-up

This should be at 6 weeks to test urine and BP. If the BP remains raised or proteinuria persists, investigate for renal or connective tissue disease with ultrasound scanning, urine microscopy, 24-hour collections and autoantibody screening. Counsel a 1 in 10 risk of recurrence.

ECLAMPSIA

Definition

Occurrence of convulsions in association with signs and symptoms of pre-eclampsia.

Incidence

An incidence of 4.9:10 000 maternities in the UK (1:2000).

PRESENTATION

About 40% occur before labour, 20% during labour and 40% after delivery (up to 7 days); 10% occur with proteinuria alone and the diastolic BP remains at or below 100 in 34%. About 60% are preceded by one or more of the following: headaches, visual disturbance and epigastric pain. Eclampsia is more likely to occur in teenagers (×3) and in multiple pregnancy (×6). The differential diagnosis includes a cerebral bleed, local anaesthetic toxicity, epilepsy, thrombotic thrombocytopaenic purpura (TTP) and metabolic abnormalities.

TREATMENT

- Summon help.
- Obtain iv access and if still fitting give diazemuls 10 mg iv.
- Check airway for obstruction and give oxygen.
- Stabilize blood pressure (as for pre-eclampsia).
- Transfer to delivery suite and inform the obstetric and anaesthetist consultants.
- Commence magnesium sulphate with a bolus dose of 4 g (20 mL of 20% solution) given over 20 minutes (if already on treatment give a further 2 g bolus unless recent levels high). Maintenance dose is 1 g/h (make up 5 g in 500 mL normal saline and run at 100 mL/h).

Magnesium sulphate causes central and therefore respiratory depression.

- **2–4 mmol/L** = therapeutic range
- **>5 mmol/L** causes loss of patellar reflexes
- **>6 mmol/L** causes respiratory depression.

Obstetrics

Respiratory rate, oxygen saturations and patellar reflexes should be recorded regularly to detect toxicity. This is more likely if renal function is poor (reduce the infusion rate if urine output is low). One gram of calcium gluconate iv over 2–3 minutes is used to reverse toxic effects.

- Once stable deliver if antenatal.
- Follow up as for severe pre-eclampsia, but with extra emphasis on monitoring oxygen saturation levels. Consider transfer to ITU with CT/MRI scan if there are neurological localizing signs or if seizures continue.
- Continue the magnesium sulphate infusion for 24 hours after the last seizure.

CLOTTING ABNORMALITIES

Normal haemostasis is dependent on intact vessels, platelets and fibrin. The intrinsic system (factors VIII, IX, XI, XII) is activated by exposed collagen and produces activated Factors VIII and IX. Together with factor VII from the extrinsic system (activated by thromboplastin) these activate factor X with which Va converts prothrombin to thrombin in the presence of calcium. Thrombin converts soluble fibrinogen to insoluble fibrin plugs which are degraded to FDP by plasmin.

APTT (activated partial thromboplastin time) measures intrinsic activity and the prothrombin time (PT) measures extrinsic activity.

In pregnancy, factors I, VII, VIII, X increase and the platelet count falls.

DISSEMINATED INTRAVASCULAR COAGULATION

Causes

- *In utero* fetal death: DIC occurs only if the fetus remains *in situ* for >3 weeks
- Amniotic fluid embolus: incidence 1 in 80 000 with 80% mortality
- Abruption
- Pre-eclampsia
- HELLP syndrome: a variant or pre-eclampsia characterized by **H**aemolysis, **E**levated **L**iver enzymes and **L**ow **P**latelet counts
- Acute fatty liver of pregnancy (AFLP)
- Massive haemorrhage (>25% blood volume)
- Septicaemia
- Transfusion reaction.

Diagnosis

The earliest haematological change is an increase in fibrin degradation products (FDPs) and decline in fibrinogen levels. Clotting times then increase and platelet counts fall. Finally, the condition becomes clinically evident with spontaneous bleeding (e.g. mucous membranes and old cannula sites) and end-organ damage from microthrombi (renal damage and gangrene).

Management

- Notify and discuss with senior haematology staff.
- Treat the underlying cause: usually involves emptying the uterus and antibiotics to cover infection (discuss with senior microbiologists).
- Prompt correction of hypovolaemia and tissue hypoperfusion.
- Deliver the fetus vaginally if possible, minimize tissue trauma, and avoid regional blocks.
- Transfuse: usually with plasma reduced blood with fresh frozen plasma (1 unit per 5 of blood) and occasionally platelets. Cryoprecipitate contains fibrinogen (unlike fresh frozen plasma (FFP)) but no anti-thrombin III and is used if fibrinogen levels are particularly low. The exact replacement will be determined by the haematological/clotting results.
- Regular clotting profiles.

THROMBOEMBOLISM

Incidence

An incidence of 1 per 1000 ongoing pregnancies and 2 per 1000 recently delivered pregnancies. Venous thromboembolism (VTE) is the commonest cause of direct maternal death.

Risk factors for thromboembolism

- immobility
- surgery (relative risk of VTE is ×10 after LSCS)
- thrombophilias (lupus anticoagulant; antithrombin III, protein S and C deficiencies and activated protein C resistance)
- multiparity
- obesity
- age over 35
- previous history of TE
- family history of TE
- infection
- pre-eclampsia.

DIAGNOSIS

Most cases present in the third trimester and up to 6 weeks after delivery with leg pain, swelling and erythema or dyspnoea, chest pain and sometimes haemoptysis. **Diagnosis on clinical features alone is unreliable.**

For suspected deep vein thrombosis arrange **Doppler flow ultrasound.** This has a high sensitivity (94%) for iliac/femoral vein thrombosis although it may not be able to distinguish external compression from occlusion and will not exclude calf vein thrombosis. **Limited venography** is the investigation of choice for suspected below knee thrombosis. The radiation dose to the fetus is small and is justifiable in view of maternal risk. If a pulmonary embolus is suspected check arterial blood gases and a chest X-ray (with shielding of the abdomen there is no risk to the fetus and it excludes other causes of chest pain). A **perfusion lung scan** should be carried out and once again the radiation risk should be considered less than the risk of missing the diagnosis.

TREATMENT

Treatment with iv heparin should commence as soon as the clinical diagnosis of a DVT or PE is made or strongly suspected. It is only stopped if the definitive test (Doppler/venogram/ventilation–perfusion (VQ) scan) proves negative. Take blood for baseline clotting, thrombophilia studies, lupus anti-coagulant and platelets. Start an intravenous infusion of 1000–1500 IU heparin/h after a loading dose 5000–10 000 IU. Check the activated partial thromboplastin time (APTT) 6 hours later and adjust to maintain a level of 1.5–2.0. Then, check clotting times every 24 hours or 6 hours after any change in treatment. After resolution of clinical symptoms convert to subcutaneous heparin 10 000 bd subcutaneously or low molecular weight heparin 2500–5000 units per day monitored by factor Xa heparin assay (appropriate range = 0.2–0.4). Check maternal platelet count at regular intervals, especially around a week to ten days after commencing treatment. Heparin can cause an immune-mediated thrombocytopenia with paradoxical thrombotic episodes.

For delivery reduce the heparin to 5000–7000 IU bd and normalize the APTT. Have FFP available for bleeding. Resume iv heparin 20 000–30 000 IU/24 h after delivery and then convert to warfarin for 6–12 weeks. Warfarin is safe to use whilst breastfeeding.

13

POSTNATAL PROBLEMS

PYREXIA

Definition

Maternal temperature of more than 37°C on more than one occasion after delivery.

Incidence

Variably reported at 1–5% of deliveries. However, postpartum genital tract sepsis is still a significant cause of maternal mortality.

CAUSES OF PUERPERAL PYREXIA

The causes are listed below, with the common organisms responsible shown in parentheses.

- **Uterine**
  - more likely if retained products of conception or prolonged rupture of membranes (mixed vaginal flora including *E. coli, Streptococcus A* or *B, Clostridium* and anaerobes).
- **Urinary**
  - 40% of hospital infections (*E. Coli, Streptococcus B/D, Proteus, Klebsiella*).
- **Breast**
  - mastitis/abscess occurs in 2.5–4.6% of mothers (*Staphylococcus aureus*). Simple breast engorgement can cause a low grade pyrexia.
- **Wound**
  - Cellulitis (*Staphylococcus*).
  - Abscess (*E. coli*).
  - Episiotomy, vaginal and cervical lacerations (mixed anaerobes, *streptococci*).
  - Necrotizing fascitis (*Staphylococcus* and *Streptococcus*).
- **Chest**
  - Aspiration pnuemonia or atelectasis following general anaesthesia.

- **Other causes**
  - Appendicitis.
  - Cholecystitis.
  - Deep vein thrombosis.
  - Pelvic thrombophlebitis.

Many of these problems can be prevented. Minimize vaginal examinations and catheterizations and use aseptic technique. Nipple care and wound hygiene are important. Antibiotic prophylaxis should be given at all Caesarean sections and manual removals of retained placentae. Antibiotic treatment should at least be considered during labour in the presence of a known potential pathogen such as group B streptococcus especially with prolonged rupture of membranes. Prophylaxis against deep vein thrombosis and pulmonary emboli should be considered in all women undergoing Caesarean section.

HISTORY

- Are there any symptoms to localize the cause of the pyrexia? Enquiry should be made for any abdominal pain, dysuria, secondary bleeding, offensive discharge, breast soreness or discharge and leg pain.
- Are there any obvious risk factors? A history of fever or offensive liquor during or prior to labour suggests possible **chorioamnionitis** which is likely to progress to endometritis. Preterm rupture of membranes and preterm delivery may be due to infection and prolonged rupture of membranes will certainly predispose to endometritis, as will prolonged labour (especially where multiple vaginal examinations have been carried out). Retained placenta and the need for manual removal further increases the risks of sepsis.
- Mode of delivery is an important consideration. Caesaerean section is associated with a 13-fold increased risk of puerperal sepsis (endometritis, pelvic abscess, urinary tract and wound infections) and an increased thrombotic risk. Forceps delivery may cause a pelvic haematoma which secondarily becomes infected.

EXAMINATION

- General examination. Is the patient unwell? If the pyrexia is associated with tachycardia and hypotension consider septicaemia.
- Check for abnormal breath sounds or reduced air entry on auscultation of the chest.
- Check the legs for any sign of thrombosis.

- Check the breasts for tenderness, erythema and nipple discharge. Is there axillary lymphadenopathy ? Remember that breast engorgement may be associated with a transient low grade pyrexia without infection.
- Examine any abdominal wounds for swelling or associated cellulitis.
- Check for other areas of tenderness especially over the renal angles and above the symphysis pubis. If the uterus is unusually tender or fails to involute normally (it is usually no longer palpable 2 weeks after delivery) suspect uterine infection and retained products. The uterus may be deviated to one side by a pelvic haematoma.
- Pelvic examination. Note any swelling or infection associated with any perineal wounds. Gently pass a speculum and take a swab from the cervix for chlamydia and gonorrhea. Does the lochia seem offensive? If the cervix still easily admits a finger more than 4 days after delivery there may be infected retained products of conception.

INVESTIGATIONS

- **Full blood count.** A rise in the white cell count normally occurs during labour and delivery, but a drop in haemoglobin out of proportion to the observed blood loss may indicate a pelvic haematoma.
- **Blood cultures.** Should be taken before starting antibiotics and include anaerobic and aerobic cultures. Do not take from an intravenous cannula.
- **Mid-stream urine sample** for culture. Urinalysis may show blood and protein because of contamination from the lochia without indicating infection.
- **High vaginal and cervical swabs** should be performed by passing a speculum.
- **Wound swabs**, **sputum samples** and any **nipple discharge** should be taken as indicated by clinical findings.
- Any suspicion of **deep vein thrombosis** should be investigated with **Doppler ultrasound** or **venography.**

MANAGEMENT

- If there are any features of septicaemia or rapidly increasing cellulitis associated with necrosis of the overlying skin (suggesting necrotizing fasciitis) seek immediate senior advice.

- Occasionally, serious infections will need surgical management with drainage or debridement.
- Intravenous fluid treatment may be necessary if the patient is nauseous, vomiting, dehydrated or hypotensive.
- Initial **antibiotic therapy** will depend on the suspected diagnosis, whether that patient has any known allergies and whether she is breastfeeding. Most antibiotics can be given to breastfeeding mothers except for tetracyclines although metronidazole may affect the taste of the milk. Where pelvic infection is suspected start treatment with ampicillin and metronidazole or augmentin (erythromycin if allergic). If a wound or breast infection seems likely consider using flucloxacillin (better coverage of staphylococci and streptococci). Do not use first or second generation cephalosporins as these do not provide adequate cover for the common puerperal infections. Antibiotics should be given intravenously in patients who are vomiting, have suspected pyelonephritis or any evidence of a severe infection especially septicaemia. If the patient **fails to respond to initial treatment** discuss the results of any cultures and review the clinical diagnosis with a senior microbiologist. Consider adding an aminoglycoside, especially if a urinary tract infection is likely. Remember you will need to check levels. A third generation cephalosporin is an alternative. A swinging pyrexia is likely to indicate a collection in either the breast, wound or pelvis which may require drainage.
- Thrombotic problems will need to be treated with heparin and then warfarin. Discuss with local haematologists which particular heparin regimes are in use in your hospital.

MENTAL ILLNESS IN THE PUERPERIUM

Definition and classification

- **Puerperal psychosis:** a group of illnesses marked by delusions, hallucinations and impaired perception of reality occurring in close temporal relationship to childbirth; usually manic or depressive.
- **Major depressive illness:** a profound and consistent lowering of mood with biological symptoms but without hallucinations and delusions.
- **Minor depressive illness:** 'understandable' symptoms of unhappiness and anxiety differing quantitatively rather than qualitatively from the 'normal' stress reaction to childbirth.

Incidence

In the 3 months after delivery up to 16% of women will have an episode of mental illness, most of whom will have been previously psychiatrically well. There is a 16-fold increase in risk of major mental illness in the puerperium. One in 500 women are admitted with puerperal psychosis; 5% have major depressive illness and a further 10% minor depressive illness.

RISK FACTORS FOR POSTPARTUM PSYCHIATRIC ILLNESS

- **Previous history**
  - previous puerperal psychiatric illness
  - previous major psychiatric illness
  - family history of major psychiatric illness
- **Present pregnancy**
  - Caesarean section
  - prolonged stay of newborn on neonatal unit
  - maternal illness
- **Other**
  - unrealistic expectations
  - other major life events.

PRESENTATION

Most women experience some lowering of mood three days after delivery ('3–day blues') which improves spontaneously within 48 hours and requires only support and reassurance.

- **Puerperal psychosis** has a relatively sudden onset between 3 and 14 days after delivery with a rapidly changing picture of *delire triste* (fear, restlessness and confusion) followed by hallucinations, delusions and disorientation.
- **Major depressive illness** tends to have a more gradual onset over the first 2 months after delivery. A third present by 4 weeks and two-thirds by 10 weeks. There is a lowering of mood with biological symptoms such as psychomotor retardation and diurnal variation, but no delusions.
- **Minor mental illness** presents mainly as depressive or anxiety states and less commonly with phobic or compulsive behaviour. The onset is more insidious usually presenting after 3 months.

MANAGEMENT

Where possible identify high risk individuals antenatally. Contact the local mother and baby unit for advice and plan care following delivery. There is often a consultant psychiatrist locally who has a special interest in postpartum psychiatric problems.

Psychoses

Refer urgently to a psychiatrist. Sedate with phenothiazines (e.g. chlorpromazine 150 mg stat and 50–150 mg tds). Beware Parkinsonian side effects and dystonias (treat with procyclidine). Admit to mother and baby unit unless rapid response at home (usually improves within 48 hours). Consider electroconvulsive therapy (ECT) if not responding within 3–7 days or in depressive psychoses (e.g. stupor). Tricyclics take 10–14 days to work. There is no evidence for the use of prophylactic medication. Lithium may be indicated for a previous history or relapse of a manic depressive illness, but breastfeeding is contraindicated. Recurrence rates for postpartum psychosis are as high as 1 in 2.

Depressive illness

Admit if suicidal or not eating. Treatment with anti-depressants (e.g. Dothiepin) should be continued for 6 months. Selective serotonin re-uptake inhibitors are best avoided in breastfeeding women. Consider ECT as above. For women with no previous psychiatric history the recurrence risk for future pregnancies is again approximately 50%.

Minor illness

Treatment is mainly supportive by reducing social isolation (contact hospital or community social work teams), teaching anxiety management techniques and allowing an opportunity to talk through feelings. Contact with support groups may help. There is a limited role for benzodiazepines in anxiety states but avoid where irritability and loss of temper is a problem.

A regime of progesterone supplementation for prophylaxis and treatment of postpartum depression has become popular in some centres although opinions vary over its benefit.

The **Edinburgh Postnatal Depression Scale** is a questionnaire designed to help highlight those women at risk of postnatal depression so that increased social support can be directed appropriately.

SECONDARY POSTPARTUM HAEMORRHAGE

Definition

Any abnormal bleeding between 24 hours and 6 weeks after delivery.

Incidence

There is an incidence of 0.5–1.5% of maternities. The aetiology is shown in Table 13.1.

Table 13.1 Aetiology of secondary postpartum haemorrhage

Type of haemorrhage	Aetiology
Uterine	Endometritis Retained products of conception Trophoblastic disease
Iatrogenic	Anticoagulants Contraceptive steroids Retained swabs
Others	Infection superimposed on lower genital tract trauma

HISTORY

- **Bleeding:** Ask about onset and length of time from delivery. The vaginal loss is normally red ('lochia rubra') for 3 days then pink for 7 days with some further white discharge ('lochia alba') for up to 6 months. Has the bleeding been continuous since delivery or started again? (the former is more suggestive of retained products and the latter infection). Ask for some estimate of the blood loss and the passage of clots or tissue.
- **Associated symptoms:** Ask about abdominal pain and symptoms of pyrexia.
- **Delivery:** What was the mode of delivery? Was there any difficulty with delivery of the third stage? Was the placenta thought to be complete?
- **Treatment:** What treatment if any has already been given for the bleeding (usually antibiotics, occasionally ergot tablets, norethisterone or tranexamic acid)? Has the patient started using oral contraception, been given Depo-Provera or had an IUCD inserted ? Has the patient been anticoagulated?

EXAMINATION

- **General condition:** Examine for pallor and signs of shock. Record pulse, blood pressure and temperature.

- **Abdominal examination:** The uterus is usually not palpable abdominally by 12 days after delivery. If the uterus is still palpable check for tenderness.
- **Pelvic examination:** Look for blood stains on the legs as a guide to the heaviness of bleeding. Carry out a gentle speculum examination. Remove any blood from the vagina and look for evidence of bleeding through the cervical os or lacerations in the lower genital tract. Remove any tissue or foreign bodies and send for histological examination. Take swabs for culture from the vagina and cervix. Do a bimanual examination to assess the size and tenderness of the uterus. The cervical os is normally closed by day 5 although the external os of a multiparous patient may admit a finger tip. Retained products of conception are unlikely if the cervix is closed and ultrasound assessment is of little value in excluding retained tissue.

MANAGEMENT

- **Prevention:** Use antibiotic prophylaxis for Caesarean sections, difficult operative deliveries and for manual removal of placentae. Ensure that the uterus is empty at the time of delivery. If there is any doubt about the completeness of the placenta or membranes arrange an examination under anaesthetic.
- **If the patient is hemodynamically stable:** Take blood for full blood count and group and save. Consider normal menstruation and iatrogenic causes. If the cervix is closed the most likely diagnosis of abnormal bleeding is endometritis which can be treated initially with antibiotics. Co-amoxiclav or ampicillin are safe in breastfeeding mothers. Metronidazole is safe but may affect the taste of the milk and consequently interfere with feeding. Do not give tetracyclines. Cephalosporins tend to be ineffective. If the bleeding persists it may respond to a progestogen (norethisterone 15–30 mg daily over 10 days) but uterine exploration and curettage may be required to exclude retained tissue first. If there is evidence of retained products (bulky uterus and open internal os) any coexisting infection should be treated first and uterine evacuation arranged 12–24 hours later.
- **If the patient is shocked:** Treat as for other causes of major obstetric haemorrhage. Summon assistance. Site an intravenous line and take blood for full blood count, clotting, blood cultures and cross match at least four units. Resuscitate and remove any clot or tissue from the vagina and cervix. If the uterus is not well

contracted give syntometrine one ampoule im or slowly iv. Insert a Foley catheter to keep the bladder empty and monitor urine output. Once the patient's condition has been stabilized and blood loss replaced, if there is still significant bleeding arrange an examination under anaesthetic by the most senior obstetrician available having informed the patient's consultant. Remember if the bleeding can not be controlled by repairing any bleeding laceration and emptying the uterus, internal iliac vein ligation or hysterectomy may be required. Otherwise treat any infection first and arrange examination in theatre after 24 hours. Even if the bleeding is due to retained products there is likely to be an element of infection. Uterine evacuation should be carried out by an experienced obstetrician as there is an increased risk of uterine perforation and bleeding in these cases.

THE URINARY TRACT IN THE PUERPERIUM

URINARY INFECTION

Aetiology

Usually due to *E. coli, Proteus* or *Klebsiella.* Increased incidence in patients catheterized during labour or prior to operative delivery or where there having problems with voiding (see below).

Diagnosis

Suspect in patients with puerperal fever, suprapubic pain or loin pain. Dysuria may not be present and routine urinalysis is unhelpful because of contamination with lochia. Send a mid-stream urine sample.

Management

Avoid catheterization if possible. Encourage a high fluid intake and check for features of retention (clinically or with ultrasound scan). Treat on the basis of urine culture results if possible but for empirical treatment ampicillin 500 mg qds, trimethoprim 200 mg bd or cephradine 500 mg tds are acceptable. If the patient is systemically unwell, there is evidence of pyelonephritis or in high risk cases (e.g. renal transplant patients) treat with intravenous antibiotics and fluids.

Note that the hydronephrosis characteristic of normal pregnancy may take a number of weeks to settle after delivery and ultrasound scans should be interpreted with caution if performed during this time.

URINARY RETENTION

Aetiology

The main causes are:

- Perineal pain due to lacerations or episiotomy, haematoma or infection.
- Pelvic haematoma (either spontaneous or, more often, after operative delivery).
- Impaired sensation of bladder distension following epidural.

Diagnosis

Lower abdominal pain associated with difficulty in voiding, frequent micturition of small volumes and a palpable bladder displacing the uterus are the cardinal clinical features. Ultrasonic scan of the lower abdomen and pelvis can be performed if there is any doubt.

Management

Adequate monitoring of micturition after delivery is essential as symptoms of retention may be masked by impaired bladder sensation. If left untreated bladder distension can result in long-term impairment of detrusor function. If the patient is not voiding adequate volumes within 12 hours of delivery, pass a catheter and if the residual exceeds 150 mL leave on indwelling catheter for further 24 hours. Treat any precipitating factors and check for urinary tract infection. If retention recurs after the catheter is removed consult a senior obstetric colleague.

URINARY INCONTINENCE

Consider urinary retention and urinary tract infection. However, the most likely cause is disruption to pelvic floor muscles and bladder neck support tissues sustained during vaginal delivery. Approximately one-fifth of women are still suffering with urinary incontinence at 3 months post delivery, with risk factors being large baby, prolonged second stage and vaginal operative delivery. Referral to a physiotherapist with an interest in the pelvic floor is advised. (Ongoing anal incontinence of flatus and/or stool is less common and is often only admitted to on direct questioning. Persistent cases should be referred for anal ultrasonography and/or physiology studies to ascertain whether the cause is sphincter trauma or perineal nerve damage.)

BREAST DISEASE

DIFFICULTY IN ESTABLISHING BREASTFEEDING

Most mothers require some assistance and many infants show some initial reluctance to feed. During the first 2–3 days the breast produces colostrum, rich in immunoglobulins but less so in fat and carbohydrate. Some weight loss is common in neonates during the first week. These changes need to be explained to mothers to reassure those women who wish to continue breastfeeding. Where there are persistent problems these may be fetal or maternal. Look for evidence of nipple disease (infection, inversion) or inflammation. Is the patient taking any medication (oestrogens, bromocriptine) that may interfere with lactation? The infant may have been feeding poorly because of congenital problems such as cleft palate, because of other illness or prematurity. If the problem is likely to be temporary consider expressing the mother's breast milk for feeding the infant by tube or bottle until breastfeeding can be commenced or resumed.

Suppression of lactation

In mothers who do not wish to breastfeed, lactation will normally cease in the absence of suckling and breast discomfort can be managed with simple analgesics and a supportive bra. Bromocriptine is no longer licensed for use as a lactation suppressant.

Mastitis and breast abscess

Cracked and sore nipples are extremely common until mother and baby have established the technique. Support and encouragement should be given by midwives. However mastitis should be treated with flucloxacillin after swabs or milk have been sent to microbiology. A breast abscess is likely to need draining. Neither condition is a contraindication to continued breastfeeding and this should be encouraged when mastitis occurs.

CONTRACEPTIVE ISSUES

(See p. 21).

14

PRACTICAL PROCEDURES

EPISIOTOMY

Indications

An episiotomy is an incision to the perineal body made during the second stage of labour to:

- Facilitate delivery when a rigid perineum delays delivery.
- Avoid a large perineal tear (previous deep 2nd degree or 3rd degree tear, or when the perineum does not have time to stretch and thin out, e.g. in instrumental deliveries, precipitous labour, breech deliveries).
- Hasten delivery in cases of suspected fetal distress.

The perineum

The perineum comprises the following:

- skin
- bulbocavernous muscle
- superficial and deep transverse perineal muscles
- levator ani
- anal sphincter.

TYPES OF EPISIOTOMY

Figure 14.1 illustrates the different types of episiotomy.

- **Medio-lateral:** Most commonly used. Usually right sided although this may vary according to the local practice. Avoids the anal sphincter completely if placed correctly but may tear medially into this structure if not made large enough. When the levator ani is involved in the incision, fat from the ischiorectal fossa may be visible. Provides more space than a medial episiotomy.
- **Medial (midline):** This incision involves severing less blood vessels and is easier to repair but is more likely to tear into the

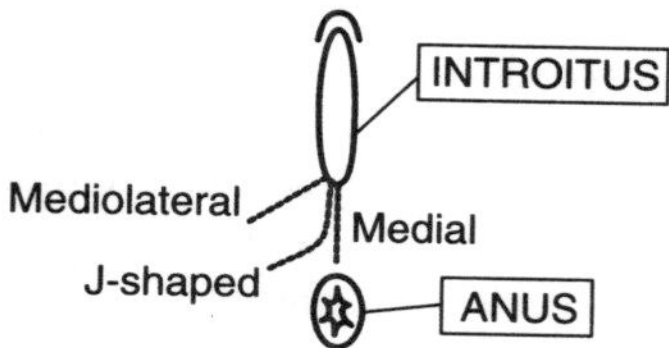

Figure 14.1 Types of episiotomy.

anal sphincter which is not formally cut. Needs experience to assess when appropriate to use. Gives less postoperative pain than a medio-lateral incision. Not recommended when large incisions are required.

- **'J'-shaped:** This incision starts in the midline and sways laterally to avoid the anal sphincter. Theoretically combines the benefits and avoids the risks of a medio-lateral and medial episiotomy.

TECHNIQUE

- **Patient:** Tell the patient what is going to happen.
- **Anaesthesia:** In emergencies an episiotomy can be placed without any analgesia at the height of a contraction when the pain caused by the episiotomy will be distracted by the contraction pain. However, proper anaesthesia such as an already existing epidural block, or a pudendal block and perineal infiltration is preferable.
- **Incision:** Two fingers (index and middle finger) are placed between the perineum and the presenting part to protect the fetus and guide the scissors. The incision is made during a contraction with scissors between the two fingers. The outline of the anal sphincter can usually be identified in the distended perineum and avoided. The incision is completed in one or, more commonly, two cuts. Multiple cuts or snips should be avoided.
- **Extension:** Should at any time the episiotomy appear to be inadequate and tearing likely, the incision should be extended, if time permits.

Pitfalls:

- **The incision is made too early:** When an episiotomy is placed, a vaginal delivery must be anticipated beyond any reasonable doubt. A Caesarean section with an episiotomy should be avoided. It is not necessary to place an episiotomy before a Kiellands forceps rotation. An episiotomy when the presenting part is not low enough and delivery imminent causes unnecessary blood loss. Under these circumstances it may be required to apply pressure on the bleeding area and/or place artery forceps on the most profusely bleeding vessels.

- **The incision is too small:** As a result delivery may not ensue or the episiotomy may tear medially and involve the anal sphincter. The latter can be avoided by looking at the perineum at all times during the delivery of the presenting part and extending the incision if tearing becomes evident. Generally it is better to make an initial generous episiotomy rather than one which may be too small.

Repair

(*See* Fig. 14.2.)

- Repeated infiltration of a local anaesthetic may be required before the repair.
- Use of nitrous oxide can significantly improve analgesia.
- Good view is essential (lithotomy, light, application of tampon in the upper vagina to stop blood flowing from uterus).
- Clean area (normal saline, disinfectants) and fashion wound edges where needed.
- Start repair with the vagina: identify apex of wound, place first suture 1 cm above the apex then continuous interlocking at 1 cm

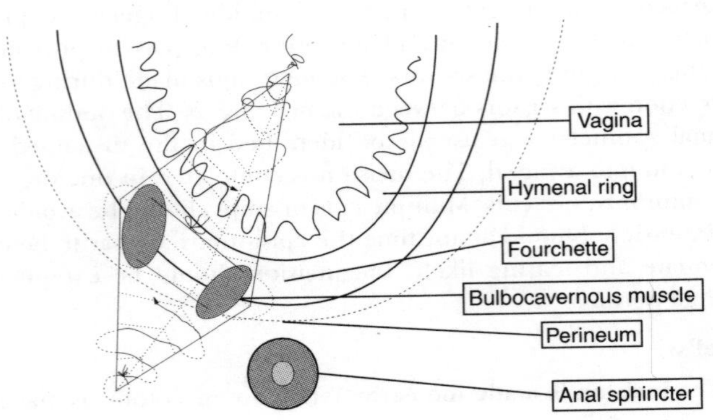

Figure 14.2 Repair of a medio-lateral episiotomy

intervals as far as the hymenal ring obliterating dead space below vaginal mucosa. Tie last suture between hymenal ring and posterior commissure. Polyglycolic acid (Dexon) or polyglactan (Vicryl) (size '0') is superior to catgut.

- The perineum is repaired by deep interrupted sutures (usually two to four) to the muscles from internal to external ('0' Dexon or Vicryl).
- The skin is repaired with interrupted or a continuous subcuticular suture ('2–0' Dexon or Vicryl) starting with the skin apex towards the vagina to avoid a 'dog ear'.
- A careful rectal examination is mandatory to exclude involvement of rectal mucosa in vaginal stitches (which may cause a rectovaginal fistula). This is an ideal time to insert an analgesic suppository (e.g. 100 mg diclofenac).

KEY POINT

Remember to take the tampon out and count the number of swabs and needles. It is the operator's responsibility to secure safe disposition of all the sharps.

FORCEPS DELIVERY

Indications

- **Poor progress during the second stage of labour:** Generally accepted time limits are half an hour of expulsive effort in multiparous women and one hour in nulliparous women. However, time limits for the second stage are arbitrary, especially with the practice of delaying active pushing in women with an epidural in place. Poor uterine activity can be a cause but also delay can be the result of cephalopelvic disproportion and malposition such as deep transverse arrest or occipito posterior position.
- **Fetal indications:** Delivery must be expedited when there is evidence of fetal distress. This will usually be based on CTG or fetal scalp blood gas abnormalities. Umbilical cord prolapse will warrant quick delivery and can, at full dilatation, be achieved by forceps. Controlled delivery of the head during a breech presentation can be achieved with forceps.
- **Maternal indications:** The commonest indication is poor maternal effort as a result of exhaustion. However, others include myasthenia gravis, hypertension, cardiac and pulmonary disease.

- **Miscellaneous indications:** Controlled delivery at Caesarean section.

KEY POINT

Dural tap (at epidural siting) without maternal headache is not an indication for an elective forceps delivery.

PRE-REQUISITES FOR A FORCEPS DELIVERY

- Valid indication
- Fully dilated cervix
- Ruptured membranes
- Suitable presentation
- Position known
- Not more than 1/5 of the head palpable abdominally
- Empty bladder
- No obvious obstruction to a vaginal delivery
- Adequate analgesia
- Lithotomy position
- Aseptic technique.

TYPES OF FORCEPS

- Forceps are primarily divided into non-rotational and rotational forceps.
- Non-rotational forceps are further divided into outlet and mid-cavity forceps.
- All forceps are made up of a blade, a shank with a lock and a handle.
- Non-rotational and rotational forceps differ in a number of ways. The former has a non-sliding lock and a pelvic curve to allow for the concave shape of the sacrum. Rotational forceps have a sliding lock to adjust for asynclitism and a minimal pelvic curve to allow straight rotation around its own longitudinal axis without allowing the maximum rotational diameter of the blades and head to supersede the diameter of the fetal head.
- Outlet forceps are lighter and have a smaller shank and handle than mid forceps. They are used when the head has reached the pelvic floor in an occiput anterior position and the presenting part can be seen, and in Caesarean sections.
- Mid forceps are used when the largest diameter of the head has passed the pelvic brim and the presenting part is at the level of the ischial spines or lower.

- Commonly used forceps are Wrigley (outlet), Neville–Barnes, Anderson, Simpson and Haig–Ferguson (mid) and Kielland (rotational).

TECHNIQUE

KEY POINT

Always explain to the patient (and her partner) what you are going to do and why you are doing it.

General

The patient is positioned in lithotomy position on an obstetric bed or operating table with adequate analgesia in the form of a spinal or epidural block or, seldom, a general anaesthetic. A pudendal block may be adequate for outlet forceps deliveries. A wedge under the mother's right side is used to avoid caval compression. The bladder is emptied. Ask the patient to push during traction.

KEY POINT

Always check before starting that both blades are a proper pair that fit and not two ill-fitting ones from different sets.

Non-rotational forceps

The left blade is inserted first. Two or three fingers of the right hand are used to guide the blade into position which follows the curvature of the head by sweeping the left hand, which holds the handle, in an arc. Only minimal force should be necessary. The right blade is inserted the same way with the opposite hands. The blades are locked in the mento-vertical line without force. The position is checked by confirming the position of the lambdoid suture, the posterior fontanelle and the occiput. Traction is performed only during contractions and in the direction of the birth canal and following it as the head descends. Progress/descent should be achieved with each pull. An episiotomy is performed in anticipation of the last pull. The head is delivered by sweeping the forceps anterior whilst preventing the perineum tearing with a pad held in the free hand.

Rotational forceps

Kielland's forceps are applied so that the markers on the lock face the occiput. In an occipito-posterior position the forceps blades are applied as a pair of non-rotational forceps. In a transverse presentation the posterior blade is applied first and the anterior blade is either applied directly or by inserting it in front of the face and gently guiding it up into position. The application should be smooth and without resistance. Once the blades are locked, slight, gentle disimpaction of the head is usually necessary to rotate the fetal head into an occiput anterior position. Rotation should be in the direction which is most logical from previous examinations; this is usually in the direction of the fetal back and should not be associated with resistance. The procedure should be smooth and without any force. Once the head is rotated to an occipito anterior position, the procedure is as for a non-rotational forceps delivery. Episiotomies can usually be made once rotation is complete and vaginal delivery is imminent.

COMPLICATIONS

Failed forceps

Unusual in experienced hands. If there is any doubt in advance regarding the success of the procedure, it should be done as a trial of forceps in the operating theatre by an experienced obstetrician with facilities for an emergency Caesarean section standing by. Consent for the trial of forceps and Caesarean section if necessary should be obtained before beginning.

Maternal injuries

- Vaginal and cervical tears; these may extend into the lower segment of the uterus.
- Spiral tears are a risk with Kielland's forceps.
- Haemorrhage.
- Bruising and lacerations of the bladder, urethra and rectum. Fistulae may ensue.

Fetal injuries

- Haematomata, abrasions.
- Intracranial haemorrhage.
- Skull fractures.
- Vertebral fractures.
- Injuries to eyes, nose, ears (all more likely to occur after incorrect application and/or too large traction forces).
- Facial nerve compression and resultant, usually transient, paralysis. Note that face marks (red imprints of the blades on both sides of the baby's head) are quite common after forceps deliveries and resolve spontaneously within days.

VENTOUSE DELIVERY

Indications

Same as for forceps plus:

- Second twin who is too high for forceps delivery.
- No regional analgesia but an urgent instrumental delivery is required.
- Urgent instrumental delivery indicated but cervix not quite fully dilated (see below).

Contraindications

- preterm fetuses
- fetal clotting disorder
- fetal distress (forceps may be quicker)
- face presentation
- delivery of the head in a breech presentation.

CONDITIONS REQUIRED FOR VENTOUSE DELIVERY

As for forceps delivery. However the ventouse can be used when the cervix is not fully dilated (9 cm dilated or more). This is best reserved for fetal distress in multiparous women who are otherwise progressing well.

Two types

- Synthetic 'soft' cup Ventouse (various diameter Silc and Silastic cups).
- Metal cup (e.g. various diameter Bird's, O'Neil, Malmstrom for central traction, and 'posterior cups' for occiput posterior positions, e.g. Bird's posterior cup).

The metal cup requires the formation of a 'chignon' (oedematous tissue sucked and shaped into the cup) for a successful outcome. This takes time to form. The Silc cup has a much larger diameter and, as it does not need any such skin moulding, it can be used almost instantaneously after its application. The Silc cup has a higher chance of slipping off.

PROCEDURE

KEY POINT

Always explain to the patient (and her partner) what you are going to do and why you are doing it.

Lubricate the cup; this will assist insertion and the air seal. All cups need to be fitted as close to the occiput as possible to enhance flexion. Use the posterior cup for occipito posterior positions as the location of the air vent on the side allows for a more correct posterior application. Digitally ensure correct position and absence of maternal tissue between the cup and the fetal scalp.

When using a metal cup, adequate chignon formation is achieved by a graded increase of the negative pressure to 0.8 kg/cm^2 over a period of 5 minutes. Only then should traction be started. With Silc cups, this negative pressure can be achieved instantaneously and traction can be commenced immediately.

Traction, aided by maternal expulsive efforts, is only applied during contractions and is exerted in the direction of the birth canal keeping the 90 degree curve in mind. Thus, the direction of traction changes with descent of the fetal head. One hand is used for traction whilst the other stabilizes cup attachment to the fetal head with one or two fingers.

An episiotomy is usually required and is performed when the fetal head is thought to be delivered during the next contraction. This may be omitted by an experienced operator when there is a lax perineum but this decision needs to be considered carefully. As soon as the baby's head is delivered the vacuum is released and the cup is removed. Further management is as for a normal delivery. With Silc cups the caput succedaneum often is exaggerated and it needs to be pointed out to the parents that this is transient in nature and will resolve within a matter of days. The same applies to the chignon created by the metal cup.

COMPLICATIONS

Failed ventouse

A Ventouse delivery should be abandoned if:

- there is no progress with each pull
- the head has not reached the perineum after three pulls
- the cup comes off twice
- delivery is not complete within 15 minutes.

Maternal complications

There may be lacerations and bleeding from the lower genital tract when tissue is trapped between the fetal skull and the cup. Anal sphincter damage occurs less frequently than with forceps deliveries.

Fetal complications

- **Subcutaneous haematoma:** Ecchymosis, bruising and minor haematomata are fairly common.
- **Scalp necrosis:** During suction the blood supply to the fetal scalp is reduced. If sustained for longer than 15 minutes ischaemia and subsequent necrosis may ensue.
- **Cephalohaematoma:** Resolves spontaneously. If large it can cause severe fetal anaemia, hypotension and even death.
- **Subgaleal or subaponeurotic haematoma:** Associated with maintaining vacuum for too long. Elevation of the whole scalp can occur and the accumulation of large amounts of blood in this very loose tissue layer may lead to hypotension and death.
- **Tentorial tears:** Shearing forces may lead to lacerations of the deep venous systems.
- **Fetal jaundice:** Increased incidence, most likely as a result from resolution of bruising and haematoma.
- **Alopecia:** In the area of cup application. Usually resolves with time.

FETAL SCALP BLOOD SAMPLING

Indications

Fetal scalp blood sampling (FBS) is used to obtain information on the biochemical status of the fetus during labour in cases where fetal hypoxia is suspected, usually on the basis of an abnormal CTG.

Contraindications

- Immediately after a transient abnormal CTG episode which has totally recovered, (e.g. a short-lived bradycardia after siting an epidural or after hypotension with caval compression). Leave for 30 minutes to allow the acid–base balance to regain its normal status. **Note: It is not appropriate to wait with an abnormal CTG and hope that it will recover.**
- If more than five samples are required, review of the situation by a senior obstetrician is mandatory and delivery should be considered.
- Hepatitis B or HIV positive mothers.
- Fetal coagulation disorders.
- In the second stage of labour an abnormality of the CTG is normally an indication to expedite the delivery rather than perform a FBS.

Shortcomings

Transient nature of the information obtained. At least two and often more samples need to be taken to allow for the identification of a trend. Sampling can be difficult or not possible (high presenting part, the cervix minimally dilated or moving parturient).

KEY POINT

Delivery is mandatory if a fetal blood sample is indicated but technically not obtainable.

TECHNIQUE

- Place the mother in left lateral position.
- Clean vulva and use sterile technique.
- Insert amnioscope through vagina and cervix using the largest size that cervical dilatation will allow.
- Remove obturator and place light source and manoeuvre so there is no cervical tissue between the amnioscope and the fetal scalp. Keep light pressure on amnioscope with the non-operating (left) hand continuously during the whole procedure to keep it in place and to ensure a water seal preventing contamination of the sample by liquor or blood.
- Clean scalp with a swab or pledgelet.
- Ethylchloride may be used to create hyperaemia of the fetal scalp.
- Apply a small amount of Vaseline or petroleum gel to the skin to enhance blood droplet formation, stab skin away from sutures and fontanelles with a specially guarded blade to avoid deep penetration in one firm push to breach the epidermal layer. Do not 'scratch' or 'slash' the skin. Re-stab only if the first stab fails to bleed.
- Remove the blade and its holder and replace with a heparinized capillary tube. Hold the tube against the droplet of blood and do not remove until the tube has filled itself with enough blood for the local blood gas analyser to perform measurements on. Avoid contamination by liquor and air bubbles. Keep the blood in the tube moving until inserted into the blood gas analyser. Take one to three samples from the same scalp wound as local practice dictates. If the scalp wound continues to bleed heavily, apply pressure with a pledgelet until it stops.

RESULTS

- Normal: pH ≥7.25, base excess ≥ –8 mmol/L;

- Suspicious: pH ≥7.20 and <7.25, base excess < –8 mmol/L and ≥ –10 mmol/L;
- Abnormal: pH < 7.20, base excess < –10 mmol/L.

ACTION

Action depends on the results and the clinical situation. If the results are 'normal' and the CTG abnormality continues then a repeat sample should be taken in 30 to 60 minutes to identify a trend. If 'suspicious' then a repeat sample should always be taken regardless of whether the CTG abnormality continues or not. If 'abnormal', immediate delivery should be considered either by Caesarean section (1st stage) or by an assisted vaginal delivery (2nd stage). A suspicious result may be acceptable in a rapidly progressing multiparous patient but may support the decision for Caesarean section in an induced primipara with slow progress in the first stage.

MANUAL REMOVAL OF THE PLACENTA

Indications

Retained placenta (i.e. third stage >60 minutes) or heavy bleeding with the placenta still attached. During a Caesarean section the placenta should separate within 1–3 minutes of the iv oxytocin being administered.

PREPARATION

This is an emergency situation as heavy bleeding may start at any time. The patient's needs are as follows:

- iv line (16 G venflon or larger)
- full blood count
- cross-match two units blood or more if acute bleeding
- monitor pv loss
- fundal height, vital signs and ensure that the bladder is empty (this may solve problem!)
- start resuscitation if required
- inform anaesthetist and theatre staff
- explain the procedure and obtain consent
- always keep parturients nil by mouth until the placenta is delivered!

KEY POINT

Visible vaginal bleeding may be minimal whilst the uterus is filling with blood. This should be suspected if the fundal height increases in size and adequate resuscitation commenced.

PROCEDURE

- Conduct in operating theatre.
- Adequate analgesia in the form of epidural, spinal or general anaesthetic.
- Place patient in lithotomy position, clean and drape.
- Stop syntocinon infusion if in place.
- Insert operating hand in vagina through cervix guided by the umbilical cord if not 'snapped' earlier.
- Cervical constriction can usually be countered by continuous pressure of the operating hand shaped into a cone.
- Uterine relaxation may be necessary (halothane, amyl nitrite, ritodrine). Use the non-operating hand to hold the uterus in place and to complement the operating hand during the procedure.
- Find the plane between placenta and uterine wall and separate with the side of the hand or digitally. This may be difficult and strenuous but perseverance will be rewarded.
- After the placenta is removed ensure it is complete and check the uterine cavity manually/ digitally so as not to leave any tissue. This is particularly important when the placenta is removed piecemeal. A large blunt curette may be used to remove any remaining fragments (this should only be performed by an experienced obstetrician).
- Give syntocinon 40 U in 500 mL normal saline over 4 hours after the procedure.
- Commence antibiotics (co-amoxiclav or a cephalosporin with metronidazole).

Pitfalls

Adherent placentae: placenta accreta or percreta. In these cases it may be impossible to separate the placenta. Conservative management may be the better option. In these cases senior help should be sought. Trying hard may do more harm in the form of initiating uncontrollable bleeding or perforation of the uterus. These are more likely in retained placentae in women with a history of previous Caesarean section/hysterotomy/myomectomy involving the uterine cavity.

RESUSCITATION OF THE NEWBORN

Approximately one-third of newborns will require some form of resuscitation, which cannot always be anticipated. Basic neonatal resuscitation skills are, therefore, imperative for any medical staff working on the labour ward. They should be able to initiate the following neonatal resuscitation and maintain it until paediatric support arrives.

PROCEDURE

- **Introduce** yourself to the parents and explain briefly what you are about to do.
- **Familiarize** yourself quickly with relevant basic information such as time of birth, gestational age, drugs given to the mother, maternal temperature, problems during pregnancy and medical history, etc.
- Ensure the **heater** is already switched on and **start the timer at the moment of birth**.
- **Dry and wrap the baby:** Oxygen need is increased when babies cool after delivery. Use a bonnet (up to 85% of heat loss may be through the head). If there is profound hypothermia wrap in aluminium foil (do not use this with a radiant heater).
- **Position:** Horizontal with head down tilt.
- **Airway:** If suction is required, use a double trap mucus extractor or automatic suction. Only the anterior nose and the mouth may be cleared blindly. Pharyngeal irritation can lead to bradycardia, hypotension and apnoea. Chest wall retraction on inspiration and poor air entry suggest a lower airway obstruction warranting suction under direct vision with a laryngoscope. Check patency of nasal passages (close off one nostril and listen with a stethoscope). In the presence of meconium the upper airway is cleared preferably whilst the head is at the perineum. Further clearance is done under direct vision with a laryngoscope. However, obsessive attention to clearance of meconium should never cause delay in IPPV in the presence of apnoea or cardiac massage in the presence of bradycardia.
- **Laryngoscopy:** This technique needs to be learned under paediatric supervision. In short, insert a laryngoscope over the tongue after proper positioning (slightly extended neck), lift the epiglottis forward and visualize the vocal cords. Intubate when there is thick meconium present below the vocal cords to aspirate the lower airways.

Table 14.1 The Apgar Score: The scores for the individual factors are added to produce the 'Apgar Score'

Factors	Score		
	0	1	2
Heart rate	Absent	<100 bpm	>100 bpm
Respiration	Absent	Slow, irregular	Good, crying
Muscle tone	Flaccid	Some limb flexion	Active motion
Stimulation	No response	Cry	Vigorous cry
Colour	Blue, pale	Body pink, limbs blue	Pink

- **Bag and mask:** When the Apgar score is 4–6 (Table 4.1), or when intubation is not possible. Proper positioning and an upper airway tube are crucial. Every IPPV system must have a blow-off safety valve to avoid too high positive pressures. Check pulmonary air entry with a stethoscope and observe chest movements.
- **Intubation:** If the Apgar score is less than 4, or when the infant does not improve after 1 minute of IPPV by bag and mask. At laryngoscopy the correct size endotracheal tube (depends on the infant's weight and gestational age: 2.0 to 2.5 for the very small and 3.5 to 4.0 for the larger neonates) is passed through the vocal cords up to the mark or the shoulder. Cricoid pressure and suction may help. IPPV is started (blow-off valve setting 30 cmH_2O or lower if <1500 g. Use 2–3 L/min of flow and perform 30 resp/min) after stabilization and removal of the laryngoscope.
- **Cardiac massage:** If asystole or heart rate <60 bpm. Mid-sternum depression of 2 cm at 100/min using two fingers, or one/two thumbs and fingers behind the chest. Ventilate at every fourth 'beat'.

KEY POINT

Obstetricians only need to be able to resuscitate to this stage and maintain it until a paediatrician arrives. The following are examples of management steps that the paediatrician may have to take subsequently.

- **Drugs:**
  - Opiate analgesia <8 hours from delivery:
    Naloxone 0.01 mg/kg im/sc.
  - Continuing asystole/bradycardia:
    Adrenaline 1:10 000 0.1 mL/kg iv or via endotracheal tube.
    Calcium gluconate 10% 1 mL/kg.

- No response:
  Adrenaline and calcium gluconate intracardially (same doses as above).
- **Blood transfusion:** O Rhesus negative blood 10–20 mL/kg in 5–10 minutes when fetal/neonatal blood loss is suspected as a cause for problems with resuscitation.
- **Stop resuscitation:** If all measures fail and no response after 25–30 minutes. Always re-check connections, settings, patency and proper positioning of endotracheal tube, etc.

SUMMARY FOR THE OBSTETRIC SHO

Advanced resuscitation techniques and measures are not the province of the obstetric SHO. In most units the obstetric SHO is not required to be involved in neonatal resuscitation apart from providing basic care until the arrival of the paediatric medical staff. Under these circumstances the obstetric SHO should adhere to the following management until help arrives:

- Heart rate >100 bpm:
  - dry, wrap and stimulate the baby if there is no regular respiration. Institute IPPV by bag and mask if baby remains apnoeic.
- Heart rate <100 bpm:
  - dry, wrap and commence IPPV (intermittent positive pressure ventilation) by bag and mask. Intubate only if adequate air/O_2 entry cannot be achieved with bag and mask. Commence cardiac massage if HR remains <100 bpm with adequate ventilation after 1 minute.

Training

All medical staff working on a maternity unit should be adequately trained in basic neonatal resuscitation techniques. All units should ensure adequate theoretical and practical training and regular (6-monthly) mandatory refresher courses for all obstetricians.

Objectives

[illegible]

- [illegible]
- [illegible]
- [illegible]

[illegible]

[illegible]

- [illegible]
- [illegible]

[illegible]

[illegible]

SECTION 2: GYNAECOLOGY

SECTION 2: GYNAECOLOGY

CONTENTS

15

PREOPERATIVE CARE

The success of surgery is as much dependent on thorough pre- and postoperative care, careful asepsis and anaesthesia as the surgery itself. The patient who has been psychologically well prepared, with normal cardiovascular and renal function, tolerates her surgery well. A patient must be capable of reacting to the stress, trauma and potential infection resulting from surgery.

GENERAL CONSIDERATIONS

A patient must have a clear understanding of the nature of the surgical procedure she is to undergo with the risks and benefits discussed. Involvement of close family members may be helpful, should the patient so wish.

Although most gynaecological procedures do not affect sexual function or response this may need to be formally and tactfully explained. These anxieties are often not expressed by patients. **There may be additional concerns that the surgery may have an effect on future reproductive capacity, especially if it involves the ovaries.**

CONSENT

The purpose of the consent is to ensure that the patient understands the nature and implication of the operation or diagnostic procedure she is to undergo. The adequacy of an informed consent is determined more by her understanding the nature and effects of the surgery she is to undergo, rather than the signing of the operative permit.

An informed consent involves the explanation of possible complications of surgery, but always in the context of the positive results to be expected from the surgery. The purpose is not to create unnecessary anxiety by discussing complications that may be catastrophic and rare, but to educate the patient and allay unfounded fears.

It ought to be normal practice for the surgeon who is to perform surgery to explain the procedure to the patient, and be present when the consent is signed, although this is commonly not the case for logistic reasons.

KEYPOINTS

- ***If you lack the knowledge to consent a patient for a particular procedure or cannot answer their queries always consult more senior staff.***
- ***A summary of the discussion with the patient should always be written in the notes.***

HISTORY AND EXAMINATION

The majority of useful information in preparation of the patient for surgery comes from the history rather than the physical examination or laboratory tests. Typically the gynaecological patient is healthy and ambulatory with a localized complaint. However a review of systems is necessary to screen for unsuspected disease. Careful note is made of current drug therapy, cigarette and alcohol intake. The date of the LMP (last menstrual period) is vitally important, as is knowledge of recent use of contraceptives. **If in doubt, perform a pregnancy test.**

The purpose of the physical examination is to assess the anaesthetic risk.

ROUTINE LABORATORY TESTS

- <40 years:
  - Haemoglobin concentration.
  - Assess need for pregnancy test.
- >40 years:
  - Haemoglobin concentration.
  - Urea and electrolytes.
- >60 years:
  - Chest X-ray; electrocardiogram.

Patients with known disease such as asthma, diabetes, hypertension, and hypothyroidism may need further assessment, and the anaesthetist should be forewarned.

Special investigations such as pelvic ultrasound may be required if pelvic masses are present, or even an IVU if there is a fixed pelvic mass or unexplained renal insufficiency.

The aim of the preoperative workup is to achieve the optimum preoperative condition of the patient to minimise operative risk.

BOWEL PREPARATION

Formal preoperative cleansing of the bowel is infrequently required in gynaecology, however anticipation of involvement by gynaecological malignancy would be an indication. Restrict to clear fluids for the day before surgery and given cathartics for a day such as GOLYTELY. This lessens the likelihood and severity of bowel complications postoperatively.

CROSS-MATCHING OF BLOOD

Most gynaecological procedures do not require cross-matching of blood, including most hysterectomies and other vaginal surgery. However potentially malignant cases, or those where technically difficult surgery is suspected, (e.g. severe endometriosis) should be cross matched especially if the preoperative haemoglobin is suboptimal.

PROPHYLACTIC ANTIBIOTICS

The aim of using prophylactic antibiotics is to reduce the number of bacteria at the operative site, and thereby decrease febrile morbidity. Commonest vaginal organisms to proliferate at wound sites are the anaerobes particularly Gram-positive cocci and Gram-negative rods such as Bacteroides. Without prophylactic antibiotics, 9–50% of women undergoing a hysterectomy will develop a postoperative infection. Presence of trichomonas or bacterial vaginosis increases the likelihood of cuff cellulitis or abscess formation.

Vaginal hysterectomy

Prophylactic antibiotics are recommended in premenopausal women, but the evidence is less clear in the postmenopausal woman. The incidence of postoperative infection is reduced from 25% to 5%, and febrile morbidity by a quarter.

Prophylactic antibiotics are not indicated in vaginal surgery where the peritoneum is not opened (e.g. repair of cystocoele or rectocoele).

Abdominal hysterectomy

Meta-analysis of published studies suggests 21% of patients undergoing an abdominal hysterectomy will have a serious postoperative infection if prophylactic antibiotics are not administered.

Regimes

Most hospitals will have their own antibiotic prophylaxis regimens. Examples include 1.2 g augmentin iv or cefuroxime 750 mg iv with metronidazole 500 mg iv or 1 g rectally on induction of anaesthesia.

Risk factors

- **Intrinsic:** e.g. diabetes, poor nutrition, valvular heart disease or compromised immunity.
- **Extrinsic:** e.g. radical cancer surgery, blood loss greater than 1000 ml and bacterial vaginosis.

Patients with valvular heart disease will require more broad spectrum antibiotic coverage.

THROMBOEMBOLIC DISEASE PROPHYLAXIS

Pulmonary emboli (PE) are a major cause of death in hospital patients, most arising from previously unrecognized non-fatal venous thrombosis.

RISK FACTORS

Risk factors for PE are age, obesity, varicose veins, immobility >4 days, pregnancy, previous DVT or PE, thrombophilia – deficiency of antithrombin III, protein C or S, anti-phospholipid antibodies or lupus anticoagulant.

- **Low-risk group:**
  - Minor surgery (<30 min); no risk factor other than age.
  - Major surgery (>30 min); age <40; no other risk factors.
- **Moderate-risk groups:**
  - Major gynaecological surgery; age >40 years or other risk factor.
  - Minor surgery in patients with previous DVT, PE or thrombophilia.
- **High-risk group:**
  - Major pelvic or abdominal surgery for cancer.
  - Major surgery in patients with previous DVT, PE or thrombophilia.

INCIDENCE OF THROMBOSIS

- **Low-risk group:**
  - risk of DVT <10%, and of fatal PE 0.01%. Prophylaxis is not indicated.

- **Moderate-risk group:**
  - risk of DVT 10–40%, and of a fatal PE 1%.
- **High-risk group:**
  - risk of DVT 40–80%, and of a fatal PE 10%.

PROPHYLAXIS

Mechanical

Graduated elastic stockings, or intermittent pneumatic compression devices. Effective in moderate risk groups and increase efficiency of prophylaxis in high-risk group. No increased risk of bleeding.

Pharmacological methods

- Low dose subcutaneous heparin (e.g. 5000 iu heparin sc bd) decreases incidence of DVT and fatal PE by two-thirds. Increased risk of wound haematoma and thrombocytopenia in 0.3%, (monitor platelet count if heparin given for >5 days). Low molecular weight heparins (e.g. clexane 20 mg od sc) have the advantage of once daily dosage and probably fewer complications.
- Dextran 70, given as a perioperative intravenous infusion, affects blood flow, platelets, endothelium and lysability of clots. More effective at preventing PE than peripheral venous thrombosis. Risk of fluid overload and allergic reaction.
- Continuous iv heparin infusions or higher dose subcutaneous regimes are used in very high risk cases.
- **Contraindications:** bleeding disorder or potential bleeding lesion.

Recommendations

- Identify risk factors
- Early mobilization
- Continue prophylaxis until discharge or beyond if high risk.

CONTRACEPTIVE PILL

There is a risk of postoperative thromboembolism of 0.96% for pill users and 0.5% for non-users.

It is usually a low risk as patients are young, fit, and early to mobilize.

- Benefits of stopping 4–6 weeks before surgery must be balanced by the risk of pregnancy.
- In emergency surgery when the risk is greater, use prophylaxis.

HORMONE REPLACEMENT THERAPY

Recent studies suggest an increased risk of thromboembolism in those women taking HRT, therefore prophylaxis should be considered in those with additional risk factors.

OTHER GENERAL PREOPERATIVE CONSIDERATIONS

- Preoperative skin preparation and douching of the vagina is often routinely performed, but their value in preventing infection has never been rigorously tested.
- Patients who are on anti-hypertensive medications should still take their medications on the day of surgery to maintain a diastolic reading of around 90 mmHg. If the diastolic BP is >110 mm Hg it is likely that surgery will be cancelled.
- Insulin dependent diabetics should be well controlled prior to surgery, and preoperatively may have insulin and glucose withheld for short operations. For longer procedures an insulin infusion with 5% dextrose titrated to blood sugars is preferred. Oral hypoglycaemic agents may need to be stopped 1–3 days before surgery depending on their half-life.

16

COMMON PROCEDURES

HYSTERECTOMY

Hysterectomy is a common surgical procedure with 20% of women in England and Wales having this operation performed by the age of 60 years. The indication for a hysterectomy should clearly be defined, and should be one for which conservative management has been or would be ineffective.

- **Total hysterectomy:** Removal of the whole uterus and cervix.
- **Subtotal hysterectomy:** A variable amount of the cervix is retained.
- **Wertheim's hysterectomy:** Removal of the whole of the uterus, a portion of the vagina, the uterosacral, cardinal and broad ligaments and the lymph nodes around the iliac vessels and on the lateral pelvic walls. The ovaries are sometimes retained in younger women.

SURGICAL TECHNIQUES

1. Total abdominal hysterectomy

The most common indications for an abdominal hysterectomy are: dysfunctional uterine bleeding, fibroids, abdominal pain (adenomyosis, endometriosis or chronic pelvic inflammatory disease) and malignant disease. The abdominal route is surgically easier and gives the surgeon the ability to remove large tumours, perform bilateral oophorectomy, accomplish adhesiolysis, omentectomy and lymphadenectomy. The usual ratio of abdominal to vaginal hysterectomies is 4:1. Many surgeons believe that this should be reversed because of the lower morbidity associated with the latter procedure. There is still an unresolved controversy as to whether the ovaries should be routinely removed at an abdominal hysterectomy in a premenopausal woman of >45 years of age. A proportion of cases of ovarian cancer will be prevented by bilateral oophorectomy. However it results in a surgical menopause and younger women should be made aware of the potential metabolic effects, the symptoms this will cause and the possible need for hormone replacement therapy (HRT).

KEYPOINT

Always discuss oophorectomy with patients who are about to undergo total abdominal hysterectomy and be clear in the consent as to what has and has not been agreed.

Operative technique

After pelvic examination, consider inserting a 14 French gauge Foley catheter to prevent immediate postoperative voiding difficulties.

Access is usually through a transverse lower abdominal incision, but may be through a vertical midline incision on occasion (most pelvic masses and suspected malignancy). The type of incision should be discussed with the patient preoperatively.

Major steps in the operation will include:

- division of the infundibulo-pelvic ligament if the ovaries are to be removed, or division between the ovaries and uterus if not
- division of the uterine arteries avoiding the ureters
- opening of the vagina
- closure of the vault (may be left open on occasions)
- closure of the rectus sheath and skin.

Complications of abdominal hysterectomy

- **Early:**
  - Mortality <0.1%.
  - 1° haemorrhage may result from a slipped ligature on the uterine or ovarian pedicle.
  - 2° haemorrhage from the vaginal vault.
  - Infection within the incision. Pelvic or intraabdominal sepsis/abscess formation.
  - Urinary retention or infection.
  - Anaesthetic complications; vomiting, respiratory infection, spinal headache.
  - Venous thrombosis leading to pulmonary embolism.
  - Incisional hernia, intestinal obstruction from adhesions.
- **Late:**
  - Adhesion formation leading to the 'trapped ovary syndrome' or intestinal obstruction.

- Hastening of the menopause.
- Increased bladder and bowel dysfunction.
- Psychosexual disorders.

2. Subtotal hysterectomy

Operative technique

The initial part of the procedure is the same as a total hysterectomy. However the uterine vessels are clamped and the uterus is divided at the level of the internal os and the defect closed.

Advantages

- Suggested but unproven decrease in bowel and bladder complications.
- Low incidence of vault haematoma, and no vault granulation tissue.
- Orgasm frequency not decreased, dyspareunia less, sense of loss not as marked.
- Reduced risk of intraoperative haemorrhage and ureteric damage in difficult cases.

Disadvantages

- Persistent menstruation in 5%.
- Continued risk of cervical cancer as cervix retained (regular smears should continue).

3. Vaginal hysterectomy

This mode of access should be preferred in the absence of any contraindications to the vaginal route for hysterectomy. However, the patient should be warned preoperatively of the small risk of conversion to an abdominal procedure.

Relative contraindications to vaginal hysterectomy

- Uterus >12 weeks
- Decreased uterine mobility
- Adnexal pathology
- Cervix flush with vagina
- Invasive carcinoma of the cervix or endometriosis

Note nulliparity and the presence of fibroids or the need to remove the ovaries, are not absolute contraindications to vaginal hysterectomy.

- Descent is physiological, and is present in most patients under anaesthesia irrespective of parity.

- Prolapse is pathological and present even when the patient is not anaesthetized.

Operation

Evaluate patients scheduled for a hysterectomy, to exclude contraindications to the vaginal route.

Assess uterine mobility, size and descent after placing patient in the lithotomy position under general anaesthesia.

The essential steps of the operation include:

- Circumferential incision of the vagina around the cervix.
- Separation and upward displacement of the bladder.
- Opening the pouch of Douglas.
- Securing the uterosacral and cardinal ligaments and, separately, the uterine vessels.
- Opening the utero-vesical pouch, securing the broad and round ligaments and removing the uterus.
- Supporting the vault by suturing the various ligaments to it.
- Closure of the vaginal skin with or without anterior and posterior colporrhaphy.

If a posterior repair is not performed it is generally not necessary to insert a pack or catheter.

Indications to convert to abdominal hysterectomy

- Band of inaccessible adhesions holding up uterus and preventing descent.
- Unsuspected adnexal pathology.
- Underestimation of uterine size.
- Inaccessible myoma.
- Inability to open the uterovesical peritoneum.
- Haemorrhage.

Complications specific to the vaginal approach

- 1° haemorrhage requiring laparotomy <0.5%.
- Increased risk of vault prolapse compared to abdominal procedure.

4. Laparoscopic hysterectomy

This encompasses all operations combining laparoscopic and vaginal surgery. The aim is to convert a difficult vaginal hysterectomy to an easier one and a proposed abdominal hysterectomy to a vaginal hysterectomy, reversing the traditional 4:1 ratio. Operating time is longer, extensive training in laparoscopic surgical skills is required and highly specialized (and expensive) equipment is needed. Recovery time and hospital stay is significantly shorter than after an abdominal hysterectomy. Most cases are in fact 'laparoscopic assisted vaginal hysterectomy' (LAVH) as laparoscopic surgery is used for only part of the procedure.

Advantage

A laparoscopy allows the surgeon to decide on the optimum route of hysterectomy based on actual pelvic pathology.

Technique

- The patient is placed in the dorsal position with legs abducted and with no (or minimal) hip flexion.
- The laparoscope is inserted through a sub-umbilical incision, with two 5 mm secondary portals.
- The pelvis is inspected and the anatomy corrected by adhesiolysis, ablation of endometriosis and and isolation of adnexal pathology.
- In most cases laparoscopic techniques are also used to divide the uterine vessels and dissect the bladder off the cervix.
- Bipolar diathermy or linear staples may be employed to divide tissues and achieve haemostasis.
- The procedure is usually completed vaginally using more traditional surgical techniques. The uterus and cervix (with or without the adnexae) are removed through the vagina.

Complications of laparoscopic hysterectomy

- Laparotomy is necessary in 5% of cases due to intraoperative haemorrhage or severe pelvic disease, beyond the scope of laparoscopic surgery.
- Venous, bowel or urological injury which may go unrecognized and present with postoperative complications.
- Injury to deep epigastric vessels by secondary trochar insertion.
- Herniae in lateral ports.

Patients recover no more quickly if there is a greater rather than a smaller percentage of the hysterectomy performed laparoscopically. The aim therefore should be to halt the laparoscopic part of the dissection as soon as it is considered possible to complete the operation vaginally.

5. Radical abdominal hysterectomy (Wertheim's)

- Indicated for patients with low volume cervical cancer confined to the cervix.

- Procedure involves dissection of the parametrial and paracervical tissue, as well as the upper third of the vagina.
- Combined with pelvic lymph node dissection, and occasionally para-aortic node sampling.
- Ovaries are usually conserved in younger women.
- There is an increased incidence of urinary tract complications (1–2%).
- It avoids the intestinal, vaginal and bladder complications of radiotherapy.
- There is a psychological benefit of tumour removal.
- The patient may still need radiotherapy if the lymph nodes contain metastases.

OPERATIONS FOR GENUINE STRESS INCONTINENCE

BURCH COLPOSUSPENSION

Indications

- Objective urodynamic diagnosis of genuine stress incontinence (GSI) with or without anterior vaginal wall prolapse. The procedure of choice in a fit patient with GSI (*see* p. 264).

Contraindications

- Foreshortened, scarred immobile vagina, where elevation of the lateral fornices is unlikely.
- Coexisting detrusor instability (DI) may lower cure rates, but a colposuspension is not contraindicated if genuine stress incontinence persists after adequate treatment of the DI.
- Voiding difficulties, as gauged by increased residual volumes and pressure/flow voiding studies. A maximum preoperative voiding pressure <15 cm water predisposes to post-operative voiding difficulties (i.e. poor flow and high residual volumes).
- Desire for future childbearing. Subsequent vaginal deliveries may reverse the benefits of the operation. An alternative is to have any other children by elective Caesarean section.

Surgical technique

Regional or general anaesthesia can be used. The patient is in the lithotomy position with legs supported in Lloyd–Davies stirrups.

KEY POINTS

- **French gauge urethral catheter in place throughout the operation.**

- **Lower abdominal transverse incision with entry into the retropubic space.**
- **Insertion of the finger into the vagina next to the bladder neck, elevating the vagina on each side to sweep the bladder medially.**
- **Insertion of two or three non-absorbable sutures between the paravaginal fascia and the ileopectoneal ligament.**
- **Suction drainage to the retropubic space and insertion of a suprapubic bladder catheter.**

Postoperative management

Remove drain at 24 hours. Leave suprapubic catheter on free drainage until day 3 or 4 and then begin intermittent clamping. Measure urethrally voided volumes and residuals (by unclamping the catheter after a urethral void). When there have been two residuals <100 ml remove the catheter. Incontinence cure rates of 80–90% have been achieved.

Complications of colposuspension

- Venous haemorrhage
- Bladder and urethral injury
- Ureteric kinking, rarely ligation
- Voiding difficulties (up to 25%)
- Postoperative detrusor instability (up to 25%)
- Postoperative enterocoele 20%.

OTHER TECHNIQUES FOR MANAGEMENT OF GSI

- **Anterior colporrhaphy:** Has the advantage of correcting concurrent anterior vaginal wall prolapse and does not commonly lead to long-term voiding difficulty or detrusor instability. However cure rates for GSI are only 60–70%.
- **Endoscopic bladder neck suspension operation (Stamey):** Needle insertion of a non-absorbable suture either side of the bladder neck secured by a synthetic buffer below the pubocervical fascia and sutured to the rectus sheath at a tension sufficient to close the bladder neck.
- **Marshall–Marchetti–Krantz (MMK) operation:** Sutures placed in the proximal half of the urethra and attached to the symphysis pubis. Osteitis pubis occurs in 0.5–5% of cases.
- **Sling procedure:** Passage of fascial strips from abdominal wall, or synthetic strips, behind the symphysis pubis to be sutured together below the urethra. Usually a secondary GSI procedure, when there is reduced vaginal capacity and mobility.

Complications: bladder injury and urine extravasation, haematoma, sepsis particularly with synthetics, and later retention, urethral stricture.

- **Peri-urethral injections:** The aim with these techniques is to increase urethral resistance. Collagen, Teflon and silicon-based compounds are injected into the bladder neck often under local anaesthetic. Useful for mild GSI. Cure rates are lower than after a colposuspension, but recovery is immediate and repeat procedures are possible.

PELVIC FLOOR REPAIR

(*See also* p. 261)

- **Posterior colporrhaphy** is employed to correct a rectocoele (bulging of the posterior vaginal wall and rectum into the vagina). It involves dissection of the rectum from the vaginal wall and the placement of 'levator sutures' to appose muscles of the levator plate. Redundant skin is excised. Significant postoperative pain is common as is urinary retention. Narrowing of the vagina should be avoided and recurrences can occur.

KEY POINT

Ask preoperatively about current sexual activity and future wishes as overzealous treatment may cause significant long-term morbidity.

- **Repair of enterocoele:** Enterocoeles are caused by the pressure of small bowel loops acting through the pouch of Douglas causing posterior wall and vault prolapse. They are often difficult to detect preoperatively and should always be considered during vaginal wall repair. Repair is usually carried out vaginally but abdominal procedures do exist. The hernial sac of peritoneum should be identified and excised to prevent recurrence.
- **Vault prolapse:** This is a relatively common complication of hysterectomy, caused by the loss of vaginal support from the cardinal and uterosacral ligaments. It can be repaired abdominally (a sacrocolpopexy) by attaching the top of the vagina to the sacrum or vaginally by suspending the vault onto the sacrospinous ligament (a sacrospinous vault fixation).
- **Anterior colporrhaphy:** *see above.*

TERMINATION OF PREGNANCY

(*See also* 'Procedures' section, pp. 310.)

In Great Britain the following are indications for termination of pregnancy (TOP):

- The continuation of the pregnancy would involve risk to the life of the pregnant woman greater than if the pregnancy were terminated.
- The termination of the pregnancy is necessary to prevent grave permanent injury to the physical or mental health of the pregnant woman.
- The pregnancy has not exceeded the 24th week and the continuance of the pregnancy would involve risk, greater than if the pregnancy were terminated, of injury to the physical or mental health of any existing children of the family of the pregnant woman.
- There is a substantial risk that if the child were born it would suffer from such physical or mental abnormalities as to be seriously handicapped.

Termination of pregnancy for any of these categories is allowed up to the end of the 24th week of pregnancy. Termination of pregnancy for severe abnormality or for grave maternal risks can be undertaken at any gestational age. Third trimester termination of pregnancy does occur, but these procedures are only performed in specialist centres and will normally involve referral to a tertiary subspecialty fetal medicine team.

Two doctors must sign the Abortion Act Form (Certificate A) prior to the patient going to the operating theatre or having any form of medical treatment to ripen the cervix. The notification form must be completed by the person carrying out the termination of pregnancy.

Approximately 190 000 terminations are performed each year in England and Wales, of which 98% are performed by vacuum aspiration. Half of the women were not using contraception at the time of conception, and a third requesting this procedure will be under the age of 20 years. The maternal mortality from a termination in developed countries is 1 in 100 000, with serious complications occurring in <1% and minor in 10% (remember psychological distress). The abortion is complete in 95–98% of cases.

EXAMINATION AND HISTORY

- Take a full medical, social, family and contraceptive history.
- Confirm dates and check that vaginal examination findings agree.
- If there is doubt organise a vaginal ultrasound examination. Take endocervical, high vaginal and chlamydia swabs for microbiological examination. (If swabs have not been performed serious consideration should be given to treating the patient prophylactically with 1 g metronidazole pr (one dose) and 7 days of doxycycline (100 mg bd po).
- Ascertain the patient's blood group. Give anti-D to all rhesus negative women (250 IU im if <20 weeks and 500 IU im if 20 or more weeks). Above 20 weeks' gestation a larger feto-maternal haemorrhage is possible at the time of the TOP and a Kleihauer test must be performed after the procedure to determine if more anti-D is required.

Counselling

This should be non-directional with constructive advice. Risks, benefits and methods of termination should be discussed as well as alternatives such as continuing the pregnancy or adoption. Consent should include the risks of uterine perforation (uncommon but usually necessitates laparoscopy/laparotomy), retained products of conception requiring further uterine evacuation (1–2%) and post-TOP endometritis (also common).

High-risk groups are teenagers with poor support, patients undergoing repeat terminations, those with a genetic risk, cases of sexual abuse and late terminations at 18–20 weeks.

METHODS

First trimester suction termination of pregnancy

- Almost all first trimester terminations are suitable for day case surgery, usually under general anaesthesia, but occasionally under local anaesthesia.
- Suction termination of pregnancy can be performed at gestations up to 12–14 weeks.
- Patients should have cervical preparation (for instance 800 micrograms of misoprostol per vaginum or cervagem pessary) at least one hour before the procedure.
- The cervix is dilated mechanically to a diameter corresponding to gestation.
- The contents are evacuated with a rigid or soft suction curette, and the uterine cavity checked to confirm completion of the procedure.

- Ten units of syntocinon may be given intravenously during the procedure to decrease the bleeding.

Second trimester termination of pregnancy

- After 12–14 weeks a medical method of terminating pregnancy is preferred .
- 1 mg gemeprost (prostaglandin E1) vaginal pessaries are inserted into the posterior fornix of the vagina every 3 hours until abortion has taken place, up to a maximum of five pessaries in 24 hours. About 80% will have aborted within 24 hours.
- Haemorrhage and infection are the commonest complications with blood transfusion being required in 0.6 % and infection reported in 10% of cases.
- If the abortion is incomplete surgical evacuation will be necessary. This will be indicated by continued heavy bleeding or an open internal cervical os.
- Discuss the case with more senior staff before ordering an ultrasound examination for diagnosis of retained products as ultrasound can be misleading in these situations.
- Remember that later terminations for fetal abnormality may require specialized investigations (e.g. karyotyping).
- Mifepristone, an antiprogesterone, can be given orally 36–48 hours prior to admission for the gemeprost. This is becoming increasingly popular. Misoprostol (not licensed) is commonly used instead of gemeprost.

Early medical termination of pregnancy

This technique is reserved for first trimester terminations of less than 63 days gestation. Mifepristone 200 mg is given orally and is followed 36–48 hours later by a gemeprost 1 mg vaginal pessary. This regime results in complete abortion in 95%, incomplete in 4% and a missed or viable pregnancy in <1% of cases. If products of conception are not identified prior to discharge, the patient must attend for a follow-up scan in 2 weeks to exclude an ongoing pregnancy or retained products.

Post-abortal bleeding can be expected for 10–12 days and return to normal menses in 5–6 weeks.

COMPLICATIONS

Early

Blood loss increases with gestation, and may be due to uterine atony, retained products, trauma to the cervix or uterine perforation.

Sepsis is uncommon and is most often caused by retained products.

Late

Psychiatric sequelae can be minimised by careful counselling, post-operative and follow-up support. Infertility following termination is uncommon. Possible cervical incompetence is avoided by the use of cervical softening agents such as prostaglandins.

FUTURE CONTRACEPTION

An intrauterine contraceptive device can be fitted at the time of the termination of pregnancy, although there is a theoretical risk of displacement of the device.

A combined oral contraceptive pill can be started on the following day.

Depo-Provera injections can be given prior to discharge from hospital.

KEYPOINT

It is essential that any patient undergoing termination of pregnancy is given adequate contraceptive advice before and at the time of termination and that a viable plan is made regarding future contraception.

GYNAECOLOGICAL ENDOSCOPIC SURGERY

This is also known as minimal access surgery. It involves major procedures carried out using minimally invasive techniques which employ the hysteroscope and laparoscope.

Advantages

- Rapid postoperative recovery
- Lower patient morbidity
- Avoidance of a laparotomy
- Shortened stay in hospital
- Reduction in postoperative pain and infective morbidity.

Disadvantages

- Heightened patient expectations of success and reduced tolerance of failure
- Need for advanced surgical training and expensive equipment
- Length of time taken to complete the operation.

LAPAROSCOPY

Equipment

Laparoscope and light source, video camera and monitors, rapid flow CO_2 insufflators with automatic pressure control and smoke evacuator, mono-polar and bi-polar diathermy forceps, saline irrigator and suction apparatus, laparoscopic operating tools (scissors, traumatic and atraumatic grasper).

Energy source

Electrosurgery, laser, ultrasonic scalpels.

Basic techniques

- **Veres needle insertion:** With the patient horizontal, the veres needle is inserted through the deepest part of a vertical umbilical incision beyond the sheath and into the peritoneal cavity, (an alternative site being suprapubically) and entry is confirmed by injecting 5 mL of normal saline. If the end of the needle is correctly placed none of this should be able to be withdrawn. The gas flow should be no more than 1 litre per minute with the intraabdominal pressure not exceeding 15 mmHg.
- **Trochar insertion:** Once an adequate pneumoperitoneum has formed the first trochar can be inserted in a similar manner, keeping in the midline to avoid the pelvic vessels. Additional trochars are inserted under direct vision with the patient then placed in the Trendelenberg position. The inferior epigastric vessels emerge from the deep inguinal ring with the round ligament and are found just lateral to the lateral umbilical ligament.

Relative contraindications to laparoscopy

- Coagulopathies
- Abdominal ileus
- Large abdominal mass
- Hiatus hernia and external herniae
- Severe medical disease
- Previous abdominal surgery.

Complications of laparoscopy

Incidence: Minor 5.2/1000; Major 1.1/1000 (haemorrhage, bowel perforation, urinary tract injury).

- **Bowel injuries:** Often unrecognized at the time of laparoscopy with most injuries presenting between the 3rd and 7th postoperative days. On examination the physical signs can be non-specific and include mild abdominal distension, lower quadrant tenderness, decreased bowel sounds, a temperature of 37.2–38.3°C, and a raised white cell count. Subdiaphragmatic gas on an erect X-ray is not helpful as evidence of bowel injury due to the previous pneumoperitoneum.

- **Urinary tract:** Common sites of ureteric injury occurring at the time of laparoscopic surgery are:
  - adjacent to the infundibulo-pelvic ligament
  - at the level of the utero-sacral ligaments
  - near the uterine artery.

Laparoscopic management of ovarian cysts

Unsuspected malignancy in an ovarian cyst is uncommon (0.04%). Cytology of cyst fluid is unhelpful with false-negatives in 10–66%. Ultrasound features which would heighten suspicion are irregular borders, thick septae, papillations, solid areas and ascites. Ca125 measurements and transvaginal Doppler further increase the sensitivity and specificity for detection of ovarian malignancy. Laparoscopic surgery should be avoided on a potentially malignant cyst.

- **Simple cyst:** Aspiration is rarely sufficient, with 40% recurring. Laparoscopic dissection and removal of an ovarian cyst causes little bleeding and the area is left to heal by secondary intention.
- **Dermoid cysts:** These are more troublesome to remove laparoscopically. The sebaceous contents are highly irritant to the peritoneal cavity and if there is spill during the procedure thorough irrigation of the pelvic cavity is required.
- **Endometrioma:** If >4 cm in diameter they are unlikely to respond sufficiently to GnRH analogues. They may be densely adherent to the pelvic side wall and time consuming to remove. Identify ureter and pelvic vessels to help prevent injury.
- **Oophorectomy:** If the entire ovary is to be removed the infundibulopelvic ligament can be secured using bipolar diathermy, staples or endo-loops.

Laparoscopic management of ectopic pregnancy (EP)

Improved and earlier diagnosis by high resolution vaginal ultrasound and human chorionic gonadotropin (HCG) measurements offers opportunity for less invasive management. Larger ectopics associated with haemodynamic compromise may be better managed with a more traditional laparotomy.

1. Salpingotomy

The procedure of choice in patients who have only one fallopian tube are haemodynamically stable and wish to preserve fertility.

- **Technique**:
  The fallopian tube is held with atraumatic forceps and a one centimetre incision is made in the anti-mesenteric border with uni-polar diathermy needle over the site of the ectopic. The products of conception are teased out with the aid of irrigation and suction. The tube heals by secondary intention. This carries the risk of persistent trophoblastic tissue (up to 10% of cases) which requires further surgery or treatment with methotrexate.
- **Postoperative follow-up**:
  - Serial serum HCG measurements on day 2 and 7. A steady fall of >15%/24 hours should be expected. Rising or static levels suggest persistent trophoblastic tissue and the need for further treatment.
  - Re-admit if the HCG is not falling or if the patient is symptomatic and consider Methotrexate therapy 50 mg/m^2 im or a repeat laparoscopy and salpingectomy.
  - Consider hysterosalpingogram (HSG) at 6 weeks to confirm tubal patency.

2. Salpingectomy

This is the procedure of choice when the contralateral tube is healthy.

There is no difference in intra-uterine pregnancy rates between salpingectomy and salpingotomy and the latter is associated with a higher repeat ectopic pregnancy rate.

- **Technique**
  Place the fallopian tube under traction and pass the EP through two endo-loops which secure the pedicle. A salpingectomy is performed with scissors.
- **Contraindications to laparoscopic surgery for EP**
  - Operator inexperience
  - Haemodynamic instability
  - Gross adhesions.

Laparoscopic management of pelvic adhesions

Their relationship to pain is poorly understood. Laparoscopic division is not to be undertaken lightly as the bowel is often involved.

However they are more easily and more effectively dealt with laparoscopically than by laparotomy and recurrence is less likely.

- **Indication for adhesiolysis**:
  - To allow access to ovaries or uterus when surgery on these is intended.
  - Dissection for infertility.
  - In patients complaining of altered bowel function and pelvic pain.

HYSTEROSCOPY

Non-operative hysteroscopy

Fine diameter hysteroscopes measuring between 2.5 to 4.5 mm are employed to inspect the uterine cavity and cervical canal. It can be performed in an out patient setting with over 95% of patients suitable.

The most common distension media are CO_2, normal saline and dextran. CO_2 insufflation pressures should be restricted to <120 mmHg and flow rates to 100 mL/min. Laparoscopic insufflators even on a low flow setting rate will still have flow rates of 200–400 mL/min. There is a potential risk of CO_2 embolism, however this is rare.

Alternative fluid distension media are normal saline or a high molecular weight dextran (e.g. Dextran 70). In the UK the former is increasingly popular when 2.5 mm hysteroscopes are employed. Dextran, when used in low volumes, does not mix with blood often improving the image however instruments must be thoroughly rinsed afterwards as the dextran will cause clogging. Anaphylactic reactions occur with dextran in 0.01% of patients.

- **Endometrial biopsy:** These are performed using endometrial aspiration devices such as the Pipelle de Cornier or with a narrow metal curette (a kevorkian) – often the most uncomfortable part of the procedure.

Operative hysteroscopy

Requires large diameter instruments up to 6–8 mm to resect pathology. The operative procedures are performed usually under general anaesthetic in a day case or inpatient setting. A distension medium of a 1.5% glycine solution is employed which has non-conductive properties and is appropriate during electrosurgical resection.

Transcervical endometrial resection (TCRE)

This is an alternative to hysterectomy for dysfunctional uterine bleeding.

- Prior preparation of endometrium with GnRH analogues for 6 weeks may make the procedure easier.
- Electrosurgical resection of the endometrium of the uterine cavity is combined with roller ball diathermy to the fundus and isthmus (laser is an alternative).
- The majority are performed as day cases under general anaesthetic although overnight stay is not uncommon.
- Overall satisfaction rates are 80–90%, with approximately half of these women becoming amenorrhoiec.
- Adequate contraception must be continued and simultaneous sterilization is often carried out.
- If HRT is subsequently desired combined preparations (oestrogen and progesterone) are necessary.

The hysteroscope can also be used to resect intrauterine and submucous fibroids, congenital uterine septae and to divide intrauterine adhesions.

Complications

- **Fluid absorption:** If large volumes of glycine solution are absorbed into the circulation, dilutional hyponatraemia may result potentially causing intravascular haemolysis, hepatorenal failure and cerebral oedema. When fluid loss exceeds 1000 mL then the procedure should be stopped unless near completion. Intra-venous fluids should be restricted and a diuretic administered (frusemide 10–20 mg).

  Excessive absorption of normal saline mainly leads to simple volume overload, but is unsuitable for electrosurgical resection because of its conductive properties. Fluid overload may be avoided by theatre staff checking the fluid balance at least every 10 minutes.
- **Uterine perforation:** This usually occurs at the time of insertion of the hysteroscope. Nulliparous women and those with an acutely anteverted or retroverted uterus are most at risk.

  It is rarely significant unless the bowel or bladder is adherent to the uterus; the procedure can be repeated after one month.

  The likelihood of uterine perforation is lessened by **always** performing a bimanual examination before hysteroscopy and inserting the instrument under direct vision. A potentially more serious complication can occur if the uterus is perforated during an endometrial resection. A laparoscopy should be performed, and if there is any doubt regarding the integrity of visceral organs, a laparotomy.

- **1° Haemorrhage:** This is rare following resections or ablative procedures. If it does occur insert an 18–20 French gauge Foley catheter and inflate slowly with 15–30 mL of saline to tamponade the vessels and then withdraw after 4 hours.
- **2° Haemorrhage:** 10–14 days later; also uncommon. May resolve with antibiotics.
- **Infection:** Active clinical signs of infection at the time of a procedure are a contraindication to hysteroscopy. Antibiotic prophylaxis for operative hysteroscopy is not routinely given.

The recent MISTLETOE[1] study of endometrial resection and laser treatment demonstrated a very low mortality rate from these procedures. However 1% of procedures were complicated by the need for emergency surgery at the time (laparoscopy, laparotomy or hysterectomy) due to complications.

MYOMECTOMY

Fibroids are very common and found in 40% of all women aged >50 years. In those still menstruating they are the reason for 33% of all hysterectomies. They are 3–9 times more common in Afro-Caribbeans than Caucasians. The risk of malignancy is very low (around 0.18%) and fibroids usually regress gradually with the onset of the menopause.

A myomectomy should be considered for women who have symptomatic fibroids but who wish to retain reproductive function and menstruation. However it is unsuitable for multiple small fibroids and those sited within the broad ligament are more vascular and removal carries an increased risk of emergency hysterectomy. There is a 5–10% recurrence rate and 20–25% of patients will have a hysterectomy eventually.

[1] The MISTLETOE study (**M**inimally **I**nvasive **S**urgical **T**echniques/**L**aser, **E**ndothermal **or** **E**ndoresection). **Reference:** Overton, C., Hargreaves, J. & Maresh, M. (1997). A national survey of complications of endometrial destruction for menstrual disorders: the MISTLETOE study. *British Journal of Obstetrics and Gynaecology* **104**, 1351–59.

Traditional surgery for fibroids

Surgery for fibroids is traditionally myomectomy and total abdominal hysterectomy.

Innovative surgery for fibroids

- Laparoscopic myomectomy
- Laparoscopic myolysis
- Laparoscopic myolysis and endometrial resection
- Vaginal hysterectomy for large fibroids
- Hysteroscopic resection.

SURGICAL TECHNIQUES

Pretreatment with GnRH analogues brings about size reduction – 36% by 12 weeks and 45% by 24 weeks. This change is only temporary however with a return to original size by 4 months after cessation of treatment. It benefits the patient by improving preoperative haemoglobin levels and by reducing blood loss perioperatively.

Abdominal myomectomy

- Initial preparation as for abdominal hysterectomy.
- Bloodless field helped by application of a Bonney's clamp.
- Shell-out as many fibroids through as few incisions as possible.
- Avoid occlusion or injury to the intramural part of the fallopian tube.
- Obliterate all cavities to avoid the creation of dead space and haematomata.
- Reperitonealize all suture lines.

Laparoscopic management of fibroids

Bipolar uterine needle treatment:

- Multiple insertions of bipolar needles into the myoma, with the aim to devascualarize. Myomata up to10 cm in diameter appropriate.

Laparoscopic myomectomy:

- Technically difficult and time consuming.
- Uterine incisions are made with unipolar diathermy as for the abdominal approach.
- Laparoscopic suturing techniques are used to repair the uterine incisions.
- Size limit of 10 cm, and no more than four myomas removed at one session.

Hysteroscopic management of fibroids

- Outpatient hysteroscopy is necessary to assess feasibility (ideally <10 cm in diameter).
- Ultrasound/magnetic resonance imaging may be necessary to assess anatomical relations.
- Pedunculated intrauterine and submucous myomas protruding into the cavity are most suitable.

Complications of hysteroscopic myomectomy

- Uterine perforation
- Intrauterine haemorrhage
- Infection
- Synaechie (13.4%)
- Uterine rupture in 3rd trimester of a subsequent pregnancy. If the cavity has been breached then elective Caesarean section is indicated.

17

ROUTINE POSTOPERATIVE CARE AND COMPLICATIONS

PAIN CONTROL

Postoperative pain control is vital for both patient comfort and to reduce the risk of other complications such as thromboembolic events and chest infections.

After major surgery the following may be used:

- Bolus injections of im morphine with anti-emetic.
- Patient controlled analgesia (PCA) pumps that combine a steady infusion of morphine under patient control as required.
- Epidural analgesia.

Most gynaecology patients will progress onto oral analgesics quickly. These should be prescribed on a regular, rather than as the occasion arises (prn), basis and sensible choices include:

- Paracetamol 1 g qds orally/rectally (po/pr).
- Diclofenac 50 mg tds po or 100 mg pr 18-hourly (avoid in patients with peptic ulcer disease, those with compromised renal function and asthmatics sensitive to aspirin).
- Codeine phosphate 30–60 mg qds po. May delay return of normal bowel function and consideration should be given to the use of lactulose or Senna tablets to combat constipation.

Combined analgesic preparations are becoming less popular with anaesthetists and pharmacists alike.

ROUTINE POSTOPERATIVE OBSERVATIONS

- Nursing observation and vital signs measured every 15 min, and then hourly until stable; then 4-hourly.
- Bed rest until morning and then begin mobilization with assistance.
- **Call house officer if:**
  - Temperature >38.5°C

  - Pulse rate >110 beats/min or <70 beats/min
  - Diastolic BP >100 mmHg or <60 mmHg
  - Respiratory rate >24 breaths/min or <10 breaths/min
  - Urine output <1/2 body weight in kg/hour.
- Monitor input and output.
- iv fluids – general principles apply. Most patients will be drinking adequately by the first postoperative day.
- Nil by mouth until bowel sounds audible. Most gynaecology patients will be taking light diet by the second postoperative day (and many sooner).
- Haemoglobin on the second postoperative day.

PULMONARY COMPLICATIONS

- **Pulmonary collapse**: Common. Risks are advanced age, smoking, obesity, prolonged anaesthesia, and pre-existent pulmonary disease. Prevention by deep breathing, coughing, chest physiotherapy, and use of bronchodilators. Prevention of collapse will decrease the risk of pneumonia and hypoxaemia.
- **Pulmonary embolus**: Characterized by sudden onset of chest pain, tachypnoea, tachycardia and dyspnoea, although the presentation may be less dramatic (e.g. unexplained tachycardia). Investigations include chest X-ray, arterial blood gases, ventilation perfusion scans and pulmonary arteriography.

If a PE is confirmed, treatment until recently has been with iv heparin for 7 days, introducing warfarin in the last 2–3 days which is then continued for 3–6 months. Newer low molecular weight subcutaneous heparins are now licensed for treatment of pulmonary emboli and discussion with medical or haematological colleagues is appropriate.

Possible differential diagnoses include myocardial infarction, pneumonia, pneumothorax or pulmonary oedema.

BOWEL FUNCTION

Rapid recovery of bowel function usually occurs when operating time has been short and confined to the adnexae. More extensive surgery leads to bowel dysfunction. Normal bowel sounds without abdominal distension suggest a patient may tolerate a light liquid diet. Until flatus or faeces are passed a more regular diet should be withheld. Early ambulation will help patients to recover bowel function more rapidly as will use of alternative analgesics to opiates.

Absence of bowel sounds associated with abdominal distension implies a **paralytic ileus.** May be treated with nasogastric (NG) suction and longer bowel rest.

If pain, nausea and vomiting accompany abdominal distension then **intestinal obstruction** should be suspected. Diagnosis may be confirmed by supine and erect abdominal X-rays. Complete obstruction requiring surgical intervention is rare; partial obstruction is more common and often resolves spontaneously. Using conservative therapy (NG tube and IVI) significant improvement or resolution should be seen within 24 hours. If not, consider whether laparotomy is necessary.

FEVER

An elevated temperature of <38°C is common in the first 24 hours; >38°C suggests a chest infection. Persistence for >48 hours suggests infection at the operative site being either a haematoma or a developing abscess. If a pyrexia occurs after 4–5 days a wound infection or DVT should be suspected. Urinary tract infections do not cause high temperatures unless pyelonephritis supervenes.

URINARY TRACT COMPLICATIONS

These are uncommon and can usually be avoided by good surgical practice. If there is any doubt at the time of surgery regarding the integrity of the urinary tract immediate intraoperative evaluation is preferable to observation.

- **Urinary retention:** Common following radical pelvic dissection or with surgery for urinary incontinence. For such procedures placement of urinary catheter (often suprapubic) intraoperatively avoids this complication.
- **Fistulae:** Vesicovaginal and ureterovaginal fistulae present with continuous postoperative dribble incontinence. They can be differentiated by inserting a Foley catheter and injecting a solution of indigo-carmine dye into the bladder. If no dye is seen in the vagina insert a tampon and mobilize the patient. If staining of the tampon occurs a vesicovaginal fistula is diagnosed. If this test is negative suspect a ureteric fistula. Confirm this with an intravenous ureterogram.
  - **Vesico-vaginal fistulae:** Repair immediately or at 2 months. However, small holes may heal spontaneously if a catheter is left in place for a longer period of time.

- **Ureteric injury:** Occurs secondary to devascularization, ligation or kinking. Unilateral hydronephrosis usually presents with loin pain and is detected with ultrasound. Insertion of a ureteric stent retrogradely or antegradely through a percutaneous nephrostomy may be possible. If not then ureteric reimplantation will be necessary.

WOUND COMPLICATIONS

- **Dehiscence:** Disruption of any layers of the surgical incision, excluding the peritoneum. Incidence 1 in 250.
- **Evisceration:** Breakdown of all levels of abdominal incision with protrusion of intrabdominal contents through the incision. Rare.

Predisposing factor:
Infection.
Symptoms and signs:
Spontaneous passage of sero-sanguinous fluid through the wound, usually on days 5–8.
Patients at high risk:
- Previous wound infection
- Diabetes
- Chronic obstructive airways disease
- Steroid therapy
- Peritonitis
- Malignancy
- Previous irradiation to abdomen and pelvis.

Treatment:
Depends on size and depth of wound. Usually healing is by 2° intention. Large defects and evisceration require formal repair in theatre.

OPERATIVE MORTALITY

- **Common causes of mortality:**
  - myocardial infarction, pulmonary emboli, infection and heart failure.
- **Common causes of morbidity:**
  - haemorrhage and sepsis.

Postoperative deaths from infection are uncommon in gynaecology, but may occur due to ruptured tubo-ovarian abscess, unrecognized bowel complications, immunosuppression and malignancy.

18

CONTRACEPTION

COMBINED ORAL CONTRACEPTIVE PILL

Since its introduction in 1961 the oestrogen content of the combined oral contraceptive pill (COCP) has fallen by seven-fold and this method of contraception is now used by 3 million women in the UK. Ovulation is suppressed by both the oestrogen and progestagen content. An overall failure rate of 0.2–0.3 per 100 woman-years is recorded. There is **no** upper age limit for non-smokers.

It is safer to take the oral contraceptive pill than to have either an ongoing pregnancy or a termination of pregnancy.

COCP contents

The COCP is taken daily for 21 days followed by a pill-free interval of 7 further days (the 'pill-free week'; PFW). A few preparations have seven inactive tablets instead of the PFW. Nearly all preparations contain ethinyl oestradiol as the oestrogen with one of three different progestagens. The newer progestagens (gestodene, desogestrel and norgestimate) which are found in 'third generation' pills have theoretical benefits over the older preparations. They give better cycle control and have a less detrimental effect on lipid profiles, blood pressure and carbohydrate metabolism (but see below).

Phasic preparations are so called because the progestagen content of the active pills varies according to the position of the pill in its packet, in theory mimicking the endogenous cycle more closely. A monophasic preparation is usually tried as first-line, changing to bi- and triphasic pills if break through bleeding is a problem.

Adverse effects

Headache, breast tenderness and irregular bleeding are the commonest side effects, but usually disappear by the end of the third cycle. If persistent then the progestagen content can be altered.

Advantages

- Reduction in menstrual disorders (dysmenorrhoea, menorrhagia, premenstrual tension, and ovulatory pain).
- Less pelvic inflammatory disease and benign breast disease.
- Fewer ectopic pregnancies and functional ovarian cysts.
- Reduction in the incidence of ovarian and endometrial cancer by 50%.
- Possible protection against thyroid disease, rheumatoid arthritis, fibroids, and osteoporosis.

Disadvantages

- A possible increase in the incidence of breast cancer (overall relative risk for current users: 1.24). The added risk of breast cancer seems to relate to the age at which the COCP is stopped rather than the actual duration of use:
  - if stopped at 25 years of age, by 35 there would be one extra case of breast cancer per 7000 original users
  - if stopped at 45 years of age then by 55 years of age there would be one extra case per 300 original users.
- Cervical cancer data is conflicting (possible doubling of risk). All women should be screened with 3-yearly cervical smears.
- Increased incidence of benign liver tumours (still rare however).
- Impaired glucose tolerance, increased cholesterol and triglycerides levels and a reduction in HDL cholesterol (all predisposing to arterial disease).
- There is an increased clotting tendency, with a rise in vitamin K dependent clotting factors, diminished anti-thrombin III activity and plasminogen levels (all predisposing to venous thromboembolic events). A number of studies have suggested that the greatest risk is with the third generation COCP (the cause of the most recent 'pill scare'). However, the risk of a thromboembolic event on any COCP is still at least half that of the risk whilst pregnant. Also, there is only a 1–2% mortality associated with these events. It seems sensible, as a rule, to prescribe a second generation pill in the first instance but, provided the patient is counselled appropriately, third generation pills may still be used if there is indication.
- Cholestasis may occur in susceptible women.
- There may be symptoms of depression, irritability and fatigue, with disturbance of sleep and libido.

Drug interactions

Concurrent use of broad spectrum antibiotics (ampicillin, tetracyclines and cephalosporins) destroy gut bacteria which recycle metabolised oestrogen, thereby reducing its efficacy. Therefore additional protection is necessary during the treatment and for 7 days afterwards. Other drugs which induce hepatic enzyme activity include carbamazepine, phenytoin, griseofulvin and rifampicin. Women on these drugs long term need to take a formulation containing 50 micrograms of ethinyl oestradiol (or take more than one pill per day) and even then efficacy may be reduced.

Absolute contraindication

Any proven arterial or venous thrombosis, ischaemic heart disease, known prothrombotic abnormality, diseases of the liver, undiagnosed genital tract bleeding, oestrogen dependent neoplasms and focal and crescendo migraines.

Relative contraindications

Hypertension, homozygous sickle cell-disease, very severe depression and inflammatory bowel disease. Certain COCPs can be used with well diabetics for short periods but the progesterone only pill (POP) or the Mirena intrauterine system (IUS) would be the contraceptives of choice.

KEYPOINTS

What to do if a pill is missed: Advice according to the British National Formulary (BNF)

If you forget a pill, take it as soon as you remember, and the next one at the normal time. If you are 12 or more hours late with any pill (especially the first in the packet) the pill may not work. As soon as you remember, continue normal pill taking. However, you will not be protected for the next 7 days and must either not have sex or use another method such as the sheath. If these 7 days run beyond the end of a packet, start the next packet at once when you have finished the present one, i.e. do not have a gap between packets. This will mean you may not have a period until the end of the two packets but this does you no harm. Nor does it matter if you see some bleeding on tablet taking days.

Actually, 7 consecutive days of pill taking 'switches off' the ovary and seven more days without the pill theoretically are needed before ovulation can take place again. Therefore pills at the end or the beginning of each packet are the most important as missing them will extend the pill free interval, seriously risking ovulation. However, missing up to three pills consecutively mid-packet is unlikely to allow ovulation so extra precautions (e.g. the sheath) are considered by some as 'overkill'. Undoubtedly though the safest advice is given in the BNF, and is still supported by the Family Planning Asssociation.

Causes of breakthrough bleeding (BTB)

- Genital tract lesion
- During the first 2–3 months of use
- Missed pills
- Vomiting (and severe diarrhoea)
- Pregnancy complications
- Liver inducing drugs
- Reduced absorption (gastrointestinal [GI] disease).

PROGESTERONE ONLY PILL

The main mode of action of the progesterone only pill (POP) is on the cervical mucus, making it hostile to sperm penetration. This effect lasts only 24 hours and hence the need for precise timing. It must be taken at the same time every day with just a 2-hour leeway. If taken appropriately it is as effective as the COCP. It has a variable effect on ovulation.

It is especially effective in women over 30 years of age with a failure rate in this group of 1.0 per 100 woman-years. There is evidence that progesterone containing contraceptives may be less effective with increasing patient weight.

The POP most commonly contains either norethisterone or levonorgestrel.

If pills are missed or vomiting occurs extra precautions should be taken for 7 days, as with the COCP.

Indications

The absence of oestrogen means that the risk of thrombosis is not increased and therefore the POP is suitable for smokers, diabetics, hypertensives or women with a history of thromboembolic disease. It is also suitable for lactating women and those with focal migraine.

Mechanism of action

There is a variable effect of progestagens on ovulation. The main mode of action is on cervical mucus penetrability and there is some effect on implantation.

Side effects

Mainly menstrual irregularities. Some women describe bloating and weight gain. However it is usually well tolerated. Over half of all users will have a normal pattern of menstruation although amenorrhoea becomes more likely in the older age groups.

INJECTABLES

DEPO-PROVERA (MEDROXYPROGESTERONE ACETATE OR DMPA)

This is a 150 mg deep intramuscular injection given within the first 5 days of menses every 12 weeks. Failure rates of 0–1 per 100 woman-years are recorded. Return of fertility is on average 9 months after the last injection. Side effects are weight gain, irregular bleeding and amenorrhoea. Cessation of menses is not harmful but may cause recurring anxieties of possible pregnancy.

CONTRACEPTIVE IMPLANTS

NORPLANT

- A minor surgical procedure is necessary to insert the six small rods subdermally into the inner aspect of the left upper arm, taking 5–10 minutes. Six capsules are inserted in a fan shape, with each containing 36 mg of crystalline levonorgestrel, releasing 30–35 micrograms each day.
- Pregnancy rates vary between 0.2 per 100 woman-years after year 1 to 1.6 per 100 woman-years after year 4. There is no associated increased risk of ectopic pregnancy.
- Removal of norplant takes 30 minutes and serum levels of levonorgestrel become undetectable within 48 hours (i.e. instant return of fertility).
- The main reason for discontinuation is disruption of the menstrual cycle, affecting 60–100%, but returning to a normal pattern by 1 year.
- The mean duration of use is 3.5 years.

INTRA-UTERINE DEVICES

Choice of coil

For example, Copper T 380 'Slimline' (Cu T 380 S) or similar, and levonorgestrel containing IUS, (Mirena intrauterine system). Inert coils are no longer in use.

Mechanism of action

Copper coils block implantation by creating an inflammatory reaction within the uterus. They also appear to affect fertilization. The Mirena IUS releases 20 micrograms/day of levonorgestrel and this continues for 3–5 years. The progestagen causes endometrial atrophy and prevents implantation. Its actions are still principally local so most women will continue to ovulate.

Effectiveness

The Cu T 380 S in the first year of use has a failure rate of about 0.4 per 100 woman years. The efficacy of the Mirena IUS is unsurpassed at 0.15 pregnancies/100 years. IUDs are more effective in the older woman with a decreased risk of infection but this may relate to life style.

Duration of use

The Cu T 380 S is approved for 8 years use. Any copper IUD licensed currently in the UK, which is fitted in a woman over 40 years of age, may remain in the uterus until the menopause. The Mirena IUS is now licensed for 5 years.

Indications

Parous women, nulliparous women where other methods are unacceptable, older women not wanting sterilization and those who are poorly compliant with other methods. The Mirena IUS should be seriously considered in women with menstrual difficulties, provided appropriate investigations have failed to find pathology.

Contraindications

Suspected pregnancy, unexplained abnormal uterine bleeding, recent pelvic infection (within the last 6 months), current or suspected STDs, HIV infections, distorted uterine cavity, immunosupression, Wilson's disease, and heart valve prostheses.

INSERTION OF INTRAUTERINE DEVICES (see also pp. 311)

- Optimum insertion time is day 4 through to day 14 (of a 28-day cycle).
- Screen for infection prior to insertion (HVS and endocervical swabs for chlamydia).
- Antiseptic to cleanse cervix.
- Local anaesthetic can be administered offered by an intra-cervical route.

- Consider mefenamic acid 500 mg whilst waiting for the procedure.
- Consider prophylactic antibiotics (metronidazole 1 g pr immediately and 7 days of doxycycline 100 mg bd) for women not screened for infection who are at high risk.
- The Mirena IUS insertion tube is 4.8 mm which means effective local anaesthesia and cervical dilatation to Hegar 5 or 6 are almost always required.
- Most IUD problems relate to the insertion. Perforation occurs in 1 in 1000. Review at week 1 and 6, (infection most likely to occur in first 20 days after insertion). If expulsion were to occur this would normally be in the first 3 months.
- Women should be taught how to check the coil threads themselves after each period.

ADVERSE EFFECTS OF INTRAUTERINE DEVICES

Intrauterine pregnancy

If conception occurs with the coil in place, the coil should be removed. Removal of the coil does not increase the risk of a first trimester miscarriage. If it is retained due to the coil threads not being visible, there is an increased risk of second trimester miscarriage (which can be septic), antepartum haemorrhage and premature labour. The coil is not teratogenic.

Ectopic pregnancy

An IUD reduces the risk of an EP but is more effective in preventing intrauterine pregnancy. Hence a patient who is pregnant with a coil in place is more likely to have an ectopic than in other cases of unplanned pregnancy.

Infection

The Mirena IUS offers protection against infection. Whilst others provide no protection against infection, they are not now thought to be the cause of infection. However, if an infection occurs with an IUD *in situ* it may be more severe due to the presence of a foreign body. This is reduced by screening all prospective users for sexually transmitted disease especially chlamydia.

Actinomyces-like organisms

Actinomyces israeli is a bacterium which is found as a mouth and gastrointestinal commensal. It is sometimes found on cervical smears from women who have coils in place for a long time. Most patients will be asymptomatic and the coil should be removed and another reinserted. Dyspareunia, discharge and tenderness suggest a symptomatic infection which is serious and will require long term penicillin.

Lost threads

If the threads cannot be seen, they are likely to be short or drawn up into the canal and can be brought down with retrieval devices. Less than 5% will need a general anaesthetic (GA). However it may also mean a woman may be pregnant or at risk of becoming pregnant. Ultrasound or a pelvic X-ray assist in location. Devices that have perforated the uterus can be removed laparoscopically.

Abnormal bleeding and pain

Important differential diagnoses include infection, ectopic pregnancy and malposition. Menstrual loss with copper coils may increase by one-third. Mefenamic acid 500 mg tds, or tranexamic acid 1 g 6 hourly daily are effective in reducing the heavier bleeding and dysmenorrhoea associated with copper coils. The Mirena IUS can reduce menstrual loss to less than 25%, but will be responsible for IMB or spotting for up to 18 days per cycle in the first 2–3 cycles. The patient must always be counselled about this early side effect. Only 10% of women with a Mirena *in situ* will complain of progestagenic side effects.

BARRIER METHODS

Condoms

Provide protection against sexually transmitted diseases (STDs) and are a barrier to HIV transmission. Failure rates of between 2–15 per 100 woman-years are reported, usually attributable to incorrect use.

Diaphragms

Use with spermicides is recommended (Nonoxynol-9). Failure rates of 4–8 per 100 years in careful and consistent users are stated. Motivation is required for successful use but there is no impairment of sexual enjoyment. Careful fitting is required and tutoring in how to use the device. The cap should be left in place at least 6 hours after the last episode of intercourse and if there is more than 3 hours delay between insertion and intercourse then more spermicide should be used. There is an increased incidence of urinary tract infection associated with their use.

POSTCOITAL CONTRACEPTION

Combined hormone method

50 micrograms ethinyl oestradiol with 250 micrograms levonorgestrel is taken as two pills and repeated after 12 hours (Yupze method). It can be used up to 72 hours after unprotected intercourse and overall prevents three out of four pregnancies that would have otherwise have occurred if no treatment had been used. The risk of teratogenesis is negligible. Up to 50% of women will experience nausea and 24% may vomit (in which case further tablets may be necessary). Some routinely prescribe an oral antiemetic to prevent this. The contraindications to the COCP mostly do not apply but a history of thromboembolism is still regarded as a relative contraindication and previous migraine with aura is still an absolute contraindication. Another method of emergency contraception is also advisable for women presenting with a simple migraine at the same time.

Copper IUD

A copper coil can be inserted not more than 5 days from the most probable calculated date of ovulation, even if there have been multiple acts of unprotected intercourse. Day 14 is the most common day of ovulation if the cycle is 28 days in total. Therefore, day 19 is the last day when coil insertion is permissible as emergency contraception.

Levonorgestrel (LNG)

Two doses of 0.75 mg LNG taken 12 hours apart has recently been shown to be as effective as the Yuzpe method and is associated with fewer side effects. It is not currently marketed in a convenient form and 25 tablets of 30 micrograms LNG (the dose used in LNG progesterone only pills) must be taken to reach this dose and repeated 12 hours later. Fortunately there are, in practice, few reasons why a woman cannot receive the Yuzpe regime.

STERILIZATION

- Around 30% of women in England and Wales will request this procedure for family planning. Most commonly perfomed via the laparoscope under GA using Filshie clips to mechanically occlude the fallopian tube.
- Indications: historically for medical reasons, (risk of uterine rupture, chronic medical conditions and grand multiparity) but

today performed mainly for social reasons and sexual convenience of the couple.

Examination

In addition to the routine screening procedures and pelvic examination, factors which might contraindicate or complicate the operation such as previous abdominal operations and gross obesity should be noted.

Counselling

- Always discuss the possible need for mini-laparotomy should pelvic or abdominal adhesions be encountered which obscure the view of the fallopian tubes. This involves a short transverse or midline incision in the abdomen and a longer hospital stay.
- Failure rates of 2–3/1000, (0.2–0.6 per 100 woman-years). See below for reasons.
- Mortality rates of between 4–15/100 000 of which half relate to anaesthestic complications.
- Avoid immediately following a pregnancy (due to higher failure rates and altered attitudes) although it may be acceptable at the time of a Caesarean section if there has been prior discussion.
- Expect an increase in menstrual loss and pain if stopping COCP. The sterilization procedure *per se* does not increase menstrual bleeding.
- Irreversibility: Couples should treat the procedure as being irreversible. Reversals can be paid for privately, but conception rates after reversal vary from 40–70% with an increase in the ectopic pregnancy rate. Counselling should always involve discussion of how the situation would change if the male partner died or was separated and a new partner was found.
- Vasectomy should be discussed as an option, mentioning the lower morbidity and mortality rate and the lower failure rate (0.02/100 women years).
- When pregnancy does occur following a sterilization the proportion of ectopic pregnancies is much higher (at least 15%).
- There should be some discussion of the risks of laparoscopy, including bowel damage.
- Consider the alternative of inserting a Mirena IUS.

METHOD

Filshie clip: A laparoscopic technique is usually employed with GA, but it is also possible with local methods. Advantages include minimal tube destruction (4 mm), no possible migration off the tube once the clip is locked and complete tubal ischemia due to constant pressure of the silicone pressure insert. Always attempt to identify the tube by the fimbrial end and ensure that the clip is placed fully accross the isthmic portion of each tube.

Other laparoscopic methods have employed silicone rings, (Fallope) and the Hulka clips but neither method is popular in the UK. Unipolar diathermy to effect sterilisation is now rarely employed and studies from the US have suggested very high failure rates.

Reversal of sterilization may be requested in 10% and is more common in the under 30s with fewer live children and more terminations.

FAILED STERILIZATION

Causes:

- The woman is pregnant at the time of the sterilization.
- The tube recanalizes or a fistula forms.
- Clips, rings or diathermy were imperfectly applied to the tube.
- The wrong structure is occluded, (e.g. the round ligament).

Most failures are due to operator error and occur within 1 year of application. After this time it is more likely to be due to natural and non-negligent causes.

Intrauterine pregnancy

As long as this is diagnosed early the patient has a choice between continuing or having an abortion. A second operation affords an opportunity to establish the cause of a failure, especially if the tubes are completely removed for histological analysis.

Ectopic pregnancy

The incidence is higher if tubal cautery was used rather than tubal occlusion.

19

THE MENOPAUSE AND HORMONE REPLACEMENT THERAPY

THE MENOPAUSE

In a woman aged more than 50 years, the menopause is a retrospective diagnosis made 1 year after the last period, when contraception is no longer required.

If the woman is less than 50 years old, 2 years amenorrhoea and other menopausal symptoms are necessary to make the diagnosis.

Two FSH levels >30 IU/L, 3 months apart strongly suggest the end of fertility. Levels from 15–30 IU/L indicate that there is a small risk of ovulation.

THE CLIMACTERIC

The climacteric is the 2–3 year transitional phase during which ovarian activity ceases and which when complete leads to the menopause.

In developed countries the menopause occurs around the age of 51 years (45–56 years). Up to one-third or more of a woman's life will be after the menopause. Climacteric and postmenopausal women will constitute 20% of the entire population. This state of oestrogen deficiency not only causes distressing symptoms, but also has implications for long-term health.

SYMPTOMS ASSOCIATED WITH THE CLIMACTERIC

Vasomotor symptoms

Hot flushes, night sweats, headaches and episodes of wakefulness occur in 50–75%. Can last >5 years in 20–25% of women. Most severe in the 2 years leading up to the menopause.

Genital atrophy and urinary symptoms

Vagina and urethra have a common embryological origin and oestrogen deficiency results in the atrophy of both.

- **Vagina:** dyspareunia, recurrent bacterial infections, vaginal bleeding.
- **Urethra:** frequency, dysuria, urgency and incontinence.

Emotional symptoms

Anxiety, forgetfulness, difficulty in concentration, feelings of unworthiness and loss of libido. Psychological disturbances may be due to oestrogen deficiency or result from coincidental but concurrent socioeconomic crises. There is no increase in the incidence of depression after the menopause.

Generalized atrophy of connective tissues

Skin thinning, osteoporosis, generalized aches and pains, loss of hair, brittle nails and bone pain.

Irregular menstrual bleeding, secondary to anovulation and relative oestrogen and progesterone deficiency

Abnormal bleeding at the time of the climacteric should be investigated as for postmenopausal bleeding. Endometrial sampling, hysteroscopy and/or transvaginal ultrasound should be employed. The postmenopausal endometrium has a thickness of 5 mm or less. If the bilayer is greater than this then endometrial hyperplasia and cancer need to be excluded. If these abnormalities are not present then treatment with cyclical progestogens, hormone replacement therapy or even low dose oral contraceptive pills in women without other risk factors will regulate the cycle.

LONG-TERM IMPLICATIONS OF THE MENOPAUSE

OSTEOPOROSIS

The peak bone mass is achieved in the fourth decade of life. After skeletal maturity, bone is lost at about 1% annually up to the menopause, increasing to 2–3% for the following 7 to10 years. Bone loss results from increased bone resorption, and loss of trabecular bone exceeds that of cortical bone. Typical sites of osteoporotic fractures are the vertebral body, distal forearm, and proximal femur.

Clinical consequences of osteoporosis

Osteoporosis causes morbidity (pain, deformities and loss of independence) and carries significant risk of death. One in seven women will suffer a hip fracture by the age of 75 and the mortality at 1 year is 33% with a further 50% of women becoming functionally dependent. The absolute risk of a fracture doubles with each decade after 50 years.

Risk factors for osteoporosis

Female, elderly, white or asian, early menopause <45 years, hypogonadism, smoking, high alcohol intake, physical inactivity, thin body type, hereditary, secondary endocrine (eg thyrotoxicosis, Cushing's disease), drugs (eg steroids).

Investigations

- Spinal X-ray. About 50% of all vertebral fractures are asymptomatic.
- Bone densitometry, by dual energy X-ray absorptiometry (DEXA). Measurements are taken in the lumbar spine and proximal femur. The relative risk of a fracture increases 2–3 times for each standard deviation of decrease in bone density from the mean.
- **Indications for bone densitometry:**
  - oestrogen deficiency, particularly after an early menopause.
  - when considering HRT in the presence of relative contraindications (risk-benefit analysis).
  - when monitoring the response of osteoporosis to treatment.

There is no evidence to support the use of widespread screening.

Treatments options for osteoporosis

Aim: Prevent the development of osteoporosis by exercise, adequate calcium intake and HRT.

- Oestrogen supplementation. Implants are the most potent, resulting in an 8.4% increase in bone density in a year. However this is becoming a less favoured route of administration (see below). Oestrogen may also replace the structural fabric of bone by increasing collagen content. Reduction in fracture risk is dose and duration dependent.
- Bisphosponates reduce fracture risk and increase bone density by 2% in the spine in the first year of therapy.
- Calcitonin (injections or nasal spray) reduces bone loss; however the effect on fracture risk is less clear.
- Calcium and vitamin D supplements are only useful in those who are obviously deficient (e.g. those in long-term institutional care).

- Fluoride causes a dramatic increase in bone mass but evidence that treatment prevents fractures is inconclusive.

ISCHAEMIC HEART DISEASE

At the age of 45 men are 5–6 times more likely to die of ischaemic heart disease (IHD) than women. After the menopause, by the age of 60 years, the incidence of IHD in women is equivalent to that in men. This is due to the increase in plasma cholesterol and triglycerides, decrease in high density lipoprotein (HDL), and increase in very low density lipoprotein (VLDL) which occur when oestrogen levels decline. In users of HRT the relative risk for IHD is 0.58, with a possible 20% reduction in stroke incidence.

Treatment

Oestrogen replacement partially reverses these unfavourable lipid changes. There are also important beneficial changes in arterial blood flow. Progestagens have a tendency to reduce HDL and elevate LDL cholesterol but the impact is marginal and likely to be of no clinical significance.

HRT is beneficial in the presence of angina, a previous myocardial infarct, hypertension, and hyperlipidaemia. A history of IHD is **not** a contraindication to HRT (unlike the COCP).

HORMONE REPLACEMENT THERAPY

Less than 15% of eligible women start treatment and even fewer continue it for more than 2 years. Results from observational studies suggest that long-term oestrogen therapy halves the risk of ischaemic heart disease and leads to a 60% reduction in osteoporotic fractures. However, no randomized trials currently exist that have evaluated the outcome of treatment in terms of clinical events such as rates of fractures or heart attacks.

Hormonal components of HRT

Natural oestrogens, including oestradiol, oestrone, oestriol, and conjugated equine oestrogens. Oestrogens should always be given on a continuous basis. Progestagens are mainly synthetically produced and include dydrosterone, medroxyprogesterone acetate, levonorgestrel, norgestrel and norethisterone.

Routes of administration

The oral route of administration is traditional, convenient and cheap. The gastrointestinal tract affects oestrogen pharmacodynamics by preferentially converting oestradiol to oestrone, but there is a greater beneficial effect on lipid profile due to the effect of oestrogen on liver metabolism. Parenteral oestrogens (e.g. patches and gels) avoid this 'first pass' of liver metabolism and therefore the induction of clotting factors and renin substrate within the liver is avoided. Parenteral routes also result in more stable serum hormone levels. Topical administration to the urogenital tract is possible via rings, pessaries or creams.

Progestagens in HRT are mainly taken orally, although patches are now available and the levonorgestrel releasing IUS (Mirena) offers an alternative route of administration which has the added advantage of fewer systemic side effects.

Benefits

Effective relief of vasomotor symptoms and those associated with urogenital atrophy. Risk of IHD and osteoporotic fractures is probably halved. There is a less predictable effect on psychological symptoms. Newer reports are suggesting a reduction in the incidence of Alzheimer's disease in users of HRT.

COMPLICATIONS AND SIDE EFFECTS OF HRT

The withdrawal bleed

Sequential preparations (i.e. progestagen for 10–12 days of every month) result in the return of regular menstruation and this may be heavy. This is the principle reason for poor compliance with HRT. Continuous combined regimes administer a lower dose of progestagen continuously (i.e. every day). They render the endometrium atrophic and over 80% of women still using the HRT are amenorrhoeic at 12 months. However users of this system must be 1 year postmenopausal before use, as any endogenous oestrogen is likely to cause continued irregular menses.

Progestagen related side effects

Bloating, breast tenderness, mood swings, tiredness, depression, irritability, skin disorders, weight gain and anxiety.

Breast cancer

The relative risk of breast cancer after 10 years use is 1.1 to 1.3. Regular mammography should be offered to those over 50 years of age (the National Breast Screening Program). Fears of breast cancer may well deter women from starting or continuing HRT. However the mortality from osteoporosis and IHD far exceeds that from breast cancer and some studies have shown a survival advantage for breast cancer patients diagnosed whilst on HRT over non-users.

Endometrial hyperplasia and carcinoma

Unopposed oestrogens lead to a 5 to 8-fold increase in the risk of carcinoma of the uterus. Progestagens taken for between 10–13 days will protect the endometrium.

Thromboembolism

The risk of developing thromboembolism is about 2–4 times higher in women on HRT than non-users. This is independent of route of administration or dose, or whether progestagens are given. The risk is however small, around 3 in 10 000 women per year and should be seen in the context of the benefits of treatment. There is only a 1–2% mortality associated with thromboembolic events.

CONTRAINDICATIONS TO HRT

There are few absolute contraindications. A woman with a past history of DVT or a family history of thrombosis should not be prescribed HRT until her coagulation screen has been checked. A history of oestrogen dependent neoplasm is traditionally considered a contraindication. However, previous early stage endometrial carcinoma is no longer thought to represent a problem and a number of studies in women with previous breast cancer are tentatively suggesting that HRT may not adversely affect outcome.

CONTRACEPTION

If the FSH is >40 IU/L, there is no need for contraception. If it lies between 15 and 40 IU/L ovulation may occur. The dose of oestrogen in most preparations will not suppress ovarian activity and some form of contraception is required.

DURATION OF USE

HRT should be continued for at least 5 years beyond the menopause to confer any benefit. The evidence is in favour of it being used for much longer, the drawback being a possible duration-related increased risk of breast cancer.

PREMATURE MENOPAUSE

Definition

Ovarian failure before the age of 40 years. Affects 1% of women.

Aetiology

- **Genetic:** If the patient is less than 30 years old check her chromosomes. XO/XY mosaics, partial deletions of the X chromosome and 47XXX are karyotypes not uncommon in these women.
- **Autoimmune:** Premature ovarian failure can be associated with rheumatoid arthritis, vitiligo, diabetes mellitus, pernicious anaemia, idiopathic thrombocytopenic purpura and myasthenia gravis. Autoantibodies, including anti-ovarian antibodies can be tested for.
- **Iatrogenic:** Chemotherapy and radiation.
- **Rare syndromes:** Galactosaemia, resistant ovary syndrome and Fragile X carriers.

Biopsy is indicated only in the oligo-amenorrhoeic group. If FSH >than 40 IU/L no viable ovarian follicles will be found on biopsy.

About 44% of women post hysterectomy develop ovarian failure by 45.4 years compared to 13% of controls, possibly due to impairment of the ovarian vascular supply.

Treatment for women with premature menopause involves long term oestrogen replacement in the form of HRT. Consider investigating skeletal integrity with DEXA scans. A few cases may respond to gonadotrophin stimulation and spontaneous recovery of ovulation has been noted in the past. Childbearing prospects are likely to rest with ovum donation however.

20

CLINIC PROBLEMS

HISTORY

KEY POINT

A full and careful gynaecological, obstetric and general history should always be taken from a new patient presenting in the clinic. A gynaecological history should include:

- Presenting complaint
- Menstrual history
  - Last menstrual period (LMP)
  - Age at menarche
  - Duration and heaviness of periods
  - Length and regularity of menstrual cycle
  - Abnormal menstrual loss
  - Intermenstrual bleeding
  - Pain associated with periods
  - Age at menopause
  - Postmenopausal bleeding.
- Previous pregnancies with outcomes
- Contraception
- Vaginal discharge
- Sexual intercourse
  - Pain
  - With subfertility ask about frequency of intercourse and whether the partner ejaculates.
- Post-coital bleeding
- Last cervical smear and results
- Hot sweats and vaginal dryness
- Galactorrhoea and hirsutism
- Urinary function
- Bowel function

- Remember also to ask about previous gynaecological history and past medical history
- Is there family history of note? (e.g. ovarian or breast cancer. Thromboembolic disease?).

ABSENCE OF MENSTRUATION

- **Primary amenorrhoea**
  - No period by the age of 14 in the absence of normal growth and development of secondary sexual characteristics **or**
  - No period by the age of 16 despite normal growth and development of secondary sexual characteristics.
- **Secondary amenorrhoea**
  - Six months amenorrhoea in a woman who has previously been menstruating.

For menstruation to occur:

- The hypothalamus must release GnRH in a pulsatile manner.
- The pituitary must respond to this by secreting the gonadotrophins FSH and LH appropriately.
- The ovary must respond to these and produce oestrogen and progesterone in a cyclical manner.
- The endometrium must proliferate and then be shed through a patent genital tract

Problems occurring at any of these steps can result in amenorrhoea.

CAUSES OF AMENORRHOEA

Physiological causes

- Before puberty
- Pregnancy
- Lactation
- Menopause.

Pharmacological causes

- Combined oral contraceptive pill.

Hypothalamic causes

- Hypothalamic dysfunction
  - dietary (including anorexia nervosa)
  - exercise induced
  - chronic illness

  - hyperprolactinaemia
  - thyroid disorders
- CNS tumours, e.g. craniopharyngioma
- Kallmann's syndrome – congenital absence of GnRH.

Pituitary causes

- Tumours: hormone and non-hormone secreting adenomas
- Sheehan's syndrome
- Infarction.

Ovarian causes

- Ovarian failure
  - chromosome abnormality
  - iatrogenic (e.g. postchemotherapy)
  - autoimmune
  - resistant ovary syndrome
- Dysgenesis
- Rare enzyme deficiencies.

Genital tract causes

- Mullerian anomalies, e.g. imperforate hymen
- Asherman's syndrome
- Androgen insensitivity.

HISTORY

- **Presenting complaint:** Patients may have a variety of concerns, e.g. infertility, absence of menstruation, possibility of pregnancy, long-term health implications.
- **Developmental history:** Have the breasts and pubic hair begun to develop yet?
- **Menstrual history:** Take note of past menstrual pattern as well as present duration of amenorrhoea.
- **Contraceptive history:** Particularly the use of depot or other hormonal contraceptives. Is there any possibility of pregnancy?
- **Past obstetric history:** Recent pregnancy or lactation may be particularly relevant.
- **Past gynaecological history:** Particularly recent surgery such as cone biopsy or uterine evacuation following miscarriage.
- **Weight:** Present weight and fluctuations in weight. What is the body mass index (BMI).
- **Diet:** Anorexia nervosa typically occurs in women under 30 and may be associated with distortion of body image, unusual

attitudes to food, denial, episodes of over-eating, self-induced vomiting, constipation, overactivity and usually does not occur in association with other psychological illness.

- **Stress:** Stress in family life or career may be very relevant as it may affect hypothalamic function.
- **Exercise:** Excessive exercise also seems to affect hypothalamic function.
- **Symptoms of ovarian failure:** Hot sweats, flushes, vaginal dryness, loss of libido.
- **Other medical conditions which might cause or be associated with ovarian failure** (e.g. autoimmune conditions).
- **Symptoms of hyperprolactinaemia:** Galactorrhoea, headache, visual disturbances, drug history.
- **Symptoms of hyperandrogenism:** Hirsutism, acne, greasy skin.
- **Family history:** A history of premature menopause, diabetes mellitus, thyroid disease, congenital adrenal hyperplasia or polycystic ovary syndrome may be important.

EXAMINATION

- Secondary sexual characteristics.
- Body mass index and height. BMI is weight in kg/height in m^2 (normal range is 20–25).
- Urinalysis.
- Blood pressure.
- Hair distribution and development.
- Presence of galactorrhoea.
- Stigmata of chromosomal abnormalities or endocrinopathies.
- Pelvic examination.

INVESTIGATIONS

The investigations that you choose will depend upon the history and signs on examination and will vary depending upon whether the problem is primary or secondary amenorrhoea.

- **Pregnancy test** if indicated.
- **Pelvic ultrasound scan:** This is useful in primary amenorrhoiecs who have secondary sexual characteristics. The presence of a uterus suggests a lower genital tract anomaly (e.g. imperforate hymen) but an absent uterus should prompt karyotyping as the patient may have testicular feminization and be 46XY.
- **FSH and LH:** Raised gonadotrophins suggest ovarian failure (agenesis, karyotype abnormality, autoimmune failure).

- **Prolactin:** If raised, re-check the drug history, and consider again the possibility of pregnancy. Check thyroid function. Hypothyroidism is a cause of hyperprolactinaemia. Repeat the prolactin level. If >1000 mIU/L or galactorrhoea present organise a CT scan of the pituitary fossa. If a macroadenoma is present, check the visual fields.
- **Thyroid function:** Hypothyroidism can cause amenorrhoea.
- **Oestradiol level** may be useful to the patient in a subsequent discussion about therapy as patients who are amenorrhoeic may be hypo-oestrogenic and thus need oestrogen replacement if menses do not occur after investigation and treatment. If the problem is primary amenorrhoea and straightforward physiological delay is suspected, **X-rays for bone age** may help.
- **Chromosome analysis** if indicated, e.g. short stature, primary amenorrhoea. If symptoms of **hyperandrogenism** are present, investigate as outlined in the section on hirsutism and virilism below.
- **Progestagen withdrawal test:** (Medroxyprogesterone acetate 10 mg daily for 5 days, following which the patient should bleed within 2–7 days). The progestagen will only cause withdrawal bleeding if the endometrium is already exposed to oestrogen and the lower genital tract is patent. This test therefore demonstrates the presence of a functional genital tract and some degree of function in the ovaries, pituitary and hypothalamus. **CT or MRI** may be indicated if a hypothalamic or pituitary lesion is suspected.

KEY POINT

Exclude pregnancy!

TREATMENT

Many patients will only require reassurance. When treatment is required it will be aimed at the cause and may be surgical (e.g. ovarian or CNS tumours, Mullerian anomalies) or medical (e.g. thyroid dysfunction, polycystic ovary disease).

A few specific points of note

1. Weight-related amenorrhoea

Normalization of body mass index will restore menstruation and fertility. Ovulation-induction in the underweight may be difficult and if pregnancy is desired, miscarriage is more common than after weight gain and spontaneous ovulation.

Psychological intervention at an early stage is recommended for anorexia nervosa.

2. Anovulation

Patients who have normal gonadotrophin and prolactin levels, normal thyroid function, a positive progestagen withdrawal test and are otherwise well can be assumed not to have serious pathology and do not require further investigation.

Treatment will depend on the desire for fertility or contraception. If fertility is not desired, treatment with the combined pill or HRT is advisable if oestradiol levels are low, to prevent early deleterious effects on the cardiovascular and skeletal systems. Ovulation can be stimulated in some cases with clomiphene or gonadotrophins. In cases of ovarian agenesis and premature menopause ovum donation should be considered.

3. Hyperprolactinaemia

Patients with idiopathic hyperprolactinaemia and microprolactinomas (i.e. tumours less than 10 mm diameter on CT scan) are treated medically.

Cabergoline (initially 500 micrograms weekly, increased by 500 micrograms according to response) is more effective and better tolerated than bromocriptine, although bromocriptine should be used if pregnancy is planned.

Most macroadenomas are treated medically and monitored by prolactin levels, CT scan and visual fields. Transphenoidal surgery or radiotherapy is indicated for macroadenomas where medical therapy has failed.

Bromocriptine is stopped in pregnancy providing satisfactory pre-pregnancy treatment has been achieved.

HEAVY AND/OR IRREGULAR PERIODS

KEY POINT

The cause of any menstrual disturbance must be determined before treatment is commenced.

Definition

Measurement of the menstrual blood loss is not usually practical. Periods may be regarded as abnormal when the blood loss and associated symptoms interfere with the patient's daily life. The development of an iron-deficiency anaemia is usually indicative that treatment is required.

Causes

- **Dysfunctional uterine bleeding**, i.e. abnormal uterine bleeding in the absence of pathology.
- **Other gynaecological causes**
  - Fibroids
  - Adenomyosis
  - Endometrial hyperplasia
  - Endometrial polyps
  - Endometrial carcinoma
  - Pelvic inflammatory disease
  - Intrauterine device
  - Hormonal therapy
  - Cervical carcinoma
  - Oestrogen-secreting tumours.
- **Endocrine disorders**
  - Thyroid disease
  - Obesity.
- **Haematological disorders**
  - Von Willebrand's disease
  - Haemophilia.
- **Drugs**
  - Anticoagulants
  - Norplant
  - Depo-Provera.

HISTORY

- **Assessment of blood loss**
  - Duration of the symptoms
  - Occurrence of clots or flooding
  - Amount of sanitary protection required
  - Duration of the periods, length and regularity of the cycle
  - Restriction of lifestyle, e.g. time off work, time confined to the house
  - Occurrence of intermenstrual bleeding.
- **Associated gynaecological symptoms:** Pain or other symptoms may indicate the presence of pathology.
- **Contraception and desire for future fertility:** A recent change in contraceptive method may account for the development of the symptoms. These factors will affect the treatment options.

- **Stress.**
- **Symptoms of thyroid disease.**
- **Symptoms of bleeding disorder:** For example excessive bleeding following dental treatment, perioperatively or following childbirth.

EXAMINATION

General examination

- Is there any evidence of systemic illness?
- Is the patient anaemic?

Pelvic examination

- Is there any uterine enlargement or pelvic tenderness to suggest gynaecological disease?
- Speculum examination of the cervix.

INVESTIGATIONS

- Full blood count.
- Thyroid function if indicated.
- Cervical smear if indicated.
- High vaginal and cervical swabs for bacteriological culture and a cervical swab for chlamydia detection.
- A pelvic ultrasound scan may be indicated to confirm a clinical suspicion of uterine or ovarian disease.

ENDOMETRIAL ASSESSMENT

In which patients is this necessary?

- Women with menstrual abnormality over the age of 40 (women less than 40 years of age have a very low risk of endometrial cancer).
- Younger women who have risk factors for developing endometrial pathology, e.g. obesity, nulliparity, polycystic ovary syndrome, breast cancer, tamoxifen therapy, diabetes mellitus.
- Younger women who have failed to respond to medical treatment.
- Younger women with abnormal findings on pelvic examination.
- Younger women with unusual symptoms.
- Women with intermenstrual bleeding.

What is the procedure of choice?

- Hysteroscopy combined with endometrial curettage is more likely than curettage alone or endometrial sampling to identify endometrial pathology.

- Hysteroscopy and endometrial curettage may be performed under local anaesthetic as an outpatient procedure or under general anaesthesia. Most parous women tolerate outpatient hysteroscopy well.
- Endometrial ultrasound is not yet an established alternative to endometrial sampling. However, if the endometrial bilayer of a post menopausal woman is less than 5 mm across then endometrial cancer or atypical hyperplasia is very unlikely.
- Pipelle sampling may miss endometrial polyps and other pathology.

MANAGEMENT

Reassurance may be all that is necessary.

Medical or surgical treatment?

- The choice of treatment is determined by underlying pathology, the success of any previous treatment, future desire for fertility, contraceptive needs, any contraindication to surgery, age of the patient and patient choice.
- In general, medical treatment will be unsuccessful in the long-term in the presence of pelvic pathology such as fibroids, adenomyosis or chronic pelvic inflammatory disease.

CHOICE OF MEDICAL TREATMENT FOR DYSFUNCTIONAL UTERINE BLEEDING

Combined oral contraceptive

- Reduces menstrual loss by around 50%.
- Not suitable for smokers over the age of 35 or women with other cardiovascular risk factors.
- If the control of bleeding is inadequate, choose a pill with a higher progestagenic content.

Levonorgestrel intrauterine device (Mirena)

- Not currently licensed for use in the treatment of menorrhagia but highly effective.
- 15% of women become amenorrhoeic within 1 year. More than 90% report reduced menstrual bleeding by 6 months.
- Also a highly effective contraceptive.

Depot progestagen

- These products may give rise to troublesome irregular bleeding in the first 6 months of use. This can be treated either by giving a

double dose of depot progestagen, or by additional use of the combined pill (for 21 days).
- The dose is 150 mg im given every 3 months, starting between day 1 and day 5 of a cycle.
- Depo-Provera is more effective than Noristerat in inducing amenorrhoea (50% vs. 25% after 1 year) but more commonly gives rise to irregular intermenstrual bleeding.

Tranexamic acid

- Inhibits tissue plasminogen activator.
- Reduces menstrual loss by around 50%.
- Contraindicated in women with a history of thromboembolism.
- Dosage 1 g 6 hourly for up to 5 days during menstruation.

Mefenamic acid

- Inhibits cyclo-oxygenase.
- Reduces blood loss by around 20%.
- Useful when pain is a significant associated symptom.
- Dosage 500 mg 8-hourly for up to 5 days during menstruation.

Cyclical progestagen

- Useful for regulating the menstrual cycle.
- Not very effective in reducing menstrual loss.
- Best saved for women with irregular, often anovulatory cycles where prolonged endometrial stimulation by oestrogen leads to heavy and irregular spotting or where the luteal phase is deficient causing pre-menstrual spotting.

Danazol

- Dosage for menorrhagia 100–200 mg daily.
- Reduces blood loss by around 80% at this dose.
- Side effects are common, notably acne, hirsutism, breast atrophy and weight gain.
- Teratogenic, and so effective contraception is essential.
- Only licensed for 6 months' use.

Medical management has a limited role to play in fibroid-induced menorrhagia. GnRH analogues may be used to reduce the fibroid size prior to surgery.

CHOICE OF SURGICAL TREATMENT

Endometrial ablation

- Useful alternative to hysterectomy in cases of dysfunctional bleeding with approximately 75% satisfaction and faster recovery time.

- Less effective in women under 35, where pain is a significant associated symptom, when the uterus is significantly enlarged (cavity length 10 cm or more), or when pelvic pathology is present.
- Contraindicated when future fertility is desired.
- Treatment usually results in light or normal periods, but may not be effective. Amenorrhoea follows in 20–45% of patients.
- Preoperative thinning of the endometrium, e.g. with danazol or GnRH analogues for 4–6 weeks prior to surgery is essential for laser ablation and advisable for resectoscope ablation.
- The procedure is not a reliable contraceptive. If contraception is required, the IUD is not recommended. Hormonal methods may be used or sterilization.
- If HRT is subsequently required, a combined preparation (i.e. with progestagen) should be used.
- Long-term morbidity is unknown, but may include problems such as urinary dysfunction

Hysterectomy (vaginal or abdominal)

- Highly effective in treating menorrhagia.
- Mortality is low (approximately 5 per 10 000).
- Operative morbidity is not insignificant (Table 20.1).
- Long-term morbidity is uncertain but probably significant, and may include premature ovarian failure, cardiovascular disease, vaginal prolapse, pelvic pain, urinary dysfunction and bowel dysfunction.
- The incidence of psychosexual dysfunction is probably not increased after hysterectomy.

Table 20.1 Approximate incidence of operative morbidity in abdominal and vaginal hysterectomy

	Abdominal hysterectomy	**Vaginal hysterectomy**
Fever	30%	15%
Transfusion	15%	10%
Wound haematoma requiring evacuation	0.3% increased to 2% by low dose heparin)	1.2%
Bladder injury	0.3%	1.6%
Bowel injury	0.3%	0.4%
Pulmonary embolism	0.3% decreased to 0.1% by low dose heparin	Rare
Ureteric injury	0.2%	Rare
Myocardial infarction	0.1%	Rare

POSTMENOPAUSAL BLEEDING

Definition

Bleeding from the genital tract 6 months or more after the cessation of menstruation.

CAUSES OF POSTMENOPAUSAL BLEEDING

- Atrophic vaginitis or cervicitis
- Temporary return of ovarian function
- Trauma e.g. sexual intercourse
- Infection e.g. associated with use of a vaginal pessary
- Endometrial hyperplasia
- Endometrial polyps
- Cervical polyps
- Endometrial carcinoma
- Cervical carcinoma
- Fallopian tube carcinoma
- Ovarian carcinoma
- Vaginal carcinoma
- Exogenous oestrogens
- Oestrogen-secreting ovarian tumours
- Bleeding from the urinary tract, anus or rectum in 1% of cases.

KEY POINT

Postmenopausal bleeding is the most common presenting symptom of endometrial carcinoma. Every patient will therefore require endometrial evaluation, most usually by hysteroscopy and endometrial curettage.

HISTORY

- Is the patient sexually active? Resumption of sexual intercourse after a period of time may result in bleeding.
- Has the patient been using HRT? This includes the use of vaginal oestrogen creams which may cause endometrial stimulation.
- Does the patient have any vaginal discharge? This may originate from atrophic vaginitis, or from a neoplasm.
- When was the patient's last cervical smear?

EXAMINATION

- Pelvic examination may be difficult in the postmenopausal patient. If so, this may be deferred until the time of hysteroscopy and endometrial curettage under general anaesthetic.

- If a diagnosis of atrophic vaginitis is made in the clinic, endometrial assessment is still mandatory.

TREATMENT

- Treatment will depend upon the underlying cause of the bleeding.
- Having excluded endometrial carcinoma, often no treatment is required.
- Atrophic vaginitis may be treated with HRT. Topical oestrogen creams are used once a day for 2–3 weeks, reducing to 2–3 times weekly, aiming to have discontinued them by 6 months. Prolonged courses of oestrogen creams can cause endometrial stimulation.
- Persistent bleeding of uncertain origin may require abdominal hysterectomy and bilateral salpingectomy to exclude fallopian tube or ovarian carcinoma.

PAINFUL PERIODS

CAUSES OF PAINFUL PERIODS

- Spasmodic dysmenorrhoea
- Dysmenorrhoea secondary to organic pelvic disease
  - Adenomyosis
  - Endometriosis
  - Chronic pelvic inflammatory disease
  - Fibroids
  - Endometrial polyps
  - Intrauterine contraceptive device

The traditional classification of primary and secondary dysmenorrhoea is potentially misleading because assumptions about the origins of the symptoms are implied.

HISTORY

- Spasmodic dysmenorrhoea typically affects younger women, and as the name implies, is due to uterine spasm. A central colicky pain develops over several hours preceding the onset of menstruation and lasts for 1 or 2 days.
- Dysmenorrhoea secondary to organic pelvic disease typically develops over days or weeks (rather than hours) leading up to

the onset of the period. Other symptoms may also be present suggesting the presence of pelvic disease such as dyspareunia, infertility, heavy periods, intermenstrual bleeding or vaginal discharge.

EXAMINATION

- Is there any uterine enlargement or pelvic tenderness to suggest gynaecological disease?
- Young teenagers with a clear history of spasmodic dysmenorrhoea may be better treated initially without prior pelvic examination. If the patient is not examined it may be prudent to request an abdominal ultrasound scan of the pelvis.

INVESTIGATIONS

- If pelvic infection is suspected, perform high vaginal and cervical swabs for bacteriological culture, a cervical swab for chlamydia detection, full blood count and erythrocyte sedimentation rate (ESR).
- If pelvic pathology is suspected, or the symptoms do not respond to treatment, consider laparoscopy and hysteroscopy.

TREATMENT

Spasmodic dysmenorrhoea and dysmenorrhoea without organic pelvic disease

- Explanation and reassurance are important.
- Analgesics, particularly prostaglandin synthetase inhibitors are first-line treatment. For those with regular cycles, starting the medication a day before the cramps are expected may help. The analgesics must be taken regularly, not on an as required basis.
- Suppression of ovulation using the combined pill is usually effective.
- Cyclical progestagen such as dydrogesterone 10 mg bd taken on days 5 to 25 of each cycle may be helpful, particularly if the combined pill is contraindicated or not desired.

Dysmenorrhoea secondary to organic pelvic disease

- Analgesics such as codeine phosphate or prostaglandin synthetase inhibitors may be helpful.
- Treatments for specific conditions are outlined below in the section on chronic pelvic pain.

Hysterectomy may be indicated if analgesics are not helpful and if the patient feels that the symptoms merit surgery. Surgery cannot be guaranteed to cure pelvic pain, but is likely to be effective if the symptoms are clearly related to the menstrual cycle, particularly if uterine tenderness is present on examination.

Make every attempt to establish from the history the difference between chronic pelvic pain and primary or secondary dysmenorrhoea.

CHRONIC PELVIC PAIN

Causes of chronic pelvic pain

- **Gynaecological causes**
  - Chronic pelvic inflammatory disease
  - Pelvic adhesions
  - Endometriosis
  - Ovarian cyst
  - Intrauterine contraceptive device
  - Haematometra
  - Premenstrual syndrome
  - Genital prolapse.
- **Non-gynaecological causes**
  - Irritable bowel syndrome
  - Constipation
  - Inflammatory bowel disease
  - Diverticulitis
  - Bowel tumour
  - Urinary infection or calculus
  - Interstitial cystitis
  - Abdominal wall pain
  - Back pain.
- **Chronic pelvic pain without organic disease.**

KEY POINT

Chronic pelvic pain is a common gynaecological problem. Often organic disease is not present and even if it is it may not be the cause of the pain.

HISTORY

Symptoms suggesting gynaecological disease:

- Dyspareunia (poorly predictive of gynaecological problems)
- Vaginal discharge

- Menstrual disturbance, intermenstrual bleeding
- Infertility.

Premenstrual syndrome

The premenstrual syndrome is defined as the regular recurrence of distressing physical and psychological symptoms in the luteal phase of each ovarian cycle that regress in the early follicular phase, e.g. breast tenderness, abdominal bloating, pelvic pain, weight gain, headache, tension, irritability and depression. Symptoms may not always be clearly related to the menstrual cycle and tend to become progressively worse.

Bowel disease

- Bowel disease is a common cause of chronic pelvic pain and a careful history of bowel function should be obtained.
- Irritable bowel syndrome is a functional disorder comprising abdominal pain and distension associated with altered bowel habit (constipation, diarrhoea or both), relief of pain with bowel action, and sometimes passage of mucus rectally.

Other factors

- Spend time questioning the patient about marital, social and occupational factors.
- Enquire about the urinary and musculo-skeletal system.

EXAMINATION

- Gynaecological pathology severe enough to produce chronic pain will usually cause detectable abnormalities on examination such as uterine tenderness, uterine immobility, adnexal tenderness, an adnexal mass or tenderness or a mass in the pouch of Douglas.
- Consider the lumbo-sacral area and anterior abdominal wall.

INVESTIGATIONS

- Full blood count (looking for a raised white count).
- ESR.
- High vaginal and cervical swabs for bacteriological culture.
- Cervical swab for chlamydia detection.
- Mid-stream urine specimen for urinalysis, microscopy and culture.
- Plain abdominal X-ray, particularly if constipation or bowel obstruction suspected.

- Pelvic ultrasound, particularly if the symptoms and examination findings do not merit laparoscopy. In such cases, the scan findings are likely to be normal, but are useful in counselling the patient.
- Diagnostic laparoscopy is essential to confirm a diagnosis, however it is not always essential in the assessment of patients with pelvic pain.

MANAGEMENT

Explanation and reassurance are important, and explanation may be all that is required.

ENDOMETRIOSIS

Endometriosis is found in asymptomatic women (e.g. those undergoing sterilization) and care must be exercised in ascribing symptoms to it. Medical treatment should be considered diagnostic as well as therapeutic.

Endometriosis may be treated medically or surgically and the choice will be determined by factors such as the extent of the disease and the desire for future fertility. **Medical treatments** are generally for 6 months and alternatives include:

- Danazol 200 mg bd, starting on the first day of the menstrual cycle, increasing monthly to tds then qds if no improvement in the symptoms occurs. Side effects include acne, hirsutism, deepening of the voice, breast atrophy and weight gain, and treatment should be stopped immediately if virilizing side effects occur. Danazol is teratogenic and reliable contraception (not the combined pill) is required.
- Gestrinone 2.5 mg twice weekly, starting on the first day of the menstrual cycle. Severe hot flushes are common with this treatment.
- Gonadorelin analogues such as goserelin (Zoladex) injection 3.6 mg every 28 days, or nafarelin (Synarel) nasal spray 200 micrograms bd starting on the second day of the menstrual cycle. Patients should be warned of an initial flare of symptoms which can occur with this treatment. Severe hot flushes are common, and treatment must not continue beyond 6 months as the hypo-oestrogenic state resulting has deleterious effects on the cardiovascular and skeletal systems. 'Add back HRT' is a relatively new concept which avoids these problems.

Less effective treatments with fewer side effects include:

- Medroxyprogesterone acetate 30 mg od taken continuously for 90 days.
- Combined oral contraceptive taken continuously allowing withdrawal bleeds every three months (do not use a phasic preparation).

Surgical treatments include laser or diathermy to endometriotic deposits, excision of endometriotic deposits, uterosacral nerve ablation and total abdominal hysterectomy with bilateral salpingo-oophorectomy. Hysterectomy without oophorectomy may allow disease to persist, and subsequent surgery may be technically difficult.

CHRONIC PELVIC INFLAMMATORY DISEASE

Analgesics and prolonged courses of antibiotics may be helpful but often surgery is required. Salpingectomy alone may relieve symptoms, but usually total abdominal hysterectomy and bilateral salpingo-oophorectomy is indicated.

PREMENSTRUAL SYNDROME

General measures include exercise, dietary modification and vitamin B_6 supplementation. Treatment should be directed towards specific symptoms. Pain may be treated with simple analgesics or prostaglandin synthetase inhibitors. Bloating may respond to diuretics. Psychological symptoms may be improved by progestagens such as dydrogesterone 10 mg bd on days 12 to 26 of the menstrual cycle. Fluoxetine and other antidepressants have proved useful in some cases.

Abolition of the menstrual cycle using the combined pill taken on a continuous basis has a varying effect on symptoms, which may even become worse in some women. Newer regimes with high-dose transdermal oestrogen and cyclical progestogen have met with some success.

Hysterectomy with bilateral oophorectomy may be indicated if pelvic pain or discomfort is a major component of the syndrome, but surgery may not improve all of the symptoms and such radical surgery should always be very carefully considered in younger women.

IRRITABLE BOWEL SYNDROME

Dietary modification with elimination of gas-forming foods and increase in fibre intake is first-line treatment. Anti-spasmodics, anti-diarrhoeal agents or tricyclic antidepressants may be useful.

CHRONIC PELVIC PAIN WITHOUT ORGANIC DISEASE

This condition is common and difficult to treat. Psychological factors such as stress or sexual dysfunction may be relevant causal factors. Psychosexual counselling may be indicated. Tricyclic antidepressants or alternative therapies such as hypnosis or acupuncture may be helpful. **Surgery such as hysterectomy is often sought by the patient but is usually not helpful and should be avoided.**

MANAGEMENT OF A PELVIC MASS

(*See also* 'Oncology and palliative care', pp. 285.)

CAUSES OF PELVIC MASS

- **Gynaecological causes**
  - Ovarian cyst (benign, malignant or endometriotic)
  - Fibroids
  - Hydrosalpynx
  - Pelvic abscess
  - Uterine sarcoma
  - Endometrial carcinoma
  - Chronic ectopic pregnancy
  - Pregnancy.
- **Non-gynaecological**
  - Diverticular mass
  - Appendix mass
  - Adhesions
  - Bowel tumour
  - Inflammatory bowel disease
  - Retroperitoneal tumour
  - Pelvic kidney
  - Urinary retention.

KEY POINT

A full and careful history will indicate the possibility of a non-gynaecological origin of a pelvic mass. A history of change in bowel function is particularly important.

HISTORY

- **Gynaecological history**
- **General medical history**
- **Timecourse?**
- **Any associated pain?**
  - Typically pain is not a major feature of most gynaecological pelvic masses.
  - Pain may develop acutely as a result of torsion or rupture of an ovarian cyst or hydrosalpinx, or fibroid degeneration.
  - Pain is not usually a feature of ovarian malignancy until late in the progression of the disease when invasion of pelvic or abdominal organs, tense ascites or rupture of a malignant cyst may occur.
  - When pain is a major feature, consider an active inflammatory process such as a diverticular or appendix mass, inflammatory bowel disease, pelvic abscess or endometriosis.
  - Pelvic adhesions are usually, but not always, painless.
- **Previous abdominal or pelvic surgery:**
  - Consider the possibility of pelvic adhesions.
- **Associated bowel symptoms:**
  - See the key point above.
- **Family history and personal fears:**
  - Patients are usually very concerned about the possibility of malignancy, particularly if a close family member has had a pelvic malignancy. An understanding of such worries is very important in the treatment of the patient.

EXAMINATION

- **General examination**
- **Abdominal examination:**
  - Is the mass palpable and what are its features?
  - Is there evidence of ascites?
  - Is the liver enlarged?
  - Are the lymph nodes enlarged?

- **Pelvic examination:**
  - Is the mass continuous or separate from the uterus? Does it move when the cervix is moved?
  - Does the mass arise from either adnexal region?
- **Rectal examination.**

INVESTIGATIONS

- **Basic investigations:**
  - Full blood count
  - Cross-match blood for surgery.
- **If malignancy considered a possibility:**
  - Urea and electrolytes
  - Liver function tests
  - Chest x-ray.
- **If ovarian malignancy considered a possibility:**
  - Ca125. If raised (greater than 35 IU/mL) and ovarian malignancy is subsequently confirmed, this may be useful for monitoring the subsequent course of the disease. Note that Ca125 is not diagnostic of ovarian carcinoma, and a normal Ca125 does not exclude ovarian carcinoma.
- **Pelvic ultrasound:**
  - Particularly useful for distinguishing ovarian from uterine and non-gynaecological masses.
  - The presence of a thickened cyst wall, solid areas, septae, or haemorrhage within an ovarian cyst or ascites suggest, but do not diagnose, malignancy. An endometrioma has many of these features also.
  - Other radiological investigations such as CT scanning or MRI may yield further information.
- **If a large bowel problem is suspected:**
  - Sigmoidoscopy
  - Colonoscopy or barium enema may subsequently be indicated.

MANAGEMENT

Expectant management

- Should be considered only once a firm diagnosis is made.
- Asymptomatic fibroids may be managed expectantly. Hysterectomy should be considered if growing rapidly (to exclude sarcoma). Most gynaecologists recommend hysterectomy once the uterus is palpable abdominally, again to exclude sarcoma. If an expectant course is planned, the patient should be

kept under review (e.g. after 3 months and a further 6 months) to exclude rapid growth.

- Asymptomatic ovarian cysts in pre-menopausal women may be managed expectantly if small (<8 cm diameter), if the ultrasound scan shows no features of malignancy and if the Ca125 is normal. Patients should be followed up with serial scans (e.g. after 3 months and a further 6 months), resorting to surgery if symptoms develop or if the cyst continues to increase in size. Cysts measuring 8 cm or more in diameter are likely to become symptomatic and should be removed. Ovarian cysts in post-menopausal women should be removed.

KEY POINT

Pre-operative discussion and counselling should be full and thorough particularly with regard to:

- ***Desire for future fertility***
- ***Anticipated surgical procedure***
- ***Possible need for colostomy.***

Minimally invasive surgery

- Laparoscopy may occasionally be useful to establish a diagnosis when it is felt that a laparotomy will not be required (particularly in young women, when the mass is small or there is some doubt about its origin).
- Ovarian cysts in premenopausal women may be removed laparoscopically or under ultrasound guidance if small (<8 cm diameter), if there are no ultrasound features suggestive of malignancy, and if the Ca125 is normal.

Laparotomy

- Cross-match blood if malignancy or difficult surgery is anticipated.
- Review with the general surgeons and consider full bowel preparation if bowel involvement is a possibility.
- Ovarian malignancy is generally treated, if feasible, by taking peritoneal washings for cytological examination and performing total abdominal hysterectomy, bilateral salpingo-oophorectomy, omentectomy and debulking of any further tumour deposits. A more conservative surgical approach is taken for younger women with ovarian masses, even if the possibility of malignancy exists. Ovarian cystectomy or unilateral oophorectomy provides a histological sample for analysis. It is accepted that such patients may require a second procedure if malignancy is confirmed. A greater

proportion of ovarian neoplasms found in younger women are germ cell tumours. Many of these respond well to chemotherapy and a hysterectomy and bilateral oophorectomy can sometimes be avoided if preservation of fertility is important. There is little or no place for frozen section or simple biopsy of an enlarged ovary in young women as the diagnosis may easily be missed.

THE ABNORMAL SMEAR

CERVICAL SCREENING IN THE UK

Objective

The objective of cervical screening is to minimize the incidence of invasive cancer of the cervix.

Current government screening policy

Current policy is that all women aged 20–64 should be screened at least every 5 years, although the most cost effective interval is 3 yearly and this should be the aim.

MANAGEMENT OF THE ABNORMAL SMEAR

Inadequate smear

- The reason for the classification of a smear as inadequate is important in determining subsequent action.
- If technically inadequate (e.g. poor cellularity, air dried, too thick, obscured by menstrual debris) repeat as soon as convenient.
- If inflammatory, identify and treat any infection, then repeat.
- Once a negative (i.e. normal) smear is obtained, return to routine recall unless previous abnormal smears dictate otherwise.
- Refer for colposcopy if three inadequate smears are obtained.

Borderline smear

- Repeat the smear (after treatment of any infection if present) within 6 months and again within a further 6 months.
- Refer for colposcopy after the third borderline smear.

Mild dyskaryosis

Repeat the smear within 6 months and refer for colposcopy on the second occurrence.

Moderate, severe and uncertain grade dyskaryosis

Refer for colposcopy and gynaecological review.

Severe dyskaryosis ?invasive disease

Urgent referral for colposcopy and gynaecological review.

Glandular neoplasia

Urgent referral for colposcopy and gynaecological review which may include hysteroscopy and endometrial curettage, depending upon the patient's age (over 40 years) and the presence of other symptoms.

Viral changes

- Action should be based on the degree of accompanying dyskaryosis.
- If no dyskaryosis is present, refer for colposcopy after 3 smears showing viral changes.

REPEAT SMEARS AFTER PREVIOUS ABNORMALITIES

Following mild dyskaryosis or borderline changes, at least two negative smears at least 6 months apart should be reported before return to routine recall.

REPEAT SMEARS AFTER TREATMENT

- Following treatment of cervical intraepithelial neoplasia (CIN), smears should be taken annually for 5 years, with two smears taken in the first year, before returning to routine recall.
- Following hysterectomy for CIN, two vault smears should be taken within the first year, before discharging from cytological follow-up.

COLPOSCOPY

(*See also* 'Procedures: loop diathermy', p. 313.)

Cervical smears detect cytological abnormalities. Abnormal cells arise from areas of neoplastic change. Fortunately these are mostly confined to the epithelial layer and are known as CIN (cervical intraepithelial neoplasia). They are premalignant and if left without treatment a proportion will progress to frank carcinoma (where the abnormal changes breach the basement membrane of the epithelium to become truly invasive). CIN is graded I, II or III depending on how many thirds of the epithelial layer is affected by cellular changes. The more abnormal the smear the greater are the chances of high-grade CIN. CIN I progresses to CIN III in 15–20% of cases and CIN III carries an 18% risk of carcinoma of the cervix over 10 years. Colposcopy is used to identify CIN (which is usually invisible to the naked eye) using acetic acid and iodine solutions and a powerful magnifying lens. CIN can be graded by its appearance under the colposcope but biopsy proves more accurate. CIN II and III can be treated simply and effectively by a number of techniques, the most common now being loop diathermy which has the added advantage that it provides a specimen for histological analysis. This does not affect fertility and long term cervical damage is extremely rare (*see* pp. 313 for technique).

The unexpected finding of cervical cancer is an uncommon event in a colposcopy clinic, however poor information means that many woman fear this news. Some clinics perform biopsies in all women prior to treatment (necessitating two visits) whilst others practice a 'see-and-treat' policy which involves only one visit but has the disadvantage of overtreatment of those with low-grade lesions that appear more serious on examination.

Follow-up after colposcopy usually involves yearly smears for the next 5 years. Persistent changes on subsequent smears may represent inadequate treatment or recurrence of the CIN. The demands on colposcopy services are too great in most areas to allow follow up with colposcopy but cytological review with smears seems as effective.

PROLAPSE

Definition

Weakness of the supporting structures of the pelvic organs resulting in their herniation through the vagina and vaginal orifice.

TYPES OF PROLAPSE (Table 20.2)

Table 20.2 Types of prolapse

Prolapse	Characteristics
Cystocoele	Prolapse of the bladder and anterior vaginal wall
Rectocoele	Prolapse of the rectum and posterior vaginal wall
Enterocoele	Herniation of the peritoneum of the pouch of Douglas between the utero-sacral ligaments through the posterior vaginal wall. An enterocoele may contain small bowel or omentum
Uterine prolapse:	
1st degree	The cervix does not reach the introitus
2nd degree	The cervix reaches the introitus
3rd degree	The uterus has passed through the vaginal opening with eversion of the vagina and cystocoele (also called procidentia)
Vaginal vault prolapse	Usually a long-term complication of hysterectomy

CAUSES OF PROLAPSE

- High parity (muscle and/or neuropathic damage)
- Menopause and oestrogen deficiency
- Postoperative, particularly after hysterectomy
- Obesity
- Raised intra-abdominal pressure (e.g. chronic cough or constipation)
- Genetic predisposition.

HISTORY

- A lump or bulge in the vagina which may give rise to discomfort and backache.
- Usually worse towards the end of the day and relieved on lying down.
- Usually gives rise to few other symptoms, but occasionally is associated with bowel or urinary dysfunction.
- Rarely gives rise to discomfort during sexual intercourse, and if present, this is usually due to another cause, e.g. psychological, vaginal dryness.
- Before surgery it is important to be aware if the patient is sexually active or may be so in the future.

KEY POINT

If the patient is sexually active or may be so in the future, any repair should allow for sexual intercourse.

EXAMINATION

- Following general, abdominal and bimanual pelvic examination, examine the patient in the left lateral or Sims position.
- The anterior vagina is inspected with a Sims speculum.
- The posterior vagina is inspected with either a Sims speculum or Rampley's sponge forceps retracting the anterior vagina.
- The degree of uterine descent may be obvious, but is most easily assessed under anaesthetic prior to operation.
- Distinction between a rectocoele and an enterocoele may be difficult, but it is not essential to achieve this in the clinic. The distinction may be made by rectal examination, and will become obvious during the course of surgical repair.

TREATMENT

Physiotherapy

- Generally only effective for mild cases
- Particularly useful for prolapse in the months following childbirth
- Consists of supervised pelvic floor exercises.

Pessaries

- Only used when a patient is unfit for surgery or when a patient feels that her symptoms do not merit surgery. In the majority of cases surgery is a more effective option.
- Polythene ring pessaries are most commonly used. The ring lies between the posterior vaginal fornix and pubic symphysis. The ring size is assessed on vaginal examination. If expelled, try a larger size. Polythene pessaries should be replaced every 6 to 12 months.
- A shelf pessary may be used when a ring fails to control the prolapse or cannot be retained. The pessary lies inferior to the cervix with the cervix in the concavity and the wings of the pessary extending into the lateral vaginal fornices. The hook is just visible at the introitus. Shelf pessaries should be changed every 3 months since they otherwise quickly become embedded in the vaginal epithelium.
- Vaginal irritation may respond to changing the pessary or a 6 to 12-week course of vaginal oestrogen cream.

Surgery

(*See also* 'Common surgical procedures', p. 195.)

- Surgery may include, as appropriate, anterior vaginal repair, posterior vaginal repair, repair of enterocoele and vaginal hysterectomy. Where some degree of uterine prolapse is present, vaginal repair is usually more effective when combined with vaginal hysterectomy.
- The Manchester operation consists of excision of the cervix and suturing the utero-sacral ligaments to the cervical stump. It is seldom performed but has the advantage of preserving fertility.
- Vaginal vault prolapse may be treated by attaching the vault to the sacrum (often performed abdominally – a sacrocolpopexy) or to the sacrospinous ligament (sacrospinous vault fixation), a vaginal procedure.

URINARY URGENCY AND INCONTINENCE (WITH URODYNAMICS)

Definitions

- **Incontinence:** involuntary loss of urine.
- **Urgency:** sudden strong desire to pass urine.
- **Urge incontinence:** involuntary loss of urine preceded by urgency.
- **Stress incontinence:** a symptom, sign and condition.
  - As a **symptom** it describes the involuntarily loss of urine when intra-abdominal pressure increases, such as with coughing, laughing or lifting.
  - As a **sign**, **'demonstrable stress incontinence'** is said to have occurred when a patient loses urine when asked to cough.
  - **'Genuine stress incontinence' (GSI)** is the name given to a number of conditions causing incompetence of the urethral sphincter.
- **Dribble incontinence:** a continuous trickle of urine, in the absence of urgency or increase in intra-abdominal pressure.

Incidence

Urinary incontinence is a very common problem in women although many do not seek medical advice. The incidence increases with increasing age and may be as high as 10% for perimenopausal women, rising to 50% in extreme old age.

CAUSES

Urgency and urge incontinence

- 'Extravesical causes'
  - Diabetes mellitus and insipidus
  - **Excessive fluid intake**
  - Caffeine
  - **Diuretics**
  - Pelvic mass and pregnancy
  - Chronic renal failure
  - Constipation
- Bladder causes
  - **Urinary tract infection**
  - Bladder stones
  - Bladder neoplasms
  - Atrophic changes
  - Bladder and urethral diverticulae

  - Interstitial cystitis
  - Radiation cystitits
  - **Genuine stress incontinence**
  - **Detrusor instability**
  - Detrusor hyperreflexia (neurological problems).

Stress incontinence

- Genuine stress incontinence (Urethral sphincter incompetence)
- Detrusor instability
- Chronic retention with overflow (see below)

Dribble incontinence

- Fistulae
  - Obstructed labour
  - Pelvic malignancy
  - Previous radiotherapy
  - Postsurgery
- Chronic retention (with overflow)
  - Neurological disease
    - Stroke
    - Multiple sclerosis (MS)
    - Parkinson's disease
    - Dementia
    - Spinal injury
  - Urethral obstruction (usually after incontinence surgery in women)
  - Pharmacological (e.g. antidepressants).

HISTORY

KEY POINT

It is very important to assess to what extent the symptoms concern the patient and interfere with her daily life. Some patients, particularly those who are presenting with another gynaecological problem, will feel that their symptoms do not merit investigation or treatment.

Symptoms suggestive of urethral sphincter incompetence

- Stress incontinence is the loss of urine associated with increase in intra-abdominal pressure such as coughing or sneezing. This symptom is not synonymous with urethral sphincter incompetence – the cough may initiate detrusor activity or give rise to overflow from an overdistended bladder.

- Incontinence due to urethral sphincter incompetence can usually be controlled by extreme effort, whereas stress incontinence due to detrusor instability is usually uncontrollable.

Symptoms suggestive of detrusor instability

- Urgency, i.e. the sudden uncontrollable desire to pass urine.
- Urge incontinence.
- Urinary frequency. Daytime frequency (the passage of urine more than six times per day) may be due to habit or excessive fluid intake, but nocturia (passage of urine more than once per night) is suggestive of detrusor instability.
- Coughing and laughing can trigger detrusor contractions and result in urgency or incontinence, mimicking GSI.

Other urinary symptoms to note

- Dysuria.
- Slow stream. Uncommon in women, but if present may become worse after surgery.
- Incomplete bladder emptying may indicate urinary retention with overflow or (rarely) a bladder diverticulum.
- Haematuria.

Other symptoms to note

- Prolapse.
- Bowel habit.
- Medications.
- Other illnesses (especially neurological and diabetes mellitus).
- Previous radiotherapy.

EXAMINATION

- Weight.
- Urinalysis.
- Stress incontinence may be demonstrated by asking the patient to cough whilst standing but is not diagnostic of urethral sphincter incompetence. The cough may have caused unwanted detrusor activity.
- Most patients empty their bladder immediately prior to the consultation and so incontinence may not be demonstrated.
- Prolapse may be present but does not necessarily imply that the patient has urethral sphincter incompetence.
- Bonney's test describes the abolition of stress incontinence by elevation of the bladder neck. It was used to demonstrate urethral sphincter incompetence but is unreliable.

INVESTIGATIONS

- **Urine culture.**
- **Urodynamic investigation** should be requested when the history gives an unclear or mixed picture, and in patients who have had previous pelvic surgery. Although regarded as the 'gold standard' it should be remembered that urodynamic investigations are not physiological. Most patients find the investigations very embarrassing.

  However if surgery is contemplated for presumed genuine stress incontinence, urodynamic assessment is mandatory.
- **Uroflowmetry** is a simple investigation with the patient passing urine into a flow meter. Although usually normal in women, a reduced flow (<15 mL/s) may indicate outflow obstruction (e.g. after surgery) or poor detrusor function.
- **Urinary residual volume** is measured after voiding by inserting a urethral catheter (normal <50 mL). It can also be measured using ultrasound.
- **Cystometry** is the fundamental urodynamic investigation in women and is performed to exclude detrusor instability. True detrusor pressure is calculated by subtracting rectal (i.e. intra-abdominal) pressure from intravesical pressure. The bladder is filled at 100 mL/min and the volumes at first sensation (normal 150–250 mL) and full bladder capacity (normal 400–700 mL) are recorded. With detrusor instability, increases in detrusor pressure exceeding 20 cm water occur during the filling phase. With the bladder full, the patient stands and coughs, and any leakage, together with the associated bladder pressure, are recorded. The pressure during voiding is noted (normal <70 cm water).
- **Videocystourethrography** may be performed in conjunction with cystometry, and may demonstrate abnormalities such as urethral sphincter incompetence, vesicoureteric reflux, bladder diverticulae and fistulae.
- **Cystoscopy** may be performed when a local abnormality of the bladder is suspected. Persistent haematuria must be investigated in the absence of a urinary tract infection as urinary tract malignancy occasionally presents through a gynaecology clinic. Urine cytology can also be helpful. Ultrasound examination of the upper renal tracts or IVU may also be indicated.

TREATMENT

1. Urethral sphincter incompetence

Non-surgical

- Weight reduction.
- Physiotherapy in the form of pelvic floor exercises may be particularly useful for the younger patient (especially postnatal patients) with mild symptoms. Physiotherapy is rarely helpful for patients with severe symptoms, or in cases of failed surgery.

Surgical

Success rates are given in brackets.

KEY POINT

Patients should be counselled carefully prior to their operation. Success rates and potential postoperative voiding difficulties should be mentioned.

(*See also* 'Common surgical procedures', p. 200.)

- **Burch colposuspension** (90%). Currently the most popular choice for uncomplicated GSI. Carries a significant risk of postoperative voiding difficulties (usually temporary), *de novo* detrusor instability and predisposition to enterocoele.
- **Stamey colposuspension** (70%): lower morbidity but lower success rate than the Burch colposuspension.
- **Anterior vaginal repair and bladder buttress** (50%), is perhaps not considered the most appropriate procedure for genuine stress incontinence. In the presence of significant uterovaginal prolapse the operation may be employed to correct the prolapse and the patient's urinary symptoms may also be improved.
- **Injectable methods** (40–50%). Various different substances (collagen, silicone and Teflon) can be injected periurethrally to increase the bulk of the bladder neck tissues, causing partial occlusion and reduction in stress leakage. Can be performed as a day case procedure but may need to be repeated. Particularly useful in women with incontinence who have had previous surgery which has failed.

2. Detrusor instability

Non-pharmacological

- Bladder drill. The patient is trained to empty her bladder by the clock, initially at very short intervals with gradual lengthening of the time interval, retraining the bladder to hold larger amounts of urine without detrusor contraction. To be effective this is best done as an in-patient, often with pharmacological support (see below).

- Restrict fluid, caffeine or diuretic intake.

Pharmacological

Anticholinergics are the mainstay of treatment, either in the form of oxybutynin, tolteridine or tricyclic antidepressants. To be effective, most patients experience side effects of treatment, e.g. dry mouth and constipation. These are less significant with the newer preparations.

Surgical

- Cystodistension with or without urethral dilatation or urethrotomy may be helpful.
- Debilitating symptoms may warrant a cystoplasty or artificial urethral sphincter.

n.b. Detrusor instability in old age is difficult to treat. Anticholinergics are poorly tolerated and a permanent urethral catheter may be necessary.

VAGINAL DISCHARGE

PHYSIOLOGICAL (LEUCORRHOEA)

Physiological vaginal discharge consists of mucus and a mixture of cells from the lower genital tract. It has the following characteristics:

- it is usually mucoid or white
- the quantity varies considerably
- it is increased at ovulation, premenstrually, in the presence of a intrauterine contraceptive device, during sexual intercourse and during pregnancy.

Occasionally the discharge may be particularly heavy in association with an ectropion.

Management

- exclude infection or other pathology
- reassure
- in specific cases where the discharge is particularly troublesome:
  - cauterize an ectropion
  - remove an IUCD
  - suppress ovulation (with the COCP).

PATHOLOGICAL

1. Infection

Infection is the commonest cause of pathological vaginal discharge in women of reproductive age.

Types of infection include:

- ***Candida albicans*:** Very common. The discharge is thick, white and intensely pruritic. Treatment is with clotrimazole (canestan) or fluconazole. (*See* Pharmacopoeia, p. 321.)
- ***Trichomonas vaginalis*:** Offensive grey/green discharge with pruritis. Treatment is with metronidazole. TV is a sexually transferable disease and contact tracing and treatment of partners should be initiated via the local genitourinary clinic.
- ***Chlamydia trachomatis*:** Common. Infections are frequently asymptomatic. This is an important cause of chronic pelvic inflammatory disease, subfertility and ectopic pregnancy. Treatment is with erythromycin or doxycycline. The patient must be referred to a genitourinary medicine clinic for contact tracing.
- ***Neisseria gonorrhoeae*:** This is a common sexually transmitted disease and is frequently asymptomatic, although it may present with a discharge. Always refer the patient to a genitourinary clinic for treatment and contact tracing.
- ***Bacterial vaginosis*:** The discharge is offensive and dirty looking. It is not necessarily sexually transmitted. It is treated with topical clindamycin or oral metronidazole but can be difficult to eradicate.
- ***Herpes genitalis*:** This is a recurring problem that is usually associated with painful ulcers, most commonly with the primary infection.

Although the history and examination findings may give some indication as to the causative agent associated with the vaginal discharge always take appropriate samples for microbiological investigations:

- high vaginal swab
- endocervical swab
- endocervical sample for identification of chlamydia
- consider urethral and rectal swabs and samples from the base of any ulcer.

2. Neoplasia

The discharge is usually blood-stained or purulent.

Think of cervical cancer and endometrial cancer (especially in the peri and postmenopausal woman).

Cervical and endometrial polyps are more likely to present with intermenstrual, postcoital or postmenopausal bleeding.

(Cervical intraepithelial neoplasia (CIN) is asymptomatic.)

Special cases

Infection may be associated with retained products of conception after pregnancy or miscarriage.

In postmenopausal women exclude infection and treat as PMB.

Urinary or faecal fistulae will present as vaginal discharge and are usually found after surgery, associated with malignancy or after radiotherapy.

COMMON VULVAL PROBLEMS

PRURITIS VULVAE

Definition

Itching of the female external genitalia. Pruritis vulvae is a symptom, not a diagnosis.

Causes

- **Vaginal discharge**
  - Candidiasis
  - Trichomonas vaginalis.
- **Urinary incontinence**
- **Vulval infections**
  - Bacteriological, e.g. furunculosis
  - Viral, e.g. herpes genitalis, viral warts, molluscum contagiosum
  - Fungal, e.g. candidiasis
  - Other, e.g. scabies.
- **Vulval dystrophy**
  - Non-neoplastic lesions of the vulva
    Lichen sclerosus
    Squamous cell hyperplasia
    Other dermatoses, e.g. lichen planus, lichen simplex, eczema, psoriasis.
  - Neoplastic lesions of the vulva
    Vulval intraepithelial neoplasia
    Cancer of the vulva
    Paget's disease of the vulva.

- **Sensitization**
- **Chemical irritation**, e.g. detergent, spermicide, perfume, synthetic materials
- **Psychogenic**

COMMON CONDITIONS AFFECTING THE VULVA

Lichen sclerosus

- **Incidence:** The incidence of this common condition is unknown.
- **Clinical features:** The disease can occur at any age but is most apparent in postmenopausal women. Symptoms usually include pruritis vulvae and dyspareunia. The appearance of the vulva is usually typical with white, thin skin which may be excoriated. The affected area may include the clitoris, labia minora and majora, perineal and perianal skin. There may be genital atrophy with fusion of the labia minora to clitoris, adjacent labium majora and opposite labium minora. **The risk of associated vulval carcinoma is approximately 5–9%** and patients should therefore be kept under long-term review with biopsy of any suspicious changes.
- **Treatment:** Potent topical corticosteroids such as Dermovate are effective. They should be applied sparingly to the affected area nightly or twice daily until symptomatic relief is obtained, or until used for 3 months, following which application should be changed to a less potent steroid preparation.

  Prior to treatment, patients should be advised that the treatment is safe because the packaging will state that Dermovate is not for use on the genital area. Dermovate may cause adrenal suppression.

  Skin biopsies should be taken if the clinical appearance is not typical of lichen sclerosus, or if the condition fails to respond to treatment. Biopsies may be taken under local anaesthetic.

Bartholin's cysts

These are located postero-laterally in the introitus. Often the cysts are asymptomatic, but if recurrent are best treated by excision of the cyst and Bartholin's gland, with marsupialization of the cavity to prevent haematoma formation and to minimize the chance of recurrence. A Bartholins's abscess normally requires incision and marsupialization. An attempt to excise the cyst should not be made at this stage.

KEYPOINTS

- ***Bartholin's cysts are uncommon in postmenopausal women and if present should always be excised to exclude malignancy.***

- ***Recurrent Bartholin's abscesses may occur in patients who are immunosuppressed; exclude HIV infection and diabetes in such patients.***

Viral warts

These are best treated by excision using diathermy or laser under general or local anaesthetic. The resulting burns are painful and prone to infection. It is usually impossible to eradicate the virus and the warts tend to recur. Patients should be screened for concomitant sexually transmitted infections, and should be up to date with cervical smear screening.

Warts may proliferate in pregnancy, but treatment by diathermy may result in heavy bleeding. Treatment should be deferred until after the pregnancy, by which time spontaneous resolution may have occurred.

Florid warts may develop in patients who are immunosuppressed; exclude HIV infection in such patients.

Vulval intraepithelial neoplasia

VIN is graded I, II and III (similar to CIN). It is a difficult condition to treat and is best managed in a specialist clinic if one is available. Patients with VIN are at risk of other intraepithelial neoplasias. Ensure that the patient's cervical smear is normal and if in doubt arrange for colposcopy of the cervix to be performed. Associated anal pruritis may point to associated AIN (anal intraepithelial neoplasia). VIN is multifocal in 70% of cases and the risk of progression to invasive carcinoma is 4–10%. Observation is most appropriate in young women but treatment may be necessary with laser or local excision in some cases.

THE INFERTILE COUPLE

Definition

Infertility is defined as the failure to conceive after one year of regular unprotected sexual intercourse. It is considered **primary** if there has never been a pregnancy and **secondary** if there have been previous successful attempts at conception.

Incidence

There is an incidence of infertility of 15–20% of all couples.

Causes and relative incidence (*See* Table 20.3)

n.b. the relative incidence of the different causes varies widely from centre to centre.

Table 20.3 Causes and relative incidence of infertility

Causes of infertility	Relative incidence
Tubal disease (including endometriosis)	20–30%
Anovulation (including endometriosis)	20–30%
Male factor	10–30%
Cervical hostility	0–5%
Unexplained	20–30%

KEY POINT

Both partners should be investigated simultaneously as disease in both partners leading to infertility is common.

HISTORY

A detailed history should be taken. Here are some pointers:

Maternal age

- The older woman has a naturally declining fertility and this will affect the timescale of investigation and treatment. A sense of 'time running out' may lead to great anxiety in the couple.
- Most gynaecologists will not investigate women over the age of 44 because of the low chance of achieving a pregnancy, the high risk of genetic problems in the fetus, and the high risk of developing medical complications during the pregnancy.

Duration of infertility

Although couples are traditionally investigated for infertility after 1 year, this should be individualized for the couple. An older woman may merit earlier investigation. If an obvious cause for the infertility is present (e.g. amenorrhoea), then immediate investigation should be initiated. Younger couples may prefer investigation only after a longer period of trying for a pregnancy.

Intercourse

- Frequency of intercourse is important. Couples who have intercourse several times per week do not need to time intercourse in relation to ovulation. Infrequent intercourse may account for the infertility.
- Does ejaculation occur during intercourse?
- Pain during intercourse may indicate the presence of pelvic disease.

Factors which may indicate tubal disease

- Pain during intercourse.
- Abdominal pain.
- Vaginal discharge.
- Previous pelvic infection.
- Previous abdominal surgery (e.g. ruptured appendix). What were the findings at that time? If possible, review the operation notes.
- Previous ectopic pregnancy.
- Secondary infertility (the patient has previously been pregnant) is weakly associated with tubal damage when compared to primary infertility (the patient has never been pregnant before).

Anovulation

- A careful menstrual history will usually indicate whether the woman is ovulatory or anovulatory.
- Regular menstrual periods with symptoms such as breast tenderness, and premenstrual pelvic discomfort suggest ovulation.
- Consider the possibility of endocrinopathy, e.g. hypothyroidism, hyperprolactinaemia.

Male partner

- Previous paternities should be noted, but note that paternity may not be certain!
- Testicular trauma, infection, or surgery (particularly for undescended testis) may be important.

Cervical factor

Previous cervical surgery, e.g. cone biopsy may have caused stenosis and poor cervical mucus production.

General history

Drug abuse, smoking and alcohol may impair fertility in either partner.

EXAMINATION

Female

Usually unremarkable, but pelvic tenderness may indicate the presence of tubal disease. Is there obvious hirsutism or evidence of any other endocrinopathy? What is the patient's BMI ?

Male

Usually unremarkable, but exclude testicular atrophy and varicocoele.

INVESTIGATIONS

The first visit

- **Semen analysis:** Should be produced by masturbation after 72 hours' abstinence, and transported to the laboratory (kept warm) within 1 hour of production. 'Normal' indices (WHO values) are shown in Table 20.4. It is important to note however that results inferior to these are still compatible with pregnancy, and also that repeating semen analyses is important as substantial variation exists over time.
- **Ovulation assessment:** A progesterone level should be measured 7 days before the expected period (e.g. day 21 in a 28 day cycle). A level >20 nmol/L normally suggests that ovulation has occurred. Basal body temperature charts may be unreliable and can be psychologically stressful for the patient.
- Rubella immunity.
- Cervical smear if indicated and endocervical swabs for chlamydia.
- Encourage all women to take folic acid supplements (400 micrograms per day).

The second visit

- **Semen analysis:** If abnormal, enquire about production (collection in a spermicide-containing condom is common!) and repeat. Check FSH, LH, prolactin and testosterone levels. Treat any infection. To confirm an abnormality, three samples at 3-monthly intervals should be analysed.
- **Ovulation assessment:** If anovulatory, check day 2 FSH, LH, prolactin and thyroid function. Also consider testosterone and serum hormone binding globulin levels and the Free Androgen

Table 20.4 WHO values of semen analysis

Semen characteristic	'Normal' value
Volume	2 to 5 mL
Sperm count	>20 million/mL
Motility	>50% progressive motility
Morphology	>30% normal forms
Liquefaction	In 30 minutes

Index (all helpful in the diagnosis of polycystic ovary syndrome [PCOS]).

Further investigations

- **Laparoscopy and dye test:** This may be deferred if ovulation-induction is required (the couple may quickly conceive once ovulatory), although laparoscopy is advisable before gonadotrophin therapy is started. Laparoscopy is inappropriate if the partner is azoospermic and artificial insemination by donor (AID) is not wanted by the couple.
- **Post-coital test (but see below):** The woman must be demonstrably ovulatory, and the test must be performed immediately pre-ovulation (assessed by cervical mucus changes – large amount of thin, clear mucus, positive spinnbarkeit, i.e. stretchable to 8 cm, positive ferning, and the cervical os should be open). The test should be performed following 72 hours abstinence and the mucus should be examined 6 to 12 hours after intercourse. A normal result is one or more motile sperm per high powered field. More sophisticated tests such as the sperm-mucus penetration test may be used if available. The most common cause of an abnormal post coital test is poor timing in the menstrual cycle. The second most common cause is oligozoospermia.
- The post coital test, sperm function tests and routine testing for antisperm antibodies in semen are not now **routinely** used but may be employed in certain cases.

TREATMENT

Ovulation induction

- See the above section on treatment of amenorrhoea, particularly with regard to body weight.
- Clomiphene citrate is a first line therapy, initially with 50 mg daily on day 2 to 6 of the cycle. Effectiveness may be assessed by day 21 progesterone levels or by 'follicular tracking' with serial ultrasound scans. If still anovulatory, the dosage is increased to 50 mg bd then tds if necessary. Once ovulatory, treatment should be continued for 6 months. Side effects include nausea and hot flushes, poor cervical mucus and multiple pregnancy. Cervical mucus may be improved using ethinyloestradiol 10 mg bd on days 8 to 12. Even with careful use of the minimum effective dose of clomiphene, twins rates are increased (15%), but rates for higher orders of multiple pregnancy are not increased. Patients

who develop follicles but do not ovulate may benefit from HCG injection when the follicle is 18 mm or more in diameter.

- Gonadotrophin therapy with or without intrauterine insemination (IUI) is indicated following failure to ovulate with clomiphene, or failure to conceive after 6 months of apparently effective clomiphene therapy.
- Patients with a raised LH may have polycystic ovary disease. Ovulation induction may be difficult. If overweight, weight reduction may be beneficial. Ovarian drilling is a surgical method used to encourage ovulation from the polycystic ovary.
- Patients with a raised FSH generally have ovarian failure, and do not respond well to ovulation induction.

Male factor

- With oligospermia check drug therapy, smoking and alcohol intake. Treat any infection and varicocoele if present. Consider assisted conception techniques such as IUI and *in vitro* fertilization (IVF).
- With azoospermia, most patients have a raised FSH, and AID (artificial insemination by donor) is the only therapy. Rarely the FSH will be normal, suggesting obstruction which may be amenable to surgery, or low which may respond to FSH therapy. Where sperm numbers are very low injection of a single sperm head into an oocyte may be possible with transfer of the resulting embryo, as with IVF. This technique is known as ICSI (intracytoplasmic sperm injection)

Tubal disease

- The choice of treatment lies between tubal surgery and IVF. Tubal surgery can be suitable for the younger woman with mild correctable tubal disease. IVF should be encouraged in women with moderate or severe tubal disease or if pregnancy has not occurred within 12 months of the surgery. Surgery may involve resection of occluded proximal fallopian tube with reanastamosis or fimbrioplasty and neosalpingostomy for a damaged distal tube. Division of tubal and ovarian adhesions may be useful.

Endometriosis

Endometriosis may cause damage to the fallopian tubes or ovaries and affect their function. It is debatable whether minimal endometriosis affects fertility – certainly medical treatment will delay conception. See the above section on chronic pelvic pain for an outline of the treatment of endometriosis. There is no evidence that medical treatment improves fertility in any group of patients with endometriosis, be it minimal or severe. Surgical ablation of endometriosis may improve fertility, but there has been no randomized comparison with assisted reproduction techniques.

Unexplained infertility

- A proportion of couples will have no obvious cause found for their infertility.
- Some couples fail to conceive on a purely statistical basis (i.e. only 25% of healthy couples conceive in 1 month and only 97% conceive within 1 year). Therefore, younger couples with only a short history of subfertility may simply need the reassurance to continue trying. Even after 2 years of trying there is still a significant chance of a spontaneous conception in younger couples with unexplained infertility.
- Treatment should be individualised, and may include referral to a specialist centre for assisted conception techniques. The average 'take home baby rate' following IVF is between 15 and 20% in the UK with some units reaching 25% (and 50–60% over three cycles). ICSI is a relatively new technique suitable for oligospermic couples. Funding for assisted reproductive techniques (ART) varies around the country with many regions not providing the funding for any couples.

HIRSUTISM

Definition

Hirsutism is the excess growth of terminal hair in sites which are normally regarded as male secondary sexual characteristics. Hirsutism is often associated with acne and greasy hair and skin. Virilism is the presence of masculine body features including hirsutism, temporal balding, clitoromegaly and deepening of the voice.

Causes

- **Common:**
  - Polycystic ovary syndrome (75–90% of cases)
  - Constitutional.
- **Other causes:**
  - Drugs (danazol, androgens, phenytoin, norethisterone)
  - Congenital adrenal hyperplasia
  - Cushing's disease

- Adrenal tumours
- Ovarian tumours.

HISTORY

Speed of progression

- Rapid progression may be indicative of an androgen secreting tumour or drug ingestion.

Menstrual pattern

- Most women with polycystic ovary syndrome (PCOS) who are hirsute will have menstrual irregularity.

Drug history

Family history

Both PCOS and constitutional hirsutism have strong familial tendencies.

EXAMINATION

- **Body mass index:**
  - Note that a normal body mass index (20–25) does not exclude polycystic ovary syndrome.
- **Blood pressure.**
- **Hair distribution.**
- **Signs of virilism.**

INVESTIGATIONS

- Testosterone. Secreted normally by both the ovary and adrenal. A level greater than twice the upper limit of normal is suggestive of an androgen-secreting tumour.
- Sex-hormone binding globulin (levels are reduced in PCOS).
- Dehydroepiandrosterone sulphate (DHEAS) (secreted by the adrenal only. Therefore if the testosterone is raised, a raised DHEAS identifies the source as adrenal).
- LH/FSH ratio on day 2 of the menstrual cycle. A ratio of greater than 2 is suggestive of polycystic ovary syndrome. Timing of this test is important – it must be done in the early part of the cycle.
- Ovarian ultrasound. With PCOS characteristic appearances are seen with enlarged ovaries (>9 cm in maximum length), 10 or more peripherally arranged cysts 2–10 mm in diameter, and increased area and density of the stroma.
- 17-hydroxyprogesterone serum concentration (raised in congenital adrenal hyperplasia [CAH]).

Congenital adrenal hyperplasia (CAH)

- Most cases present at birth with ambiguous genitalia.
- Late onset or mild disease is uncommon. The most common, 21 hydroxylase deficiency, is suggested by a raised 17 α-hydroxy-progesterone level (taken in the follicular phase of the menstrual cycle), however the diagnosis may need to be confirmed by ACTH stimulation testing.

Cushing's disease

- Suggested by truncal obesity, striae and hypertension.
- Diagnosed by elevated 24-hour urinary free cortisol and dexamethasone suppression test.

Androgen secreting tumours

These are very rare. If the testosterone level is more than twice normal and an ovarian or adrenal tumour is not obviously palpable, the ovaries and adrenals should be imaged with CT.

TREATMENT

Reassurance and explanation is very important. Many patients are worried that they have a tumour.

Cosmetic measures

- Bleaching
- Waxing, shaving
- Electrolysis.

Medical treatment

- Weight reduction is important for overweight patients with PCOS.
- Cyproterone acetate, an anti-androgen, given in combination with ethinyl oestradiol. The contraceptive Dianette contains 2 mg cyproterone acetate and 35 micrograms ethinyl oestradiol (cyproterone is teratogenic and so contraception is essential). Improvement in hirsutism may take 6 months to develop. Cyproterone acetate 25–50 mg may be added to the first 10 days of each pack of Dianette, in which case regular monitoring of liver function, blood count and electrolytes is necessary due to potential liver toxicity.
- The combined pill is less effective than Dianette for treating hirsutism, but may be useful to follow a course of Dianette for maintenance therapy.
- Low-dose dexamethasone is used in patients with CAH.

RECURRENT MISCARRIAGE

Definition

Recurrent miscarriage is defined by three or more consecutive miscarriages. Between 10 and 15% of all clinically recognized pregnancies end in miscarriage. About 1% of women will have three or more consecutive miscarriages.

- This is three times the rate expected by chance.
- Two-thirds of these patients will have an underlying cause for their miscarriages.

CAUSES

1. Genetic

Approximately 4% of individuals investigated for recurrent miscarriage (male or female partner) carry a chromosomal abnormality; for example, a balanced translocation.

Management

- Karyotype both partners
- Refer to a clinical geneticist if an abnormality is found
- After counselling use of donor gametes may be appropriate or invasive prenatal testing for ongoing pregnancies.

2. Autoimmune conditions

There is an association between the presence of antiphospholipid antibodies and recurrent miscarriage.

Management

- Measure anticardiolipin antibodies
- Measure lupus anticoagulant
- Platelet count may be low
- Two tests must be positive at least 6 weeks apart
- Treat with low dose aspirin
- Consider heparin therapy.

3. Thombophilic defects

Antithrombin III, protein C and protein S deficiencies along with activated protein C resistance are all more common in recurrent miscarriers. The mechanism is unclear and there is no current evidence that thromboprophylaxis will reduce the miscarriage risk.

4. Hormonal conditions

Polycystic ovarian syndrome (PCOS) is commonly found (50%) in cases of early recurrent miscarriage. LH hypersecretion may be the cause of the increased miscarriage risk however manipulation to reduce LH levels has failed to improve ongoing pregnancy rates.

Ovulatory problems leading to subfertility are a major risk factor for subsequent recurrent early miscarriage.

- **Low progesterone levels in early pregnancy are an effect rather than a cause of pregnancy loss.**
- Treatment with progestogens is ineffective.
- **The effect of treatment with HCG is uncertain.**
- Poorly controlled diabetes mellitus is a cause of miscarriage, potentially recurrent.
- Poorly managed thyroid disease may be a cause of recurrent miscarriage.

Management

Pelvic ultrasound to identify PCOS. Glucose tolerance test and thyroid function tests are only appropriate when there is a clinical suspicion of disease.

5. Infections

Infections are unlikely to be a cause of recurrent miscarriage.

- TORCH screening is of no value.
- Bacterial vaginosis (BV) may be a cause of recurrent second trimester miscarriage.

Management

Identify and eradicate BV.

6. Cervical incompetence

Diagnosed on the basis of a history of second trimester miscarriage preceded by:

- spontaneous rupture of membranes and
- painless dilatation of the cervix.

Spontaneous miscarriage after regular painful contractions is <u>not</u> due to cervical incompetence.

Management

Cervical cerclage may be appropriate, although there is no proven effect on fetal survival.

7. Anatomical causes

Uterine abnormalities, e.g. bicornuate uterus or uterine septum, are common amongst women with normal reproductive histories and those with recurrent miscarriage. They can be diagnosed by hysteroscopy or transvaginal ultrasonography; however their relationship to miscarriage is unclear. There is no good evidence that their detection and treatment improves reproductive outcome and indeed some of the surgical methods of correction may actually reduce the chances of a successful pregnancy.

Management

- Pelvic ultrasound and hysteroscopy are preferable to hysterosalpingography.
- Hysteroscopic surgery may help in selected cases.

GENERAL MANAGEMENT

- Karyotype both partners.
- Consider karyotyping fetal products that are available.
- Pelvic ultrasound.
- Tests for:
  - Lupus anticoagulant
  - Anticardiolipin antibodies
  - Other investigations are only indicated when there are other clinical reasons to perform them (e.g. thyroid disease, symptoms of glucose intolerance).
- Treatment depends on finding a cause.
- There is evidence that reassurance alone is of value.

21

ONCOLOGY AND PALLIATIVE CARE

CANCER SERVICES IN THE UK

The joint working group of the Royal College of Obstetricians and Gynaecologists and the British Gynaecological Cancer Society, in response to the Department of Health report 'A Policy Framework for Commissioning Cancer Services', has recommended that most gynaecological cancers be treated in designated 'Gynaecological Oncology Centres' (GOCs). Uncomplicated endometrial and ovarian cancer surgery may be performed in hospitals other than GOCs, but normally patients requiring radical surgery for cancer of the cervix or vulva, as well as complicated cases of endometrial or ovarian cancer and uterine sarcoma should be referred to the GOC for primary treatment.

See p. 348 for FIGO staging systems for the various malignancies.

OVARIAN CARCINOMA

Mortality

A total of approximately 3500 deaths in England and Wales each year.

Treatment

Staging is surgical, performed at the time of laparotomy. Surgery is the mainstay of management, normally consisting of taking peritoneal washings for cytological examination, total abdominal hysterectomy and bilateral salpingo-oophorectomy, omentectomy and removal of any other tumour deposits. So called 'debulking' of the tumour to reduce the maximum deposit size to <1 cm has been shown to improve survival, perhaps by enhancing the response to chemotherapy. Surgery is normally followed by chemotherapy, except in cases of stage 1A tumours and borderline tumours. Conservative surgery consisting of washings for cytological examination, unilateral oophorectomy, and biopsy of the omentum and remaining ovary may be performed in young women with well-differentiated tumours who want to preserve their fertility. Following completion of their family, these patients should have the remaining ovary removed.

Chemotherapy must be administered in conjunction with a medical oncologist. Treatment usually involves platinum containing drugs such as cisplatin or carboplatin, although agents such as taxol and its derivatives are becoming more commonly used. Typical treatment regimens involve six courses of therapy at monthly intervals. When recurrence occurs further chemotherapy may be given but with decreasing returns. Follow-up is best performed in a joint oncology clinic with a medical oncologist, but typically patients are seen at 3-monthly intervals; more frequently if they develop problems.

Preoperative work-up is as described in the section on management of a pelvic mass (p. 255). Ca125 levels are raised in over 80% of epithelial ovarian malignancies and are useful in diagnosis, monitoring treatment and recognizing recurrence. Germ cell tumours are more common in young women and other serum markers such as AFP (alpha fetoprotein) and HCG (human chorionic gonadotrophin) may be raised. Surgery is usually more conservative in those wishing to preserve fertility and combination chemotherapy regimes involve bleomycin, etoposide and platinum-based drugs.

PROGNOSIS

Survival rates for epithelial ovarian cancer and borderline ovarian tumours are shown in Tables 21.1 and 21.2 respectively.

Table 21.1 Prognosis for epithelial ovarian cancer

Stage	5-year survival rate
I	60%
IA	65%
IB	50%
IC	50%
II	40%
III	5%
IV	3%

Table 21.2 Prognosis for borderline ovarian tumours

Stage	5-year survival rate
I	99%
II	95%
III	75%

Familial ovarian cancer

- A woman's lifetime risk of dying from ovarian cancer is approximately 0.8%. If one first-degree relative has had ovarian cancer, the risk is increased to 2.5%. With two first-degree relatives affected by ovarian cancer, the risk is increased to 30–40%.
- Occasionally, families may be identified in which a tendency to develop cancers including ovarian cancer is inherited in an autosomal dominant fashion with variable penetrance, notably:
  - Ovarian cancer alone
  - Breast and ovarian cancer
  - Colorectal and ovarian cancer.

Referral to a family cancer genetics specialist should be considered to help define risks and organize potential genetic screening.

Screening for ovarian cancer

- 5-year survival rates for advanced stage ovarian cancer are poor. Screening for ovarian cancer assumes that earlier detection will improve survival. Serum Ca125 and pelvic ultrasonography have been used to screen for early ovarian cancer. Unfortunately the sensitivities and specificities of these tests are low, giving unacceptable false-negative and false-positive rates when applied to the general population.
- Screening has been advocated for women with two or more first-degree relatives with ovarian cancer, and for women from families with familial ovarian cancer or multiple cancer syndromes. Screening by means of a Ca125 level and pelvic ultrasound scan is carried out annually from the age of 25. There are, however, no randomized controlled trials published to provide evidence that screening reduces mortality from ovarian cancer, and many gynaecologists would recommend prophylactic oophorectomy for these women once their family was complete, rather than screening.

CARCINOMA OF THE UTERUS

Mortality

There are approximately 1000 deaths in England and Wales from uterine carcinoma each year.

TREATMENT

Staging is surgical, which normally requires laparotomy. The mainstay of treatment for stage I and II disease is surgical, consisting of taking peritoneal washings for cytological examination, total abdominal hysterectomy and bilateral salpingo-oophorectomy. Some surgeons perform lymph node sampling in all but the low-risk cases. Surgery for stage I and II disease is followed by radiotherapy if there is a high risk of lymph node metastasis (e.g. poorly differentiated adenocarcinoma or deep myometrial penetration). Stage III and IV disease is normally treated by radiotherapy alone.

PROGNOSIS

Survival rates according to stage for adenocarcinoma of the uterus patients are shown in Table 21.3.

Prognosis depends upon many factors other than stage, including histological type, histological differentiation, uterine size, depth of myometrial invasion, peritoneal cytology and lymph node metastasis. Other uterine cancers (e.g. sarcomas) have a poorer prognosis and surgery is the mainstay of treatment.

Table 21.3 Prognosis for adenocarcinoma of the uterus

Stage	5-year survival rate
I	75%
II	55%
III	30%
IV	10%

CERVICAL CARCINOMA

Mortality

There are approximately 1500 deaths in England and Wales from cervical carcinoma each year.

TREATMENT

Unlike cancer of the ovary and endometrium, staging is clinical rather than surgical and includes:

- Chest X-ray.
- Intravenous pyelogram to exclude ureteric obstruction and to document any developmental anomalies of the urinary tract.
- Examination under anaesthetic, including rectal examination.
- Cystoscopy (sometimes omitted with stage I disease).

Treatment normally consists of cone biopsy for stage IAi disease (invasion less than 3 mm deep and 7 mm wide), radical hysterectomy and pelvic node dissection for stage IAii, IB (and occasionally stage IIA) disease, and radiotherapy for stages II, III and IV.

PROGNOSIS

Survival rates according to stage for cervical cancer patients are shown in Table 21.4.

Table 21.4 Prognosis for cervical cancer

Stage	5-year survival rate
IA	99%
IB	90%
IIA	80%
IIB	60%
III	40%
IV	15%

FOLLOW-UP

The GOC will have written a protocol for the follow-up of the asymptomatic patient. About 75% of recurrences occur within the first 2 years after treatment. During this critical period the asymptomatic patient will normally be seen 3-monthly in the first 2 years for clinical and pelvic examination including a vaginal vault smear sometimes. Following treatment with radiotherapy, a progressive pelvic fibrosis may develop which may be difficult to distinguish from recurrent tumour. This fibrosis is however smooth compared with the irregular knobbly feel of tumour. In doubtful cases, needle biopsy under general anaesthetic may be required. The prognosis for patients with recurrent or persistent disease is poor, with 90% dying in the first year.

CARCINOMA OF THE VULVA

Mortality

There are approximately 400 deaths in England and Wales from vulval carcinoma each year.

TREATMENT

Treatment will be individualized to the patient. Most will have a radical vulvectomy and bilateral inguinal node dissection with postoperative radiotherapy if lymph node metastasis has occurred. Selected patients may be treated with less extensive surgery.

MOLAR PREGNANCY AND GESTATIONAL TROPHOBLASTIC DISEASE

- **Molar pregnancies** occur when fertilization of the ovum occurs abnormally. They cause first or second trimester bleeding and may on occasion be associated with hyperemesis and rarely pre-eclampsia or hyperthyroidism. In most cases the diagnosis is made before these complications develop because of early ultrasound scanning. Trophoblastic pulmonary emboli can occur, however a hydatidiform mole is not truly metastatic and treatment involves emptying the uterus and close follow up with HCG levels to exclude persistent trophoblastic disease.
- **Gestational trophoblastic disease** (GTD) may occur after any form of pregnancy (i.e. **molar pregnancy**, miscarriage, ectopic, or normal pregnancy). Most commonly, GTD arises following a molar pregnancy, and may either consist of persistent trophoblastic disease or choriocarcinoma. GTD is usually highly sensitive to chemotherapy, such that virtually all patients are cured. GTD produces HCG which is useful as a tumour marker and to assess response to chemotherapy.

Incidence

Hydatidiform mole incidence is currently 1.5 per 1000 live births in England and Wales.

In the UK, following hydatidiform mole, approximately 3% of patients develop choriocarcinoma, and a total of approximately 8% of patients require chemotherapy for GTD (persistent trophoblastic disease or choriocarcinoma).

Choriocarcinoma following term pregnancy occurrence is 1 in 50 000 in England and Wales.

Registration

A registration system exists in the UK for patients with hydatidiform mole with three registration centres (Charing Cross London, Sheffield and Dundee) and two treatment centres (Charing Cross and Sheffield). All patients should be registered.

TREATMENT

Hydatidiform mole

The initial treatment of hydatidiform mole is suction evacuation of the uterus. In patients with persistent bleeding, a second evacuation may be required. Information required for registration includes the initial serum HCG level and ABO and Rh blood group of both the patient and her partner. Subsequent follow-up is coordinated by the registration centre with serum and urine samples for HCG assay sent by post. The registration centre liases with the patient, GP and hospital. Any further treatment (e.g. for persistent bleeding) should **not** be undertaken without reference to the treatment centre.

Patients should ensure that they do not become pregnant during the follow-up period until advised that it is safe to do so by the reference laboratory. A pregnancy occurring during the follow-up period will make the detection of GTD extremely difficult. A reliable contraceptive should therefore be used. There is some concern that the combined pill may make the development of GTD more likely and the reference laboratory will be able to advise individual patients about the appropriateness of this method of contraception.

Patients whose HCG level becomes normal (<5 IU/L in serum) within 56 days of uterine evacuation, and those who have a partial hydatidiform mole are at low risk of developing GTD.

Follow-up for patients who do not develop GTD will normally be between 6 months and 2 years, with further HCG levels assayed after any subsequent pregnancy. Any patient who has had a molar pregnancy before is at a slightly higher risk in a subsequent pregnancy. Therefore an early scan is warranted in subsequent pregnancies to check that a viable intrauterine pregnancy is present and following the delivery of that child serial HCG levels should be taken to ensure that gestational trophoblastic disease does not occur again.

Gestational trophoblastic disease

Choice of treatment for GTD depends upon prognostic scoring which is based on a number of factors including the age of the patient, the size of the tumour and the number and type of metastases together with the HCG levels. Low-risk GTD is usually treated with methotrexate. High-risk GTD usually requires combination chemotherapy, and surgery may also be indicated.

PALLIATIVE CARE

During the terminal course of gynaecological cancer, most patients will have physical or psychological symptoms requiring therapy. This will normally be provided by the patient's local palliative care team in conjunction with her GP. Below are some comments relating to the particular problems encountered with terminal gynaecological cancer:

Pain

Analgesics should be taken on a **regular** basis for best effect. Try simple analgesics, such as paracetamol, progressing through to weak opiates such as codeine and finally onto stronger opiates such as morphine. Oral morphine is given 4-hourly with the initial dose depending on the patients previous treatment; 5–10 mg every 4 hours is usually sufficient to replace a weaker analgesic. If ineffective, the dose should be increased in a stepwise manner by 50% each time. Twice daily modified release preparations can be used when the effective dose is reached. Parenteral opiates may be required, and this may be most comfortably administered using an indwelling subcutaneous cannula (e.g. butterfly) giving bolus doses or by continuous infusion (diamorphine 15–400 mg per 24 hours subcutaneously, depending upon the previous dose of oral opiates). Refer to the 'Prescribing in Palliative Care' section of the BNF for conversion tables.

Non steroidal anti-inflammatory agents such as diclofenac are useful for painful bony metastases and may be given in addition to opiates. Radiotherapy can provide excellent relief from bone pain.

Neuropathic pain may improve with a corticosteroid such as dexamethasone 8 mg daily, a tricyclic antidepressant such as amitryptiline 25 to 75 mg nocte, or with carbamazepine 200 mg tds. Transcutaneous nerve stimulation may be very helpful. Intractable neuropathic pain may require long-term epidural analgesia or nerve destruction.

Intestinal obstruction

Delineate the level of the obstruction with radiological imaging (which may include plain X-rays, water-soluble contrast imaging or CT scanning). If feasible, and if the patient's condition allows, surgical bypass or resection will usually be the appropriate treatment. Partial obstruction can be managed more conservatively. Medical therapy includes attention to fluid and electrolyte balance, antiemetic drugs (see below) and a low residue diet. A nasogastric tube or gastrostomy may be helpful.

Nausea and vomiting

The cause of the nausea and vomiting should be sought. Intestinal obstruction should be excluded. Antiemetics should be given on a **regular** basis for best effect and given parenterally if oral ingestion is uncertain.

Opiate-induced nausea may be treated with prochlorperazine 12.5 mg 8-hourly. The need for this often resolves after several days of opiate therapy.

Vomiting caused by obstruction may be treated by subcutaneous infusion of cyclizine 150 mg/24 hours or haloperidol 2.5 to 10 mg/24 hours.

Constipation

Laxatives should be prescribed regularly if opiate analgesia is required. Combinations of stimulants with faecal softeners are most effective. For example co-danthramer or lactulose with senna.

Ascites

May require repeated drainage to ease abdominal discomfort and improve breathing.

Ureteric obstruction

With advanced disease, treatment may be inappropriate. If treatment is indicated, percutaneous nephrostomy tubes will bypass the obstruction. Treatment of unilateral ureteric obstruction in the terminal patient is rarely indicated.

Bleeding

Tranexamic acid 1 g 6-hourly and vaginal packing may stop acute bleeding.

Bleeding from the vaginal vault usually responds rapidly to radiotherapy, but this is not usually an option in patients who have previously undergone radiotherapy treatment.

Medroxyprogesterone acetate 200 to 400 mg daily may improve bleeding from endometrial carcinoma.

Fistulae

These may be related to treatment (radiotherapy or surgery) or recurrent disease. The choice of treatment will be determined by the life-expectancy of the patient.

Rectovaginal fistulae may be simply treated by a defunctioning colostomy even in the terminally ill patient.

Leakage of urine from a fistula may be controlled by a urethral catheter or a nephrostomy. A surgical repair or urinary diversion may be indicated.

22

GYNAECOLOGICAL EMERGENCIES

BLEEDING IN EARLY PREGNANCY

Definition

Bleeding from the genital tract in the first half of pregnancy.

Causes

- **Miscarriage or variant (83%)**
  - threatened miscarriage
  - incomplete miscarriage
  - complete miscarriage
  - missed abortion
  - septic abortion
  - blighted ovum.
- **Ectopic pregnancy**
  - tubal implantations
  - ampullary
  - isthmic
  - fimbrial
  - cornual
  - cervical, ovarian and abdominal pregnancies.
- **Trophoblastic disease**
  - hydatidiform mole
  - choriocarcinoma.
- **Other causes**
  - implantation bleed
  - cervicitis
  - genital tract tumours
  - trauma
  - other sites of bleeding: bladder or bowel.

HISTORY

Last menstrual period

Establish date of LMP and whether it was normal in nature and timing. If there is any doubt go back to the period before to help establish if the LMP was normal or abnormal in time or character.

Pregnancy test

Establish when and where a pregnancy test was done. Most urinary pregnancy tests become positive at the time of the first missed period (about 4 weeks' gestation). Serum HCG values will be elevated a few days after fertilization.

Nature of the bleeding

A little bleeding (dark red) at less than 8 weeks of pregnancy may represent an ectopic pregnancy while a miscarriage presents with bright red fresh blood, sometimes heavier than a period. A history of passing tissue per vagina suggests a complete/incomplete miscarriage. An organized blood clot may be wrongly mistaken both by doctor and patient as a piece of fetal or placental tissue so suggesting a miscarriage when an ectopic may in fact be present.

Associated pain

'Period like' pains, i.e. bilateral, low abdominal or suprapubic cramping pains are typical of a miscarriage. Ectopic pregnancies are more often associated with peritoneal irritation and present with unilateral pain exacerbated by movement. A ruptured ectopic results in haemoperitoneum which may irritate the diaphragm causing referred shoulder tip pain.

Risk factors

These should be eluded from the history – a history of recurrent miscarriages may raise the possibility of further miscarriage when bleeding occurs early in a pregnancy. Risk factors for ectopic pregnancies are listed below:

- previous ectopic pregnancy
- previous tubal surgery
- IUCD *in situ*
- history of PID
- use of the progesterone only contraceptive pill.

Common symptoms of pregnancy

Nausea and breast tenderness may be excessive in trophoblastic disease but may suddenly disappear in cases of miscarriage.

Miscellaneous points

Bleeding from the cervix may be mistaken for a miscarriage so the results of the most recent smear should be established. Other sources of bleeding such as rectum or bladder should be excluded.

EXAMINATION

General points

Is the patient shocked and pale? If the patient is tachycardic and hypotensive, but visible bleeding is minimal a ruptured ectopic pregnancy should be suspected. Women with a haemoperitoneum usually lie still and don't move around. If there is excessive bleeding with pain a speculum examination should be performed to exclude products lodged in the cervical canal.

Abdominal examination

- **Palpation:** If there is tenderness is it diffuse, unilateral or bilateral? An ectopic may be suggested by true peritonism. Masses should be palpated for.
- **Auscultation:** A ruptured ectopic may cause an ileus.

Pelvic examination

- **The cervix:** Gentle movement may cause severe pain (cervical excitation) if there is adnexal pathology such as an ectopic.
- **The external cervical os:** If this is closed the diagnosis is more likely to be that of a missed or threatened abortion or an ectopic pregnancy. With incomplete abortion the cervix will be soft and partially open.
- **The uterus:** The size of the uterus is important. If it is small for dates this may indicate a failing pregnancy (missed abortion, blighted ovum or ectopic pregnancy). A large for dates uterus may indicate trophoblastic disease. A tender uterus may indicate a bleeding miscarriage (myometrial irritation).
- **Adnexal masses:** These are most likely to occur with ectopic pregnancies

The speculum examination

This is important to exclude vaginal and cervical causes of bleeding and to see tissue coming through the cervical os. This tissue should be removed with sponge forceps to reduce pain and bleeding and then sent to histology.

INVESTIGATIONS

- **A full blood count** should be performed. A low result in the absence of heavy external bleeding may indicate an ectopic pregnancy with significant intraperitoneal bleeding.
- **A group and save** should be performed to establish if the patient is Rhesus negative. It may be helpful if the patient requires a blood transfusion later.
- **Serum HCG level:** This investigation need not be performed where a diagnosis has already been made. However, in more difficult cases it can help establish a diagnosis in a number of ways.

Each laboratory will have their own established level of serum HCG which defines a 'positive pregnancy test' and this varies from lab to lab. HCG is produced by ongoing intrauterine pregnancies, incomplete abortions, blighted ova, missed abortions, ectopics and trophoblastic disease. In an ongoing intrauterine pregnancy the HCG level can be expected to double every 2–3 days. Hence, a series of HCG measurements with static or falling levels are unlikely to occur with a normal pregnancy. However, a proportion of normal pregnancies show a rise less significant than the doubling every 48 hours mentioned above and furthermore ectopic pregnancies **do** sometimes show this pattern. Ectopic pregnancies can rupture even with a falling HCG.

It is also true that after complete miscarriage, evacuation of the uterus or removal of an ectopic pregnancy, the HCG level should halve approximately every 2 days. If this does not happen either the diagnosis is wrong or inadequate treatment has taken place.

Isolated HCG measurements used in conjunction with ultrasound can also help in deciding management.

Ultrasound

The important points are as follows:

1. The presence of an intrauterine pregnancy sac

With a transvaginal scan (TVS), an intrauterine gestation sac should be visible in a normal pregnancy by 5 weeks' gestation. If the uterus is empty consider wrong dates, an ectopic pregnancy or a complete miscarriage. A pseudo sac, which represents the decidual reaction to a pregnancy developing elsewhere (i.e. ectopic), may masquerade as an intrauterine pregnancy. Because the LMP may be uncertain the gestational age may also be unclear. Studies have shown that when the serum HCG value is >1500 IU/L then an intrauterine sac should be visible on TVS. Unless there is a significant possibility of a complete miscarriage (e.g. history of heavy PV bleeding with tissue loss) then a laparoscopy is indicated if the uterus is empty and the HCG exceeds this value.

2. Shape of the intrauterine sac

The intrauterine sac should be regular in outline. A crumpled sac may indicate a failing pregnancy.

3. The presence of a fetal pole

A fetal pole will be visible with a transvaginal scan by 6 weeks' gestation. When the gestation sac is over 2.0–2.5 cm in diameter it should also be visible. A blighted ovum is diagnosed by the absence of a fetal pole in a sac greater in size than this. If there is any doubt repeat the scan in 7–10 days. If there has been no change in the scan findings, the diagnosis can be made confidently. Pseudo sacs generally appear only a few mms in size and do not have the definite bright rim around them of a true intrauterine sac.

4. Presence of a fetal heart beat

The presence of a fetal heart beat within the uterus is indicative of an ongoing pregnancy. Fetal pulsations can usually be visualized as soon as the fetal pole is big enough to measure and their absence with a fetal pole >6 mm indicates a missed abortion.

5. Intrapelvic masses

A pelvic mass is seen on scan in only a proportion of ectopic pregnancies.

6. Free fluid

This is not diagnostic of an ectopic pregnancy but if present may represent bleeding into the pouch of Douglas. It may also represent bleeding or fluid from a ruptured ovarian cyst. It is important not to ignore this finding.

Other investigations such as vaginal swabs, cervical smear and urine for culture will be guided by clinical features and history.

MANAGEMENT

An ectopic pregnancy is easily missed. It should always be excluded before a final diagnosis is made.

The collapsed patient

If a patient is bleeding excessively, or has collapsed, urgent action is required;

- Call for senior help.
- Establish good iv access.
- Cross-match blood: 2–4 units may be sufficient to start with.
- Administer oxygen and raise the foot of the bed.
- Correct hypovolaemia with blood and colloids. Haemaccel is a good choice but it may be necessary to use uncrossmatched O Rh negative blood.
- If the bleeding is heavy per vagina or the patient is bradycardiac, perform a speculum examination to see if there are any products of conception in the cervical os. If present they should be removed with sponge forceps. This often reduces the haemorrhage and pain.
- If a ruptured ectopic is suspected arrange theatre immediately and warn the anaesthetic staff. Do not wait for blood to arrive or to be given to the patient before operating.

SUSPECTED MISCARRIAGE

Before acting on the diagnosis, be certain. Serum HCG levels and ultrasound scans should be interpreted with great care. If ectopic pregnancy has not been definitely excluded but the patient is well and has no pain or tenderness outpatient management with serial HCG measurements can be considered. Always warn the patient to report a change or any new symptoms. If an intrauterine sac has been visualized but doubt remains over the viability of the pregnancy, then a repeat scan one week later may add certainty to the diagnosis. Be honest with the patient about your fears and uncertainty.

A suboptimal rise in HCG levels and/or absence of a fetal pole strengthens the diagnosis of a blighted ovum or missed abortion.

Management options once diagnosis is certain are given below:

1. Expectant

Complete miscarriage can occur without heavy bleeding or excessive discomfort although it is impossible to predict when a spontaneous loss will occur and how significant the symptoms will be. However some women wish to avoid more active management and there is minimal risk to them if they choose this option. Always give ward contact numbers to facilitate access to medical help should this be desired at a later date.

2. Medical

The use of 400 micrograms of misoprostol may bring about complete uterine evacuation. This method of medical management is not practised in all centres.

3. Surgical

Dilatation and curettage is commonly used (more accurately known as 'evacuation of retained products of conception'). If the patient is bleeding heavily she should be taken to theatre immediately. If the bleeding is slight a more convenient time can be arranged often allowing the patient to go home and return for theatre at a later time. See 'Practical procedures' section (p. 316) for help with consent.

Other points

Rhesus negative mothers will require anti-D (usually 250 IU im) administered within 48 hours of the bleeding starting. Recurrent bleeding does not necessitate anti-D more often than every 6 weeks.

Although a common problem, miscarriages are associated with considerable psychological upset. In most cases you will not be able to provide an explanation for why it has happened. One in every 6–7 conceptions will miscarry and it is sometimes helpful to stress how commonly it occurs. Having one, or even two, miscarriages does not significantly increase the risks of it occurring next time. Patients suffering three or more miscarriages should be considered for investigation at a recurrent miscarriage clinic.

SUSPECTED ECTOPIC PREGNANCY

Most patients with an EP will be haemodynamically stable and emergency laparotomy will not be necessary. A number of treatment options then exist, both surgical and medical.

Surgical management

The diagnosis is usually confirmed laparoscopically. Increasingly, ectopics are also being removed laparoscopically, however this depends on surgical skills and local equipment. Recovery is faster and hospital stay shorter than with the traditional 'open' approach. Using either method, the ectopic can either be removed together with the fallopian tube (**salpingectomy**) or it can be extracted through a linear incision in the tube called a **salpingotomy.** Unless the contralateral tube has been removed or damaged, salpingectomy is the treatment of choice. It is associated with a lower subsequent ectopic pregnancy rate without decreasing the intrauterine pregnancy rate significantly. If the tube is conserved, postoperative serial HCG measurements are required to ensure complete removal of all the trophoblastic tissue. A persistently raised HCG level will require further treatment.

It is important when consenting a patient that these different possibilities are discussed.

Medical management

This option is not available in all centres. It uses **methotrexate** and is associated with very few side effects. Provided cases are selected carefully it is proving to be a safe and successful way of treating the ectopic and conserving the tube. HCG monitoring is crucial with early recourse to surgery if symptoms supervene or HCG levels fail to fall. Methotrexate can also be used to eradicate persistent trophoblast following incomplete surgical treatment after salpingotomy or when the ectopic is sited in a surgically difficult site (e.g. cornua or cervix).

HYPEREMESIS

This is the presence of excessive vomiting in pregnancy such that the patient becomes dehydrated.

Causes

- normal pregnancy
- multiple pregnancy
- molar pregnancy.

History

- Establish the date of the last menstrual period.
- Ask about the time and amount of vomiting.
- Exclude the presence of any infection such as chest, urine or bowel.
- Is the vomiting a new phenomena or has the patient had nausea throughout the pregnancy? e.g. is this just gastroenteritis?

EXAMINATION

- **General:** How dehydrated is the patient. Is her breath ketotic? Is there anything to suggest a GI or urinary tract cause?
- **Uterus:** Does the uterine size match the gestation? A large for dates uterus may suggest a molar or multiple pregnancy.

INVESTIGATIONS

- **Full blood count:** A very raised white cell count may be a sign of infection.
- **Urea and electrolytes:** To see how dehydrated the patient is and exclude significant electrolyte imbalance.
- **Urine:** To look for ketones.
- **Scan:** To establish an ongoing single or multiple pregnancy and exclude a molar pregnancy.

MANAGEMENT

- **Expectant:** Complete bed rest with iv fluids. Pay particular attention to the sodium and potassium values and replace salts as necessary. Severe hyponatraemia can result in seizures and coma and can occur in more serious cases. Do not rush the reintroduction of food and drink.
- **Active:** As expectant but with anti-emetic drugs such as prochlorperazine, metoclopramide or promethazine. None are licensed for use in the first trimester, but extensive use over a number of years has failed to show any harmful effects.
- **Parental feeding:** May be required, but the help of specialist staff should be sought. Thiamine deficiency can occur in the most severe cases resulting in Wernicke's encephalopathy. Serious consideration should be given to intravenous B vitamin supplements in prolonged cases.

A **molar pregnancy** requires evacuation of the uterus, performed by an experienced operator. All patients with trophoblastic disease must be registered with one of the three specialist centres who will organize appropriate follow-up (*see* p. 290).

PAIN AND POSITIVE PREGNANCY TEST

CAUSES

- **Ectopic pregnancy**.
- **Incomplete miscarriage:** An early miscarriage often presents with bleeding and lower abdominal pain. The pain is caused by the passage of clots through the cervix and once a diagnosis is made (see above) the treatment is usually an evacuation of uterus in theatre under general anaesthetic.
- **Bleeding corpus luteum:** The presence of an early intrauterine pregnancy confirmed on ultrasound can be complicated by pain

if the corpus luteum of that pregnancy is bleeding into the abdominal cavity. To establish such a diagnosis a laparoscopy has to be performed and the bleeding stopped.

- **Coincidental pathology:** e.g. UTI or appendicitis.

PELVIC PAIN AND NEGATIVE PREGNANCY TEST

KEYPOINT

Despite the negative pregnancy test are you sure that this is not an ectopic pregnancy?

Urinary pregnancy tests have a false negative rate and if there is any doubt perform a serum HCG before finally excluding an ectopic pregnancy.

GYNAECOLOGICAL CAUSES

- Primary dysmenorrhoea
- Acute or chronic pelvic infection
- Exacerbation of endometriosis
- Complications of ovarian masses:
  - rupture of a cyst
  - bleeding into a cyst or tumour
  - ovarian torsion
  - ovarian hyperstimulation syndrome.
- Complications of fibroids:
  - degeneration (generally seen in pregnancy)
  - extrusion of fibroid polyp through cervical os.

NON-GYNAECOLOGICAL CAUSES

- **Bowel related:**
  - appendicitis
  - diverticular disease
  - constipation
  - irritable bowel syndrome
  - bowel perforation
  - bowel obstruction.
- **Urinary:**
  - calculi
  - pyelonephritis
  - cystitis.

INITIAL ASSESSMENT

Assess the situation:

- How ill is the patient?
  - is this an 'acute abdomen'?
  - is active resuscitation or urgent intervention required?
- How long has the patient had the pain for?
- Has she had it before?

HISTORY

- **Symptoms suggesting a gynaecological cause will include:**
  - bilateral lower abdominal and pelvic pain
  - dyspareunia
  - menstrual disturbance
  - presence of menstruation or vaginal bleeding.
- **Symptoms suggesting a non-gynaecological cause:**
  - urinary symptoms
  - disturbance of bowel habit
  - loss of appetite
  - nausea and vomiting (this may be present with some gynaecological conditions).

CLINICAL EXAMINATION

Most signs are non-specific and may occur with gynaecological or non-gynaecological conditions. These include fever, tachycardia, signs of peritonism such as tenderness, guarding and rebound tenderness, abdominal distension and masses.

In general, pelvic masses and/or tenderness are more likely to be gynaecological in origin, particularly if cervical excitation is present.

SPECIAL INVESTIGATIONS

These will depend upon the presentation, the potential causes and the apparent urgency of the situation. When pelvic infection is suspected appropriate microbiological specimens must be taken before starting treatment.

In most cases a full blood count and pelvic ultrasound are necessary. Always consider non gynaecological causes and involve other specialties where necessary.

OVARIAN HYPERSTIMULATION SYNDROME

The ovarian hyperstimulation syndrome is an iatrogenic condition that is an important unwanted effect of fertility treatment. It can occur after stimulation of ovulation with gonadotrophins, gonadotropin-releasing hormone (GnRH), HCG or clomiphene. Multiple large follicles appear in the ovaries and there is accumulation of fluid in body cavities.

Patients most at risk

- Women who have been hyperstimulated before
- Young women (<35 years)
- Women who have required a long course of gonadotrophins.

Presenting complaints

- Abdominal pain
- Oedema
- Abdominal distension
- Breathlessness.

EXAMINATION

Look for hypovolaemia (hypotension and tachycardia), ascites, pleural and pericardial effusions and evidence of thromboembolic events. Measure the abdominal girth to help monitor progression and resolution of any ascites.

INVESTIGATIONS

- Ultrasound scan
  - size of ovaries
  - presence of ascites
  - pleural or pericardial effusions
- Haemoglobin and haematocrit
- Urea and electrolytes
- Clotting screen
- Serum albumin and LFTs
- Chest X-ray.

TREATMENT

All cases require careful assessment by experienced staff. Treatment should aim to provide symptomatic relief, reverse haemoconcentration, prevent thromboembolism and to maintain cardiorespiratory and renal function. In mild to moderate cases of ovarian hyperstimulation syndrome the patient should be monitored by serial ultrasound scans, sometimes at home and with bed rest until the cysts resolve. In severe cases where the ovaries are enlarged and full of cysts the patient must be:

- Admitted to hospital.
- Placed on bed rest.
- Given intravenous fluids and albumin.
- Given analgesics.
- Monitored with serial urea and electrolytes, platelets, ultrasound scans and serum protein levels.
- Consideration should be given to anticoagulating the patient with sc heparin or at the very least using anti-thrombotic stockings.
- Termination of pregnancy is only necessary in exceptional cases.
- Embryo transfer should be delayed as rising HCG levels from a successful implantation will serve only to fuel the condition.

23

PRACTICAL PROCEDURES

URETHRAL CATHETERIZATION

Urethral catheterization can either be performed with the patient anaesthetized prior to an abdominal operation or with the patient awake to empty the bladder post operatively when the patient is unable to void.

The operator should observe sterile procedures, having washed their hands with hibitane and donned gloves. In the sterile pack there should be:

- A sterile aqueous solution (chlorhexidine).
- A sterile catheter (either a Foley catheter or a Quill).
- Sterile drapes.
- Sterile swabs.
- A sterile kidney dish.
- A catheter bag is also required if a Foley catheter is to be left *in situ.*

PROCEDURE

- The patient is placed in the dorsal position, the knees flexed and hips extended.
- Standing on the right hand side of the patient a sterile drape is placed below the buttocks and across the lower abdomen.
- A sterile swab dipped in chlorhexidine is used to clean the pubis and urethra in an anteroposterior direction.
- The left hand is now used to expose the urethra and the process repeated.
- Without moving the left hand the sterile catheter is placed into the urethra and bladder.
- The urine is drained into the kidney dish.
- If using a Quill catheter, the catheter is removed while pressure is applied suprapubically and the bladder is empty.
- If a Foley catheter is to be left *in situ,* the balloon of the catheter

is filled with 20 mL water for injection via its port and a catheter bag is attached and the catheter and bag is taped to the leg.

HORMONE IMPLANTS

Hormone implants are available as oestrogen or testosterone in a pellet form. The size of the pellet varies with the dose. Oestrogen is available in 25, 50 and 100 mg. Testosterone is available in 100 mg form only, but by cutting it in half a lesser dose can be obtained.

The aim of the implant is to raise oestrogen or testosterone levels in the patient to relieve symptoms of the menopause. (Testosterone is thought to improve libido.)

The site of implants can be the lower anterior abdominal wall or buttock (upper outer quadrant).

Equipment

A sterile pack contains:

- Local anaesthetic (2 mL 1% lignocaine)
- Mediswabs × 2
- Sterile drape
- Sterile glove
- Green needle
- Orange needle
- Scalpel
- Catgut suture.

THE PROCEDURE

- Wash hands and don sterile gloves.
- Expose the area destined for the implant.
- Clean the skin over an area of 6 × 6 cm with the Mediswabs.
- Make a hole in the sterile drape and place that over the cleaned area.
- Draw up the local anaesthetic with a green needle with a 2 mL syringe.
- Change the needle to a small orange needle and inject local anaesthetic just under the skin over an area of about 1 cm.
- Wait for one minute.
- During this time ask the assistant to open the implant required and place the pellet onto the sterile pack.
- With the scalpel blade make a small (0.5 cm) skin incision through the area which has been anaesthetized with the local anaesthetic.

- With the trocar and cannula together push this through into the skin incision into the subcutaneous fat about 1 cm.
- Remove the trocar.
- Place the implant onto the shelf on the cannula and push it into the subcutaneous fat with the blunt trocar provided.
- Remove the trocar and cannula together.
- Swab the incision.
- Place one catgut stitch across the incision and tie securely.
- Cut the suture with the scalpel blade.
- Cover the wound with a sterile dressing or plaster.

PROSTAGLANDIN-INDUCED TERMINATION OF PREGNANCY

Termination of pregnancy can be legally carried out in Britain up until 24 weeks' gestation and there is no limit if there is a very serious congenital abnormality. Most are performed much earlier. At less than 9 weeks' of pregnancy a medical termination can be performed using 200 mg RU 486 (mifepristone) followed by a prostaglandin 48 hours later (such as Gemeprost (PGE_1) or misoprostol). The highest success rates occur at <7 weeks' gestation. Between 9 and 12 weeks a surgical termination is usually required by using a general anaesthetic and vacuum extraction of products from the uterus.

Beyond 12 weeks when the fetus is getting too large for vacuum extraction, prostaglandins once again become the method of choice.

Once all the necessary legal paperwork has been completed and the patient has signed a consent form the prostaglandin-induced termination of pregancy (PG-TOP) can be commenced in two forms:

- Extramniotic PG-TOP
- Gemeprost/misoprostol TOP.

EXTRAMNIOTIC PG-TOP

This method is becoming less popular and may not be used in your unit.

Before starting make sure the patient is not allergic to penicillin. A sterile solution of 500 mg ampicillin, 1 mg of prostaglandin E2 and 40 units of syntocinon is mixed together with normal saline. The total volume is 50 mL and this is put into a 50 mL syringe and connected via a fine tube to the Foley catheter, which is primed with the fluid.

With the patient in the dorsal position, the legs flexed at the knee and abducted at the hips, a sterile Cuscoe speculum is put into the vagina and opened to expose the cervix. The cervix is cleaned using an aqueous solution of hibitane on a sterile swab by use of a sponge holder. Using a no-touch technique and holding the Foley catheter gently with the sponge forceps the catheter is introduced through the cervix until the tip and the part holding the balloon is well into the uterus. The balloon of the catheter is then blown up with the air in its reservoir. The prostaglandin solution is then ready for it to be infused into the uterus via a syringe pump. The patient is allowed to eat and drink normally initially. Once pain is experienced analgesics are administered as necessary until the patient aborts spontaneously. This process can take between 12 and 72 hours, the infusion being replaced as necessary.

GEMEPROST/MISOPROSTOL TOP (SECOND TRIMESTER TOP)

When Gemeprost or misoprostol are used the same premise of consent and legality has to be satisfied. Most practioners now 'prime' the uterus with 200 mg of mifepristone. Ensure that the consent has been obtained prior to giving it as it occasionally will induce abortion on its own. Forty-eight hours later the patient is admitted and a vaginal examination is performed. Gemeprost pessaries or misoprostol tablets (not licenced for this use) are then placed in the posterior fornix. This process is repeated every 3 hours until a spontaneous abortion occurs. If after five doses no abortion has taken place, the patient should be re-examined. If the cervix is still closed the same dosing protocol can be repeated the following day or an intravenous infusion of syntocinon is started. If after another 24 hours there has been no progress on vaginal examination extramniotic prostaglandins should be considered (see above).

Once an abortion has occurred, if it is complete and the patient is not bleeding no further action is required. If however the abortion is thought to be incomplete the patient is taken to theatre for evacuation of uterus. Remember to administer 250 IU of anti-D to Rhesus negative patients <20 weeks and perform a Kleihauer test and give 500 IU of anti-D to those ≥20 weeks.

INSERTION AND REMOVAL OF INTRAUTERINE CONTRACEPTIVE DEVICE

There are many different intrauterine contraceptive devices (IUCDs). The most frequently used are the copper containing devices which have individual intrauterine lifespans. Copper containing IUCDs are thought to alter the endometrial millieu and prevent implantation. Other IUCDs are plastic and are coated with a progestogen. This also prevents implantation but has the added benefit of reducing menstruation.

TO INSERT AN IUCD

Firstly, establish that the patient is not pregnant. An IUCD should be inserted during the first 10 days of the cycle. If there is any doubt perform a pregnancy test and/or scan to establish the non-pregnant state.

Equipment (all sterile)

- Cuscoe speculum
- Drape
- Single toothed vulsellum
- Long scissors
- Sponge forceps
- Cotton wool buds
- Uterine sound.

PROCEDURE

- With the patient in the dorsal position, flexed knees and hips abducted, a vaginal examination should be performed to establish the size and position of the uterus, i.e. anteverted or retroverted.
- Place a sterile Cuscoes speculum in the vagina and visualize the cervix.
- Clean the cervix using a sterile swab gripped in a sponge forceps and dipped in aqueous hibitane.
- Grip the anterior lip of the cervix with the single toothed vulsellum and gently pull in the vaginal axis to correct any flexion of the uterus.
- Sound the uterus to measure its length.
- Push the IUCD into the uterus as per instructions on the packet of the IUCD (every IUCD manufacturer has different methods of insertion).
- Use the sound to ensure that the IUCD is not lying in the cervical canal.
- Remove the vulsellum and cut the strings of the IUCD to a length of about 1–2 cm from the cervix.
- Remove the speculum.

The patient is allowed to feel the redundant IUCD threads so she knows what to feel for when she examines herself to make sure the IUCD is still in place. The patient is asked to return to have the position of the IUCD checked in 2 months' time.

TAKING A CERVICAL SMEAR

All women over the age of 20 who have been sexually active (with a uterus) should have smears performed every 3 years. This practice should continue to about 60 years of age, but the frequency and duration of cervical smears may alter depending on results. A smear is best taken when the patient is not menstruating as reading the smear can be more difficult.

Before taking a smear the date of the last menstrual period should be ascertained so the pathologist knows the day of the cycle.

Equipment

- Cuscoe speculum
- Aylesbury spatula
- Glass slide
- Fixing solution.

PROCEDURE

With the patient in the dorsal position, knees flexed, hips adbucted, a Cuscoes speculum is inserted into the vagina to expose the cervix. With the Aylesbury spatula in the right hand, the most distal portion of it (the more pointed end) is inserted into the cervical os and rotated through 360 degrees and then back through 360 degrees. The spatula is then withdrawn and both sides of it wiped over the glass slide. The fixative solution is then dropped over the glass slide and the slide is then allowed to dry in air.

CERVICAL CRYOCAUTERY AND LOOP DIATHERMY

Cervical cryocautery and loop diathermy are both methods of treating cervical abnormalities. Cervical cryocautery is usually used to treat a cervix with an ectropion which has a normal cytology.

Loop diathermy is either performed in the colposcopy clinic under local anaesthetic or in theatre under general anaesthetic.

CERVICAL CRYOCAUTERY

Procedure

- Establish the patient is not pregnant.
- Place the patient in the lithotomy position.
- Insert a Cuscoe speculum into the vagina to expose the cervix.
- Chose a cryocautery attachment to fit the shape of the cervix.
- Apply the cryocautery apparatus to the cervix and switch on.
- Keep the apparatus applied to the cervix for 2 minutes.
- Turn off the cryocautery machine.
- Remove the probe carefully from the cervix as it often 'freezes' to it and can denude the treated area if time is not allowed for it to separate spontaneously.
- Remove the Cuscoe speculum from the vagina.

LLETZ (LARGE LOOP EXCISION OF THE TRANSFORMATION ZONE)

Procedure

With the patient in the lithotomy position in the colposcopy clinic and where all the abnormal area of the cervix is visible a loop excision can be performed under local anaesthetic.

- A Cuscoe speculum is placed into the vagina and the cervix is visualized.
- 10 mL of local anaesthetic (Citanest) is injected into both lateral aspects of the cervix using a dental syringe and needle.
- With the patient anaesthetized and a suction apparatus attached to the Cuscoe speculum, the loop diathermy cautery is placed onto the cervix lateral to the abnormal area.
- The diathermy is switched on and is pulled laterally to cut off a cone-shaped area of cervix. This is removed using a sponge forceps.
- The base of the area is cauterized using ball diathermy.
- When the bleeding has stopped the Cuscoe speculum is removed and 20 mL Sultrin cream is put into the vagina to prevent infection.

ENDOMETRIAL BIOPSY

Endometrial biopsy is a procedure to establish the presence or absence of endometrial pathology or to determine the effect of various hormones on the endometrium. It can either be performed blindly or under direct vision. It is possible to take an endometrial biopsy in outpatients with no pre-medication or anaesthetic. A number of different devices are available but the Pipelle and Z-samplers are used more frequently than Vabra.

PROCEDURE

With the patient in the dorsal position, knees flexed and abducted at the hips, a vaginal examination is performed to establish the size and position of the uterus.

- A Cuscoe speculum is placed in the vagina to expose the cervix.
- The sampling device is introduced through the cervix into the uterine cavity.
- The internal os is often closed and traction on the cervix with the single toothed tenaculum often helps and is usually tolerated well.
- A negative vacuum is then applied by withdrawing the inner core and a piece of endometrium is sucked into the pipelle.
- This is placed in a pot containing formalin and analysed in histopathology.
- The pipelle and speculum are then removed from the vagina and the patient is allowed to rest (sometimes this procedure is painful due to the minimal cervical dilatation).

OUTPATIENT HYSTEROSCOPY

Using a hysteroscope an endometrial biopsy can be obtained under direct vision.

- With the patient in lithotomy position the patient is examined to establish the size and position of the uterus.
- A Sims' speculum is placed in the vagina to expose the cervix which is grasped gently with a single toothed vulsellum.
- 15 mL of local anaesthetic (Citanest) is introduced into both para cervical ligaments using a syringe.
- The cervix is gently dilated using the gas hysteroscope.
- Through the hysteroscope the endometrium can be visualized.
- Any abnormal area is then noted and the small biopsy forceps are introduced along the hysteroscope and the biopsy taken under direct vision.
- The biopsy and hysteroscope are removed. The biopsy is sent off for analysis. The vulsellum and Sims' speculum are removed.
- The patient is allowed to rest prior to being allowed home.

DILATATION AND CURETTAGE

This procedure, although commonly undertaken, is now being superceded by hysteroscopy. Dilatation and curettage (D&C) is a blind procedure to explore the uterine cavity. It is used in cases of postmenopausal bleeding and menstrual irregularity after the age of 40.

- It is usually performed under a general anaesthetic in theatre.
- The patient is placed in the lithotomy position and the vulva and vagina are cleansed with aqueous chlorhexidine.
- A vaginal examination is performed to establish the size and position of the uterus.
- A Sims' speculum is placed in the vagina to expose the cervix.
- The anterior lip of the cervix is grasped using a double toothed vulsellum.
- A uterine sound is pushed gently through the cervix in the line of the uterus, i.e. anterior for an anteverted uterus and posterior for a retroverted uterus.
- When resistance is met the length of the uterine cavity can be established from the marks on the sound.
- Having established the length and position of the uterus, the cervix is gently dilated using the Hagar dilators, gradually from size 3 to 8.
- Care must be taken to avoid damage to the cervix with over-enthusiastic pressure with the Hegar dilators.
- Perforation of the uterus must also be avoided by ascertaining the correct size of the uterus and taking care.
- A curette is then inserted gently into the uterine cavity to reach the fundus.
- Firm pressure can then be used when drawing the curette back toward the internal os across the endometrium.
- This manoeuvre is repeated a number of times along different areas of the endometrium.

SECTION 3: APPENDICES

SECTION 3: APPENDICES

CONTENTS

appendices

SECTION [illegible] APPENDICES

CONTENTS

APPENDIX I

A PHARMACOPOIEA OF COMMONLY PRESCRIBED DRUGS IN OBSTETRICS AND GYNAECOLOGY

Drug	Dosage	Route	Notes
Aciclovir (**Zovirax**)	200 mg 5×/day	po	For treatment of buccal and vaginal herpes simplex.
	5–10 mg/kg tds	iv	For complicated varicella-zoster infections in pregnancy.
	5% cream ×5/day	top	For labial and genital herpes simplex.
Aluminium hydroxide (suspension)	5–10 mL qds	po	Between meals and before bedtime. Tendency to cause constipation.
Ampicillin	0.25–1.0 g qds	po	Broad spectrum antibiotic but *Staphylococcus aureus*, *E. coli*
	usually 500 mg qds	im/iv	and *Haemophilus influenzae* may be resistant.
Amoxycillin	250 mg tds	po	Double dose in severe infections. Better oral absorption than
	500 mg tds	im/iv	ampicillin.
Anusol cream	twice daily	top	Apply to haemorrhoids.
Arachis oil enema	130 mL single dose	pr	Faecal softener. Warm before use.
Azithromycin	1 g single dose	po	Treatment of genital chlamydia.
Betamethasone	2× 12 mg doses 24 hours apart	im	For promoting fetal lung development. To be effective give at least 24 hours prior to delivery if possible. Evidence supports its use between 24 and 34 weeks' gestation and possibly up to 36 weeks.
Bromocriptine	2.5 mg on 1st day then bd for 14 days	po	For prevention of lactation in selected situations. Seek advice prior to its use. See BNF for use in prolactinomas and acromegaly.
Cabergoline	1 mg first day postpartum	po	A one-off dose for suppression of lactation. Also used in hyperprolactinaemia.

Drug	Dosage	Route	Notes
Carboprost (**Haemabate**)	250 micrograms stat	Deep im	For PPH secondary to uterine atony when other measures fail. Dose can be repeated every 15–90 min to maximum of 8 times (total permissible dose 2 mg).
Cefotaxime	usu 1 g bd	im/iv	Moderate to severe infections.
	2 g qds	im/iv	Life-threatening infections.
	1 g single dose	im/iv	For gonorrhoea.
Ceftazidime	usually 1 g tds	im/iv	
Cefuroxime	usually 750 mg tds	im/iv	1.5 mg iv for surgical prophylaxis. Give on induction ± 2 post op doses of 750 mg 8 and 16 hours later.
Cephalexin	250 mg qds or 500 mg tds	po	
Cephradine	250–500 mg qds	po	
Chlorpheniramine maleate (**Piriton**)	4 mg 4–6 hourly	po	
Chlorpromazine	25–50 mg stat then tds	po/im	For short-term management of violent/agitated patients. Wait 20 min to judge effect and give further dose if needed.
Ciprofloxacin	250–750 mg bd	po	
	100–400 mg bd	iv	(over 30–60 min)
	750 mg single dose	po	60–90 min prior to procedure for surgical prophylaxis.
Clomiphene (**Clomid**)	50–100 mg od d2–d6 of cycle	po	For anovulatory infertility. See 'The infertile couple'.
Clotrimazole (**Canestan**)	500 mg pessary	pv	Single one-off dose for vaginal candidiasis.
	1% cream 2–3 ×/day	top	Stronger creams available with shorter treatment regimes.
Co-Amoxiclav (**Augmentin**)	375 or 675 mg tds	po	
	600 mg–1.2 g tds/qds	Slow iv	
	1.2 g at induction	Slow iv	For surgical prophylaxis.
Codeine phosphate	30–60 mg prn or 4 hourly	po/im	Max dose =240 mg/day.
Co-codamol	1–2 tabs every	po	

Drug	Dosage	Route	Notes
Co-dydramol	4–6 hours		
Co-proxamol			
Cyclizine	50 mg tds/prn	po/iv/im	Commonly used in hyperemesis.
Danazol	200–800 mg daily in up to 4 divided doses	po	For endometriosis. Usually for 6 months. Begin during menses. Effective contraception required Aim to achieve amenorrhoea.
Diamorphine	5–10 mg 4 hourly	sc/im	For acute pain.
Diazepam	2 mg tds	po	For anxiety (starting dose).
	10 mg over 2 min	iv	For seizure control.
Diclofenac	Max 150 mg/day		
	25–50 mg tds	po	For regular pain control.
	75 mg od	deep im	For severe pain control. Max. 2 days.
	100 mg 18 hourly	pr	For post-op pain relief.
Dihydrocodeine	30 mg 4–6 hourly	po	
	30–50 mg 4–6 hourly	im	
Dinoprostone	1 and 2 mg doses (posterior fornix)	pv	For induction of labour.
Doxycycline	100 mg bd	po	For genital chlamydia treatment needs to be 14 days.
Dydrogesterone (**Duphaston**)	10 mg bd d11–d25	po	For dysfunctional uterine bleeding.
	10 mg 2–3× daily d5–d25	po	For endometriosis.
	10 mg bd d5–d25	po	For dysmenorrhoea.
Ergometrine	500 micrograms stat	im/iv	For treatment of PPH or prevention in high risk cases. Give only after delivery of shoulders. See also **Syntometrine**.
Erythromycin	250–500 mg qds	po	
Ferrous sulphate	200 mg 1–3×/day	po	For treatment of iron deficiency anaemia. Dose may be limited by SE.
Flucloxacillin	250 mg qds	po/im	
	250 mg–1 g qds	iv	
Fluconazole (**Diflucan One**)	150 mg capsule stat	po	For recurrent/acute vaginal candidiasis.

Drug	Dosage	Route	Notes
Folic acid	400 micrograms od	po	To prevent first occurrence of NTD. Take before conception and until 12 weeks' gestation.
	4–5 mg od	po	To prevent recurrence of NTD. Take when trying for pregnancy and until 12 weeks' gestation.
Frusemide	20–40 mg	slow iv/po	Dose can be repeated and increased but caution.
Gaviscon	10–20 mL qds	po	After meals and before bedtime.
Gemeprost **(Cervagem)**	1 mg pessary (posterior fornix)	pv	For softening and ripening the cervix prior to first trimester transcervical procedures. Administer 3 hours before. For use in second trimester termination (see p. 205.)
Gentamicin	2–5 mg/kg/day in three divided doses	im/slow iv	Pre and one hour post dose levels should be performed. Max peak conc.=10 mg/L and max. trough conc.= 2 mg/L. If the peak level is too high, reduce the dose. If the trough is too high reduce the frequency. See BNF for endocarditis prophylaxis.
Gestrinone	2.5 mg twice weekly	po	Start on first day of the cycle. Treatment for endometriosis.
Glycerol suppositories	1 supp. prn	pr	
Haloperidol	5–10 mg stat	im/po	For violent or agitated patients. Wait 20 min to judge effect. Give further dose if needed.
Heparin – prophylaxis (give first dose 1–2 h prior to surgery)			
(Calciparine)			
Heparin calcium	5000 units bd	sc	Unfractionated heparin.
(Clexane)			
Enoxaparin	20 mg od	sc	Low molecular weight heparin (LMWH).
	40 mg od	sc	If high risk.
(Fragmin)			
Dalteparin	2500 u od	sc	LMWH.
	5000 u od	sc	If very high risk.

Drug	Dosage	Route	Notes
Heparin – treatment of DVT/PE			
(**Calciparine**)	Load with 5000 u iv then 1000–2000 u/h iv or 15 000 units sc bd for 5 days at least (DVT and PE). Aim to keep APTT 1.5–2.5		
(**Clexane**)	1 mg/kg sc bd for at least 5 days (DVT only).		
(**Fragmin**)	10 000–18 000 units sc od for at least 5 days (DVT only).		
(**Tinzaparin**)	175 u/kg sc od for at least 6 days (DVT and PE).		
Hydralazine	5–10 mg (over 10 minutes) 25–75 mg tds/qds	Slow iv po	For hypertensive crises. Can be repeated 30 min later if necessary. Side effects include tachycardia and headache.
Hyoscine (**Buscopan**)	20 mg qds	po/im/iv	For acute spasm.
Ibuprofen	1.2–1.8 g daily in 3–4 divided doses	po	Take after food. The dose can be further increased with caution.
Indomethacin	50–200 mg/day in divided doses	po	For rheumatic disease.
Ispaghula Husk (**Fybogel**)	1 sachet bd	po	Dissolve in water.
Labetalol	100 mg bd – 500 mg tds	po	Avoid abrupt withdrawal.
Lactulose	15 mL bd	po	
Magnesium trisilicate (5% oral suspension)	10 mL tds	po	Antacid which may cause diarrhoea.
Mebeverine	135 mg tds	po	For treatment of irritable bowel syndrome.
Mefenamic Acid	500 mg tds	po	Preferably after food. For dysmenorrhoea begin taking drug 24–48 h prior to the anticipated onset of bleeding and continue regularly until the menstrual flow is settling.
Methyldopa	250 mg bd to 1 g tds	po	Increase dose gradually as required.
Metoclopramide	10 mg tds or prn 8 hourly	po/im/iv	

Drug	Dosage	Route	Notes
Metronidazole	400 mg tds	po	For anaerobic infections.
	400 mg bd	po	For bacterial vaginosis.
	500 mg tds	iv	For surgical prophylaxis give 500 mg iv shortly before surgery ± 2 or 3 post op doses at 8 hourly intervals.
Microlette microenema	5 mL dose	pr	
Mifepristone	200 mg once	po	See p. 205 for its use in first trimester terminations etc.
Morphine sulphate	10 mg up to 4 hourly	sc/im	Intravenous doses are a quarter to a half of intramuscular doses.
	5–20 mg 4 hourly	sc/im/po	For chronic pain.
(**MST Continus**)	30–60 mg bd	po	Modified release preparation used in the management of chronic pain. Doses can be further increased with 25–50% increments.
Nifedipine			The use of nifedipine 'crunches' to acutely reduce blood pressure is to be avoided. Use modified release preps.
(**Adalat Retard**)	10–40 mg bd	po	Note the different preparations. Begin with the lowest doses and increase as required.
(**Adalat LA**)	30–90 mg od	po	
Norethisterone	5 mg tds – 10 days	po	To arrest heavy bleeding.
	5 mg bd, d19–d26 of cycle	po	To prevent heavy bleeding.
	5 mg tds, d5–d24 of cycle	po	To prevent dysmenorrhoea, 3–4 cycles only.
Nystatin	1–2 pessaries for 14–28 nights	pv	For vaginal candidiasis.
Ondansetron	8 mg bd	po	For a maximum of 5 days.
	8 mg	iv/im	For treatment of post op nausea and vomiting.
Ortho dienoestrol	0.01% dienoestrol cream od	top	For short-term relief of atrophic vaginitis. Use daily for 1–2 weeks and then reduce to 1–3 times weekly attempting to stop treatment after 3–6 months.

Drug	Dosage	Route	Notes
Oxprenolol	80–120 mg bd-qds	po	Commonly used in hypertensive postnatal patients. Contraindicated in asthmatics.
Oxybutynin	2.5–5 mg 2–3 times daily	po	For detrusor instability. Dose is often limited by the side effects (dry mouth).
Oxytocin	see Syntocinon		
Paracetamol	0.5–1.0 g every 4–6 h	po	Suppositories also available.
Penicillin			
Benzylpenicillin	300–600 mg qds	im/slow iv	High dose regimes exist for certain infections.
Phenoxymethylpenicillin	250–500 mg qds	po	
Peppermint oil	1–2 caps tds	po	Before meals.
Pethidine	25–100 mg 4 hourly	sc/im	For acute pain.
	50–100 mg stat	sc/im	For pain relief in labour. Repeat 1–3 h later if needed. Max. dose in 24 h is 400 mg. Beware its use in the later stages of labour (see prescribing in pregnancy).
Potassium citrate	10 mL tds	po	Take well diluted with water for relief of mild dysuria.
Prochlorperazine (**Stemetil**)	5–10 mg 2–3 ×/day	po	For prevention of nausea and vomiting.
	12.5 mg	deep im	For acute attack of nausea and vomiting.
Promethazine (**Avomine**)	25–100 mg daily in divided doses	po	
Ritodrine (infusion)	150 mg (3 ampoules) in 35 mL of 5% dextrose. Begin at 1 mL/h and increase by 1 mL/h every 10 min until contractions cease or maternal pulse reaches 120/min or more. Max. dose = 6 mL/h. Use a syringe driver.	iv	Used for the suppression of uterine contractions to delay the establishment or progression of labour so that *in-utero* transfer or prolongation of steroid action can be achieved. See 'Antepartum emergencies' for more information (p. 139).
Salbutamol			
aerosol	100–200 micrograms 3–4 ×/day	inh	
nebulizer	2.5–5.0 mg 3–4 ×/day	neb	

Drug	Dosage	Route	Notes
Schering PC4	see 'Contraception' for prescribing information (p. 227)		
Senna tablets	15–30 mg od (2–4 tablets)	po	Preferably at bedtime.
Sodium Picosulphate (**Picolax**)	1 sachet twice	po	First sachet early morning day before theatre and second sachet mid-afternoon.
Syntocinon			
Post delivery, TOP or miscarriage	10 units stat dose	iv/im	Bolus doses can be given to prevent PPH or encourage uterine contraction. Never give boluses before delivery.
Augmentation of labour	15 units in 500 mL normal saline (30 milliunits/mL)	iv	Protocols vary. Always start with low infusion rates and build up over time depending on the frequency of contractions. Start at 1 milliunit/min (2 mL/h) and increase in steps every 15–20 min to a maximum of 48 milliunits/min (96 mL/h). See 'Problems during labour' for more detail (p. 100).
High dose infusion	30–50 units in 500 mL normal saline to run over 4 h	iv	Used to maintain tonic contraction of the uterus following atonic PPH or to prevent PPH in high-risk cases. Beware water intoxication with very high doses.
Syntometrine	1 mL (500 micrograms ergometrine with 5 units oxytocin)	im	For the routine management of third stage of labour. Give only after delivery of the shoulders and avoid in hypertensive patients (use 10 units of iv syntocinon instead).
Tamoxifen	20–40 mg od	po	For breast cancer. Also used as an alternative to clomid in a similar way.
Temazepam	10–30 mg nocte	po	
Terfenadine (**Triludan**)	60 mg bd	po	
Tetracycline	250–500 mg qds	po	
Thiamine	25–50 mg tds	po	Used in hyperemesis patients who risk Wernicke's encephalopathy if replacement is not provided.
	100 mg in 100 mL normal saline over 60 min once per week	iv	

Drug	Dosage	Route	Notes
Tolteridine	1–2 mg bd	po	A newer treatment for detrusor instability.
Tranexamic acid	1.0–1.5 g bd-qds	po	Take only during menses for menorrhagia.
Trimethoprim	200 mg bd	po	

Routes – po: oral; iv: intravenous; top: topical; im: intramuscular; pr: rectal; sc: subcutaneous; pv: vaginal; inh: inhaled; neb: nebulizer. Dosage – tds, three times a day; qds: four times a day; bd: twice a day; od: once a day; prn: as required; stat: one-off dose.

APPENDIX II

THE USE OF DRUGS DURING PREGNANCY AND BREASTFEEDING

The following lists include a number of drugs that are commonly prescribed to women of child bearing age. Information as to their safety in pregnancy and breastfeeding in many cases is limited. In only a few is there good scientific evidence for complete reassurance (e.g. amoxycillin), or conversely convincing evidence of harm which means that they must always be avoided (e.g. tetracyclines). For the rest, the relative risks and benefits must be considered with each individual women and the issues discussed with her where possible. There are a number of drugs which have gained acceptance in pregnancy and breastfeeding because extensive use has not shown obvious harm (e.g. methyldopa).

Useful principles to follow are:

- Make greater effort to avoid drugs in the first trimester when teratogenesis is most likely.
- Avoid long courses of medications where possible and use the lowest possible dose.
- Consider alternatives with a better track record (e.g. change ACE inhibitors for methyldopa or labetalol in essential hypertension).
- Inform the paediatricians at delivery if there has been maternal use of a drug with potential neonatal side effects (e.g. tricyclic antidepressants, carbimazole).

To simplify the following tables the drugs have been divided into only three categories, represented by the following symbols:

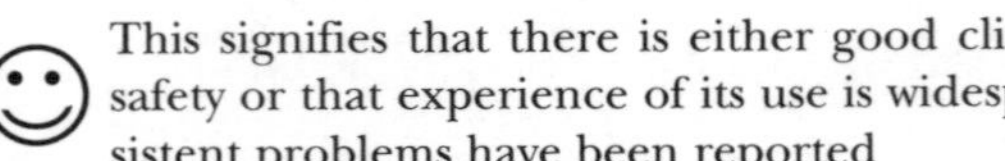

This signifies that there is either good clinical evidence for safety or that experience of its use is widespread and no consistent problems have been reported

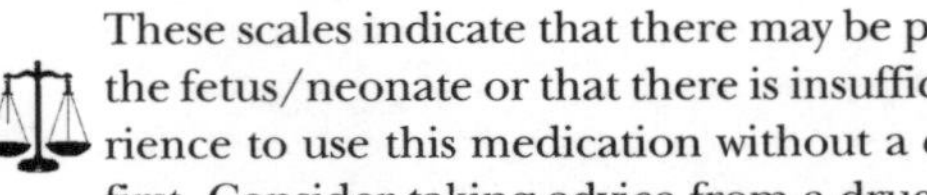

These scales indicate that there may be potential side effects on the fetus/neonate or that there is insufficient evidence or experience to use this medication without a careful risk assessment first. Consider taking advice from a drug information service.

 This symbol indicates that definite harm to a pregnancy or newborn has been shown when this drug has been used and that the risks always outweigh the benefits. Avoid.

Always take advice when asked to prescribe a drug in pregnancy or lactation if you have not previously had to consider its safety in these situations. These tables are meant only as a guide and information is constantly being updated.

USE OF DRUGS DURING PREGNANCY

Drug name	Safety (see key)	Comments
ACE INHIBITORS	⊘	Basically contraindicated. Adverse effects on fetal and neonatal blood pressure control and renal function. Possible skull defects and oligohydramnios.
Aciclovir	⚖	Safety not established. Use in life threatening infections can be justified but prophylaxis or treatment of genital herpes in pregnancy are less secure indications. No harm has been found with topical preparations.
Adenosine	⚖	Has been used to treat arrhythmias in pregnancy
Aminophylline	⚖	Safety not established. Use with caution. Monitor levels closely in pregnancy.
Amiodarone	⊘	Basically contraindicated. Potential neonatal goitre. Use in exceptional circumstances only.
Amitriptyline	⚖	Widespread experience of its use in pregnancy. One of the first line choices for depression in pregnancy. The dose of all tricyclic antidepressants should be minimized in the third trimester and paediatricians should be informed as tachycardia, muscle spasms and irritability have all been noted in neonates.
Amoxycillin	☺	Clinical studies have proven safety in humans.
Ampicillin	☺	As for amoxycillin.
Aspirin	see notes	At low dose (75 mg od) there is epidemiological evidence for its safety. At higher, regular, doses it may impair fetal/neonatal platelet function with risk of haemorrhage and also may cause early ductus closure. It competes for albumin binding sites and therefore increases risk of kernicterus. Such dosage regimes are to be avoided.
Azathioprine	⚖	A theoretical risk of chromosome abnormalities in the germ cells of the offspring has not been seen in practice. Often the indication outweighs this risk.

Drug name	Safety (see key)	Comments
BENZODIAZEPINES	⚖	Some evidence suggests teratogenicity for diazepam and temazepam although the effect of simultaneous substance/alcohol abuse are difficult to separate. All hypnotics have the potential to depress neonatal respiration and produce withdrawal phenomena.
BETABLOCKERS	⚖	No evidence of animal or human teratogenicity but IUGR, increased IUD and premature delivery reported with some, probably secondary to reduced placental perfusion. Hypoglycaemia, hypothermia and bradycardia possible in neonate. Avoid where possible (labetalol is an exception). Propranolol and sotalol are used sometimes in serious cardiac conditions.
Bezafibrate	⊘	Avoid. Theoretical risk of effect on growth and development.
Benzylpenicillin	☺	Use in pregnancy is appropriate.
Bromocriptine	☺	Although apparently safe, its use in pregnancy is to be avoided if possible. However, if the prolactinoma is large or expanding it should be maintained or resumed.
Carbamazepine	⚖	A possible human teratogen with studies showing a slight excess risk of congenital anomalies and learning difficulties. Folic acid supplementation advised. Vit K supplementation for mother near term. Monitor levels through pregnancy.
Carbimazole	⚖	Uncontrolled thyrotoxicosis is probably more harmful to the fetus than the drug, although aplasia cutis has been reported and there is potential for goitre and hypothyroidism.
CEPHALOSPORINS	☺	Possible excess of congenital malformations with 1st trimester use of cefaclor, cephradine and cephalexin. Not observed with cefuroxime or ceftriaxone. Poor information exists for use of cefotaxime and ceftazidime.
Chloramphenicol	⊘	Risk of 'grey baby syndrome' if used in third trimester. No evidence of harm for earlier use.
Chloroquine	⚖	Possible fetal eye and cochlear damage at high doses. However benefit of prophylaxis and treatment may outweigh risk.
Chlorpheniramine	☺	No teratogenicity observed but possible increase in retrolental fibroplasia in premature infants if given in last two weeks of pregnancy.

Drug name	Safety (see key)	Comments
Chlorpromazine	⚖	Lethargy, hyperexcitability, tremor, low Apgar and even seizures reported in neonates following 3rd trimester use.
Clofibrate	⊘	See bezafibrate.
Clomipramine	⚖	Potential neonatal effects. See chlorpromazine.
Ciprofloxacin	⊘	The 4-quinolones have been shown to cause arthropathy in immature animals and its use in pregnancy is not recommended.
Codeine	☺	Concern exists only for prolonged use of high doses.
Corticosteroids	⚖	High doses (>10 mg prednisolone/day) may cause fetal and neonatal adrenal suppression. Consider steroid cover in labour and inform paeds.
Co-trimoxazole	⚖	A folate antagonist so best avoided in 1st trimester. Potential neonatal haemolysis and kernicterus with third trimester use.
Cyclizine	☺	Safety not established but no evidence of harm following widespread use in first trimester.
Cyclophosphamide	⊘	
Cyclosporin A	⚖	The risks are usually outweighed by the strength of the indication. Levels must be monitored.
Danazol	⊘	Contraindicated. Being a weak androgen it can virilize a female fetus.
Diclofenac	⚖	Avoid if possible, especially the third trimester when regular doses may predispose to premature ductus arteriosus closure and pulmonary hypertension in the fetus. No evidence for teratogenicity.
Digoxin	⚖	Dose may need to be increased in pregnancy due to increased renal clearance. Overdose does pose a risk to the fetus.
Diltiazem	⚖	Possible teratogenicity.
Disopyramide	⚖	But may have oxytocic effects.
Dothiepin	⚖	See amitryptiline.
Doxepin	⚖	Safety not established. See amitryptyline.
Droperidol	⚖	Extrapyramidal effects in neonate occasionally reported.
Ergotamine	⊘	Basically contraindicated due to its oxytocic properties. Some feel it can be used sparingly with extreme caution.

Drug name	Safety (see key)	Comments
Erythromycin	☺	
Ethosuximide	⚖	No obvious teratogenicity and considered anticonvulsant of choice for petit mal epilepsy in 1st trimester.
Etretinate	⊘	Teratogenic. Avoid. Risks to fetus last many months after the end of a course of treatment.
Fansidar	⚖	The risks of malaria to pregnant mothers outweigh the possible risks of taking most antimalarials. Fansidar is a folate antagonist so supplementation is necessary. There is possibly an increased risk of kernicterus in the newborn.
Flucloxacillin	☺	
Fluconazole	⚖	Safety not established.
Fluoxetine	⚖	Safety of SSRIs has not been established in pregnancy. Use a tricyclic antidepressant if possible.
Flupenthixol	⚖	Safety not established. See droperidol.
Frusemide	⚖	Evidence of safety in third trimester. Avoid if possible.
Gentamicin	⚖	No evidence of animal teratogenicity. Theoretical risk of fetal auditory or vestibular nerve damage not observed with in utero exposure. Use justified in life threatening infections.
Haloperidol	⚖	See droperidol.
Heparin		Risks are of maternal osteoporosis, thrombocytopaenia and haemorrhage. Now considered anticoagulant of choice in pregnancy.
Hydralazine	☺	
Hyoscine	⚖	Possibly embryotoxic at very high doses.
Ibuprofen	⚖	Not obviously teratogenic but avoid third trimester use (see diclofenac).
Imipramine	⚖	No firm evidence of teratogenicity. CNS disturbance reported in neonates. See amitriptyline.
Indomethacin	⚖	Has been used as tocolytic agent and to reduce liquor volume but serious concerns exist for fetal renal compromise and premature ductus constriction.
Labetalol	☺	Used extensively for treatment of hypertension in pregnancy but be aware of possible perinatal and neonatal distress including hypoglycaemia, hypotension and bradycardia.

Drug name	Safety (see key)	Comments
Lamotrigene	⚖	Weak inhibitor of dihydrofolate reductase. Theoretical risk of NTD. Folic acid supplementation advised.
Lithium	⚖	Teratogenic with neonatal goitre and possible toxicity in the newborn. If unavoidable monitor serum levels closely through pregnancy.
Lofepramine	⚖	Safety not established. See amitriptyline.
Loperamide	⚖	
Mefenamic acid	⚖	No teratogenicity reported but see diclofenac. Not recommended.
Mefloquine	⚖	Possible teratogenicity but benefits may outweigh risks if travel to certain areas is unavoidable.
Methadone	⚖	See opioids.
Methotrexate	⊘	
Methyldopa	☺	
Metoclopramide	☺	
Metronidazole	⚖	Controversial. Certainly advisable to avoid in 1st trimester and high doses if possible. Topical clindamycin is an alternative treatment for bacterial vaginosis in pregnancy.
Nifedipine	☺	Reserve for use in severe hypertensives unresponsive to more usual agents.
Nitrofurantoin	☺	Safe in pregnancy but avoid in labour and delivery as it may cause neonatal haemolysis.
Omeprazole	⚖	Possible toxicity in animal studies. Avoid.
Ondansetron	⚖	Safety not established. An alternative is usually available.
OPIOIDS	See notes	No evidence for teratogenicity or harm to the pregnancy but beware neonatal respiratory depression and withdrawal effects on the neonates of dependent mothers.
Oxybutynin	⚖	Toxicity in high dose animal studies.
Paracetamol	☺	
Paroxetine	⚖	See fluoxetine.
Penicillin G	☺	
Phenobarbitone	⚖	Teratogenicity. Neonatal bleeding tendency. Prophylactic Vit K for mother prior to delivery. Neonatal withdrawal symptoms possible.

Drug name	Safety (see key)	Comments
Phenytoin	⚖	Congenital malformations. Folic acid supplementation and Vit K prior to delivery. Monitor levels closely.
Primaquine	⚖	Risk of haemolysis in G6PD deficient infants.
Prochlorperazine	☺	Isolated cases of congenital defects but evidence is in favour of its safety if used only occasionally and in low doses.
Proguanil	☺	Considered safe for prophylaxis.
Promethazine	☺	
Propylthiouracil	⚖	Considered the drug of choice for hyperthyroidism in pregnancy but monitor for fetal goitre and neonatal hypothyroidism.
Quinidine	⚖	Considered relatively safe but high doses may have oxytocic effect.
Quinine	⚖	High doses are teratogenic but benefit may outweigh risk in malaria prophylaxis.
Ranitidine	☺	
Salbutamol	☺	
Senna	⚖	
Sulphasalazine	☺	Risk of neonatal haemolysis. Maternal folate supplementation advised.
SULPHONAMIDES	⚖	Theoretical risk of neonatal kernicterus or haemolysis. Septrin (Trimethoprim-sulphamethoxazole) is still warranted for PCP prophylaxis in HIV.
SULPHONYLUREAS	⚖	Neonatal hypoglycaemia.
Terfenadine	⚖	
TETRACYCLINES	⊘	Contraindicated. Congenital abnormalities and adverse effects on teeth and bones reported.
Theophyllines	⚖	Safety not established. Neonatal irritability and apnoea reported. Use in severe asthma is usually justified.
Thioridazine	⚖	No adverse effects apparent. Probably safe. See droperidol.
Thyroxine	☺	
Trimethoprim	⚖	Folate antagonist. Theoretical teratogenic risk. Avoid in 1st trimester.

Drug name	Safety (see key)	Comments
Ursodeoxycholic acid	⚖	Safety not established but increasingly prescribed in cholestasis of pregnancy.
Valproate	⚖	Increased risk of NTDs (folate supplementation and screening advised) and cardiac abnormalities. Neonatal bleeding and hepatotoxicity reported.
Vancomycin	⚖	Significantly higher doses may be required to reach therapeutic levels. Administer doses over 60 minutes and measure levels.
Verapamil	⚖	Has been used to treat arrhythmias in pregnancy.
Vigabatrin	⚖	Manufacturer advises toxicity in high doses and does not recommend for use in pregnancy.
Warfarin	⚖	Congenital malformations and fetal/neonatal bleeding tendency. Heparin is probably the anticoagulant of choice, certainly for first and third trimesters.

USE OF DRUGS DURING BREAST FEEDING

Drug name/class	Safety (see key)	Comments
Aminophylline	☺	
Amiodarone	⊘	
Amitriptyline	⚖	Concentration in milk too small to be harmful but manufacturers advise to avoid.
Amoxycillin	☺	
Ampicillin	☺	
Androgens	⊘	May masculinize female infant or cause precocious development.
Antipsychotics	⚖	Small quantities only in breast milk but manufactureres advise to avoid if at all possible due to theoretical risks on CNS development (sulpiride especially).
Aspirin	⊘	Risk of platelet dysfunction and Reye's syndrome.
Atenolol	⚖	Possible toxicity although levels in milk low. Monitor infant.
Baclofen	☺	
BENZODIAZEPINES	⚖	Repeated high doses can result in neonatal lethargy.
Benzylpenicillin	☺	

Drug name/class	Safety (see key)	Comments
Bromocriptine	⊘	Suppresses lactation.
Captopril	⚖	Manufactureres advise to avoid.
Carbamazepine	☺	
Carbimazole	⚖	Use the lowest dose possible as neonatal thyroid function may be affected.
CEPHALOSPORINS	☺	Appropriate to use but caution.
Chloramphenicol	⊘	Use another antibiotic if possible. Possible bone marrow toxicity in infant.
Chloroquine	☺	
Chlorpheniramine	⚖	Small quantities in milk. May inhibit lactation. Drowsiness in infants noted.
Chlorpromazine	⚖	Drowsiness reported in the infants.
Cisapride	☺	But manufacturers advise to avoid.
Clomimpramine	⚖	See amitriptyline.
Cimetidine	☺	But manufacturers advise to avoid.
Ciprofloxacin	⊘	Little data..
Codeine	☺	
Corticosteroids	⚖	High regular doses may case neonatal adrenal suppression.
Co-trimoxazole	⚖	Competes with bilirubin for albumin binding sites so increasing risk of kernicterus in jaundiced babies. May cause haemolysis in G6PD deficient infants.
Diclofenac	☺	
Digoxin	☺	
Diltiazem	⚖	Not recommended by manufacturers.
Domperidone	☺	
Dothiepin	⚖	See amitriptyline.
Doxepin	⚖	See amitriptyline.
Droperidol	⚖	See antipsychotics.
Enalapril	☺	
Ergotamine	⊘	Avoid where possible.
Erythromycin	☺	But manufacturers advise caution.
Ethosuximide	⊘	May cause irritability and poor suckling – avoid.

Drug name/class	Safety (see key)	Comments
Etretinate	⊘	
Flucloxacillin	☺	
Fluconazole	⚖	Manufacturers advise to avoid.
Fluoxetine	⚖	Possible accumulation in infant.
Flupenthixol	⚖	See antipsychotics.
Fluphenazine	⚖	See antipsychotics.
Frusemide	☺	
Gentamicin	⚖	Use with caution.
Haloperidol	⚖	See antipsychotics.
Heparin	☺	
Hydralazine	☺	
Hyoscine	☺	
Ibuprofen	☺	
Imipramine	⚖	See amitriptyline.
Indomethacin	⚖	Manufacturers advise to avoid.
Insulin	☺	
Iodine	⊘	Breast feeding contraindicated as the iodine is concentrated in the milk and may cause hypothyroidism and goitre. Amiodarone is to be avoided similarly.
Isotretinoin	⊘	
Ketoconazole	⚖	Manufacturers advise to avoid.
Lamotrigene	⚖	Limited data.
Labetalol	☺	Consider monitoring of infant if doses high.
Lithium salts	⚖	Low incidence of effects on infants but monitor the baby for evidence of toxicity.
Lofepramine	⚖	See amitriptyline.
Mefanamic acid	☺	
Mefloquine	⚖	Safety not established.
Methyldopa	☺	
Metoclopramide	⚖	
Metronidazole	⚖	Manufacturers advise to avoid large doses.

Drug name/class	Safety (see key)	Comments
Naproxen	☺	Manufacturers advise to avoid.
Nifedipine	☺	Small amounts only but the manufacturers advise to avoid.
Nitrofurantoin	⚖	May cause neonatal haemolysis in G6PD deficient infants.
Nystatin	☺	
Oestrogens (e.g. OCP)	⊘	They suppress lactation.
Omeprazole	⚖	Manufacturers advise to avoid.
OPIATES	☺	Only a concern in dependent mothers where breastfeeding should be discouraged and controlled infant withdrawal supervised.
Paracetamol	☺	
Paroxetine	⚖	
Phenobarbitone	⚖	Use with caution. Potential for causing drowsiness.
Phenytoin	☺	Although manufacturers advise to avoid.
Prochlorperazine	⚖	See antipsychotics.
Progestogens	☺	These do not suppress lactation except in high doses but should not be started as conraceptives until after 3 weeks following delivery.
Proguanil	☺	However doses in milk are not high enough to adequately cover the baby.
Propylthiouracil	⚖	As small amounts are present only, the risk of neonatal hypothyroidism is low, but should be remembered.
Quinidine	☺	
Quinine	☺	
Ranitidine	☺	
Senna	⊘	
Sulphasalazine	⚖	Potential risk of neonatal haemolysis. Rashes and bloody diarrhoea reported.
Sulphonamides	⚖	Small risk of kernicterus and G6PD deficient haemolysis.
Sulphonylureas	⚖	Caution. Potential to cause neonatal hypoglycaemia.
Sulpiride	⊘	Present in large quantities in milk.
Terfenadine	⚖	See chlorpheniramine.
Tetracyclines	⊘	Risk of teeth discolouration.

Drug name/class	Safety (see key)	Comments
Theophylline	⚖	Caution. Neonatal irritability reported.
Thioridazine	⚖	See droperidol.
Thyroxine	☺	Theoretically may interfere with neonatal Guthrie screening.
Trimethoprim	☺	Short-term use acceptable.
Valproate	☺	
Vancomycin	⚖	Manufacturers advise to avoid.
Warfarin	☺	

APPENDIX III

BIOCHEMISTRY AND HAEMATOLOGY REFERENCE RANGES

The non-pregnant ranges are values widely quoted and are not necessarily derived from non pregnant women of child bearing age. The ranges given in the pregnancy column are taken from individual studies of healthy pregnant women. All pregnancy ranges are two standard deviations from the mean unless otherwise stated.

HAEMATOLOGY

Variable	Non-pregnant range	Pregnancy
Haemoglobin	11.5–16.0	10.6–12.8 (g/dL)
White cell count	4.0–11.0	In pregnancy the upper normal range extends to 14×10^9/L and during labour very high transient increases are commonly seen.
Packed cell volume (Haematocrit. L/L)	0.37–0.47	0.31–0.38
Mean cell volume (fL)	76–96	Values are slightly lower in pregnancy 74.4–95.6
Platelet count ($\times10^9$/L)	150–400	Platelet counts are slightly lower in pregnancy Values between 100 and 150 $\times10^9$/L are very common in the absence of pathology.
Plasma ferritin (μg/L)	20–300	Ferritin levels decline in 'normal' pregnancies, sometimes even below the lower limit of the nonpregnant range. Any value below 20 μg/L is indicative of deficient iron stores.
Serum iron (μmol/L)	11–30	Serum iron levels normally decline in pregnancy and continue to do so even if supplements are given. In iron deficiency iron levels will usually be below 10 μmol/L.

Variable	Non-pregnant range	Pregnancy
Red cell folate (μg/L)	160–640	The range quoted is wide. Folate deficiency is likely in pregnancy if the level is <150 μg/L.
Vitamin B_{12} (ng/L)	>150	A value of <100 ng/L is felt to be diagnostic of B_{12} deficiency in pregnancy.

BIOCHEMISTRY

Variable	Non-pregnant range	Pregnancy
Alanine amino transferase (ALT)	5–35 IU/L	5–31 IU/L
Albumin	35–50 g/L	22–40 g/L
Alkaline Phosphatase	30–300 IU/l	Higher levels are not always a sign of pathology – the placenta is a rich source of alkaline phosphatase.
Aspartate-amino transferase (AST)	5–35 IU/L	8–29 IU/L
Bilirubin	3–17 μmol/L	3–14 μmol/L
Calcium(ionized)	1.0–1.25 mmol/L	No significant change from non-pregnant values.
Calcium (total)	2.12–2.65 mmol/L	Pregnant values remain within the non-pregnant range but do decline a little during the first and second trimesters.
Chloride	90–105 mmol/L	Remain basically unchanged.
Total cholesterol	3.9–7.8 mmol/L	Levels can double in a normal pregnancy.
Creatinine	70–150 μmol/L	Values do fall during pregnancy and rise again in the last few weeks. 34–82 μmol/L
Glucose (fasting)	4.0–6.0 mmol/L	Plasma glucose levels do fall with advancing gestation with the majority of the drop occurring in the first trimester. 3.0–5.0 mmol/L A blood glucose of >6 mmol/L if fasted or more than 2 h from last food is abnormal, as is a glucose of >7 mmol/L at any time. Both should prompt further investigation for diabetes.
Glycosylated haemoglobin	6.0–8.5%	Remains basically unchanged.

Variable	Non-pregnant range	Pregnancy
Osmolality	278–305 mOsm/kg	Total osmolality falls by the end of the first trimester to a low of 8–10 mOsm/L below non-pregnant values.
Potassium	3.5–5.0 mmol/L	Remains basically unchanged.
Protein (total)	60–80 g/L	Total serum protein levels do fall in pregnancy. 55–73 g/L
Sodium	135–145 mmol/L	Remains basically unchanged.
Free T_4	11.0–22.9 pmol/L	Remain basically unchanged, although some assays can detect a fall in late pregnancy. 11.4–21.8 pmol/L (first trimester) 7.3–15 pmol/L (third trimester)
Triglyceride	0.55–1.9 mmol/L	There is a 3-fold increase in TG levels over the course of a pregnancy, peaking at 36 weeks.
TSH	0.5–5.7 mU/L	In the third trimester TSH levels increase so the upper limit of the normal reference range is raised to 7.0 mU/L.
Urea	2.5–6.7 mmol/L	Levels do fall in pregnancy. 2.4–4.3 mmol/L
Uric acid	150–390 umol/L	Levels fall during the first trimester and rise from 12 weeks onward. This normal rise is crucial to appreciate when interpreting results in the light of pre-eclampsia. A useful rule of thumb is that the gestation ×10 is the upper range of normal for that gestation.

APPENDIX IV

ENDOCRINOLOGICAL REFERENCE VALUES

Below are the reference ranges for hormones regularly encountered in obstetrics and gynaecology. These values do differ between individual laboratories somewhat and it is useful to annotate this table if significant differences exist with your own hospital. Note that these are non-pregnant values and that the units differ between the various hormones.

CYCLICAL HORMONES

Hormone	Early cycle (Follicular phase)	Midcycle (Periovulatory)	Late cycle (Luteal phase)	Menopausal
Oestradiol (pmol/L)	70–250	150–800	70–300	10–40
Progesterone (nmol/L)	<6	–	6–64 (>30 highly suggestive of ovulation)	
LH (IU/L)	5–10	50–95	2–8	
FSH (IU/L)	4–8	10–20	1–4	>40

NON-CYCLICAL HORMONES

TSH	0.5–5.7 mIU/L
Thyroxine (T_4)	70–140 nmol/L
Prolactin	<600 IU/L
Testosterone – women	<3.5 nmol/L
Androstenedione – women	3.5–7.0 nmol/L

APPENDIX V

SPERM PARAMETERS

(The World Health Organization 'normal' values)

Concentration	$>20\times10^6$/mL
Motility	>50% progressive motility
Morphology	>30% normal forms
Volume	2–5 mL
Liquefaction time	within 30 minutes
White blood cells	$<1\times10^6$ mL

Total motile sperm/ejaculate

Count × Motility × Volume

n.b. Sperm counts falling outside these ranges are not necessarily incompatible with spontaneous conception. Furthermore, more than one sample should be tested before it is concluded that sperm production is suboptimal.

appendices

APPENDIX VI

RISK OF DOWN'S SYNDROME PREGNANCY ACCORDING TO MATERNAL AGE

Maternal age at delivery	Risk of Down's Syndrome at delivery
15	1 : 1578
20	1 : 1528
25	1 : 1351
30	1 : 909
31	1 : 796
32	1 : 683
33	1 : 574
34	1 : 474
35	1 : 384
36	1 : 307
37	1 : 242
38	1 : 189
39	1 : 146
40	1 : 112
41	1 : 85
42	1 : 65
43	1 : 49
44	1 : 37
45	1 : 28
46	1 : 21
47	1 : 15
48	1 : 11
49	1 : 8
50	1 : 6

From Cuckle, H.S., Wald, N.J. & Thompson, S.G. (1987) Estimating a woman's risk of having a pregnancy associated with Down syndrome using her age and serum AFP level. *British Journal of Obstetrics and Gynaecology* **94**, 387–402.

APPENDIX VII

FIGO CLASSIFICATION OF GYNAECOLOGICAL MALIGNANCIES

CERVICAL

STAGE I

The carcinoma is strictly confined to the cervix. Note that extension into the body of the uterus does not alter staging.

Stage Ia

Invasion is not clinically obvious, identified only at microscopy.

- **StageIa1**: Depth of invasion is no greater than 3 mm and no wider than 7 mm.
- **StageIa2**: Depth of invasion is greater than 3 mm but no more than 5 mm and no wider than 7 mm.

Stage Ib

Clinically obvious lesions or preclinical lesions with invasion greater than 5 mm and/or wider than 7 mm.

- **Stage Ib1**: Clinical lesions no greater than 4 cm
- **Stage Ib2**: Clinical lesions gretater than 4 cm

STAGE II

Extension of the carcinoma beyond the cervix (not including corpus uteri) but not onto the pelvic side wall and/or the carcinoma involves the vagina but only the upper two-thirds.

Stage IIa

Vaginal involvement of the upper two thirds but no extension into the parametrium.

Stage IIb

Obvious parametrial involvement but not onto the pelvic side wall.

STAGE III

The tumour is included in this stage if:

- the carcinoma has extended to the pelvic side wall
- the tumour involves the lower third of the vagina
- the tumour involves the ureters causing hydronephrosis or impaired kidney function.

Stage IIIa

No extension onto the pelvic side wall but involvement of the lower third of the vagina.

Stage IIIb

Extension onto the pelvic side wall or hydronephrosis/non-functioning kidney.

STAGE IV

Extension of the carcinoma beyond the true pelvisor, there is mucosal involvement of the bladder or rectum.

Stage IVa

Spread of the tumour onto adjacent pelvic organs

Stage IVb

Spread to distant organs.

VULVAL

STAGE I

Lesion must be 2 cm or smaller and confined to the vulva or perineum with no lymph node metastases.

Stage Ia

The above with stromal invasion of 1.0 mm or less.

Stage Ib

The above with stromal invasion greater than 1.0 mm.

STAGE II

Lesion is greater than 2 cm in its largest dimension but confined to the vulva/perineum with no nodal metastases.

STAGE III

Lesion is any size but has:

- spread to the lower urethra and/or the vagina or anus and/or
- associated unilateral regional lymph node involvement.

STAGE IV

Stage IVa

The tumour has invaded the upper urethra, bladder mucosa, rectal mucosa, pelvic bones and/or has associated bilateral regional lymph node metastases.

Stage IVb

Any distant metastases including pelvic lymph nodes.

EPITHELIAL OVARIAN

STAGE I

Growth is limited to the ovaries.

Stage Ia

Growth limited to one ovary. No ascites present.

- **Stage Ia1**: No tumour on external surface of the ovary. Capsule intact.
- **Stage Ia2**: Tumour on the external surface and/or capsule ruptured.

Stage Ib

Growth limited to both ovaries. No ascites present.

- **Stage Ib1**: No tumour on external surface of the ovaries. Capsules intact.
- **Stage Ib2**: Tumour on the external surface of one or both of the ovaries and/or capsule ruptured.

Stage Ic

Stage Ia or Ib with ascites or positive peritoneal washings.

STAGE II

Pelvic extension.

Stage IIa

Extension or metastases to the uterus and/or fallopian tubes.

Stage IIb

Extension to other pelvic tissues.

Stage IIc

Stage IIa or IIb with ascites or positive peritoneal washings.

STAGE III

- One or both ovaries affected and
  - intraperitoneal metastases outside the pelvis and/or
  - positive retroperitoneal nodes.

Or

- Tumour limited to the true pelvis with histologically proved malignant extension to the small bowel/omentum.

STAGE IV

- Tumour involves one or both ovaries with distant metastases.
- If pleural effusion is present there must be positive cytology to allocate this stage.
- Parenchymal liver metastases justify stage IV.

ENDOMETRIAL

STAGE I

Confined to the body of the uterus.

Stage Ia

Tumour is limited to the endometrium.

Stage Ib

Invasion of less than half the thickness of the myometrium.

Stage Ic

Invasion of greater than half the thickness of the myometrium.

STAGE II

Involvement of the cervix.

Stage IIa

Involvement of the endocervical glands of the cervix only.

Stage IIb

Cervical stromal invasion.

STAGE III

Pelvic extension.

Stage IIIa

Tumour invasion to the serosa and/or adnexa and/or positive peritoneal cytology.

Stage IIIb

Metastases to the vagina.

Stage IIIc

Metastases to the pelvic and/or para-aortic lymph nodes.

STAGE IV

Extrapelvic extension.

Stage IVa

Tumour invasion of the bladder and or bowel mucosa.

Stage IVb

Distant metastases including intra-abdominal and/or inguinal lymph nodes.

APPENDIX VIII

CHARTS

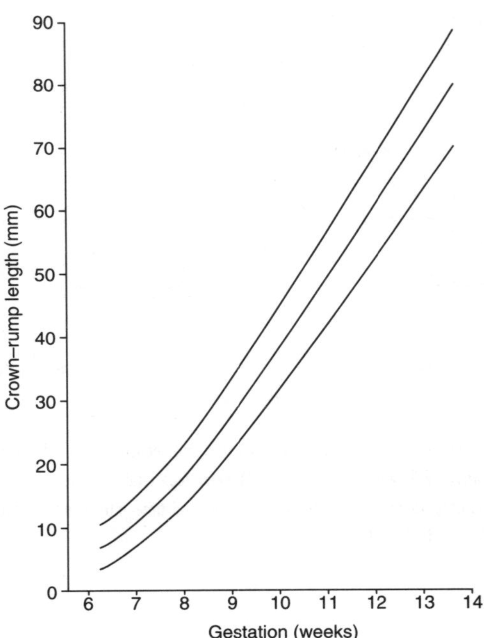

Figure A.1 Relationship between crown rump length and gestational age. (From Robinson, H.P. and Fleming, J.E.E. (1975) *British Journal of Obstetrics and Gynaecology*, **82**: 702, with kind permission of the authors and publishers).

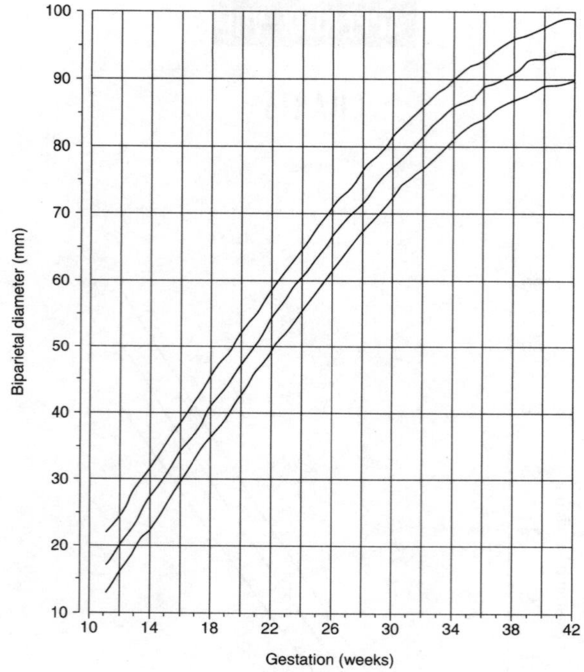

Figure A.2 Relationship between biparietal diameter and menstrual age. (From Hadlock, F.P., Deter, R.L., Harrist, R.B. and Park, S.K. (1982) Fetal biparietal diameter: a critical re-evaluation of the relationship to menstrual age by means of real-time ultrasound. *Journal of Ultrasound in Medicine*, **1**: 97–104.

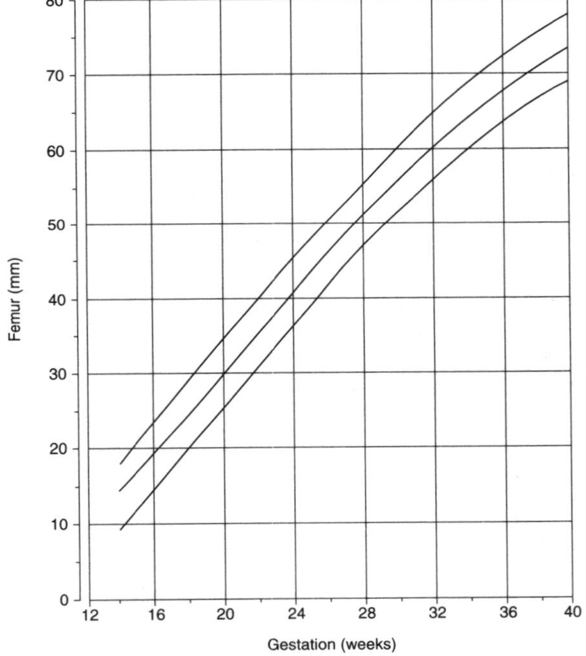

Figure A.3 Growth of the femur with gestational age. (From Warda, A.H., Deter, R.L. and Rossavik, I.K. (1985) Fetal femur length: a critical re-evaluation of the relationship to menstrual age. *Obstetrics and Gynaecology*, **66**: 69–75.

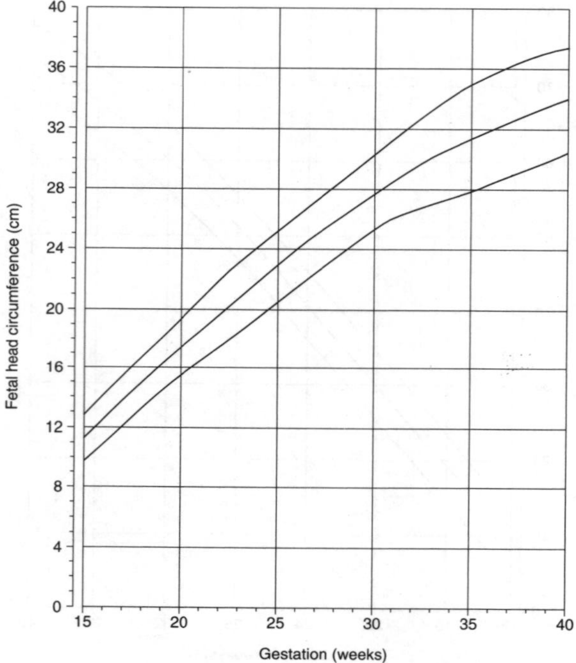

Figure A.4 Relationship between head circumference and menstrual age. (From Hadlock, F.P., Deter, R.L., Harrist, R.B. and Park, S.K. (1982) Fetal head circumference: relation to menstrual age. *American Journal of Radiology*, **38**: 647–53).

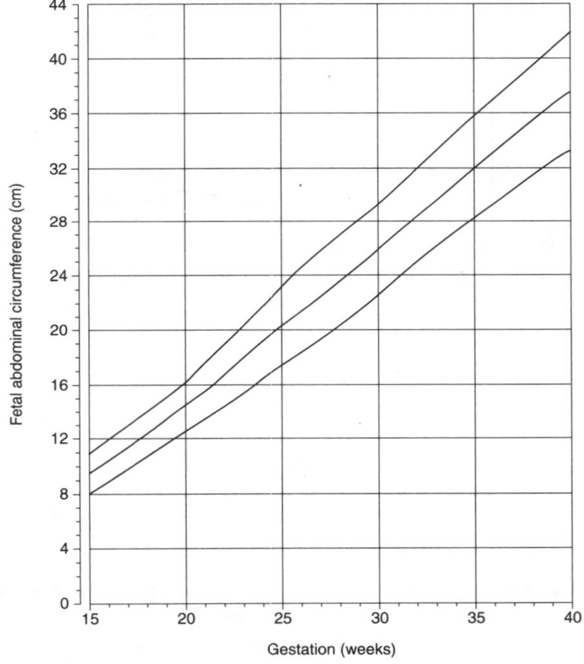

Figure A.5 Growth of the abdominal circumference with gestational age. (From Deter, R.L., Harrist, R.B., Hadlock, F.P. and Carpenter, R.J. (1982) Fetal head and abdominal circumferences: II a critical re-evaluation of the relationship to menstrual age. *Journal of Clinical Ultrasound*, **10**: 365–72.)

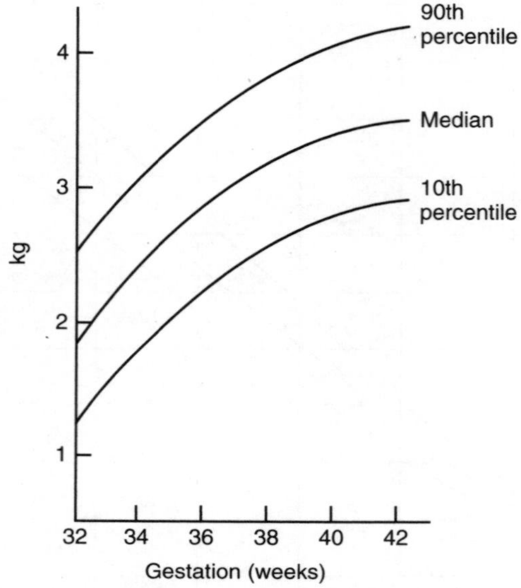

Figure A.6 Relationship between birth weight and gestational age. These data are taken from a study of Scottish newborns between 1948 and 1964. Equivalent data varies between populations for genetic and socioeconomic reasons. This has to be borne in mind when using it to assess the weight of a baby from a different population group. (From Thompson, A.M., Billewicz, W.Z. and Hytten, F.E. (1968) The assessment of fetal growth. *Journal of Obstetrics and Gynaecology British Comm.*, **75**: 903–16).

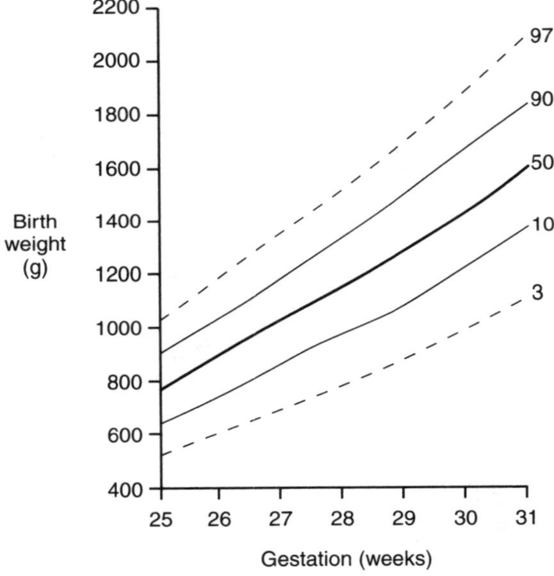

Figure A.7 Birth weight centiles for babies of 25–31 weeks. From *Handbook of Neonatal Intensive Care*, H.L. Halliday, G. McClure and M. Reido. Published by Baillière Tindall.

Table A.1 Imperial to metric weight conversion table

Pounds	Ounces															
	0	1	2	3	4	5	6	7	8	9	10	11	12	13	14	15
1	0.46	0.48	0.51	0.54	0.565	0.595	0.625	0.65	0.68	0.71	0.74	0.765	0.795	0.825	0.85	0.88
2	0.91	0.935	0.96	0.99	1.02	1.045	1.075	1.105	1.13	1.16	1.19	1.2	1.245	1.275	1.305	1.33
3	1.36	1.385	1.415	1.445	-1.47	1.5	1.53	1.555	1.585	1.61	1.64	1.67	1.695	1.725	1.755	1.785
4	1.81	1.84	1.87	1.895	1.925	1.955	1.98	2.01	2.025	2.065	2.095	2.12	2.15	2.18	2.21	2.235
5	2.27	2.29	2.32	2.35	2.375	2.405	2.435	2.46	2.5	2.53	2.555	2.585	2.605	2.635	2.66	2.69
6	2.72	2.745	2.775	2.8	2.83	2.86	2.885	2.915	2.945	2.975	3	3.03	3.06	3.085	3.115	3.145
7	3.17	3.2	3.225	3.255	3.285	3.31	3.34	3.365	3.395	3.425	3.455	3.48	3.51	3.54	3.565	3.595
8	3.63	3.65	3.68	3.71	3.735	3.765	3.795	3.82	3.85	3.88	3.905	3.935	3.965	3.99	4.02	4.05
9	4.08	4.105	4.135	4.16	4.19	4.22	4.245	4.275	4.305	4.335	4.36	4.39	4.42	4.445	4.475	4.5
10	4.53	4.56	4.585	4.615	4.645	4.67	4.7	4.73	4.755	4.785	4.815	4.84	4.87	4.9	4.925	4.955
11	4.99	5.01	5.04	5.065	5.095	5.125	5.155	5.18	5.21	5.29	5.265	5.295	5.325	5.35	5.38	5.41
12	5.44															

From *Handbook of Neonatal Intensive Care* H.L. Halliday, G. McClure & M. Reid. Published by Baillière Tindall.

APPENDIX IX

LIST OF SUGGESTED POSTGRADUATE TEXTS

1. Enkin, M., Keirse, M. J. N. C., Renfrew, M. & Neilson, J. (1995) *A Guide to Effective Care in Pregnancy and Childbirth* (2nd edition). Oxford University Press.
2. James, D. K., Ramsay, M. M., Steer, P. J., Weiner, C. P. & Gonik, B. (1999) *High Risk Pregnancy: Management Options.* London: W. B. Saunders.
3. Gibb, D. & Arulkumaran, S. (1992). *Fetal Monitoring in Practice.* Oxford: Butterworth-Heinemann.
4. de Swiet, M. & Chamberlain, G. (Editors) (1992) *Basic Sciences in Obstetrics and Gynaecology: A Textbook For MRCOG Part I (2nd edition).* Edinburgh: Churchill Livingstone.
5. Chudleigh, P. & Pearce, J. M. (1992) *Obstetric Ultrasound: How, Why and When (2nd edition).* Edinburgh: Churchill Livingstone.
6. Briggs, G. G., Freeman, R. K. & Yaffe, S. Y. (1998) *Drugs in Pregnancy and Lactation. (5th edition).* Williams and Wilkins.
7. Loudon, N. (Editor) (1991) *Handbook of Family Planning (2nd edition).* Edinburgh: Churchill Livingstone.
8. Clements, R. V. (1994) *Safe Practice in Obstetrics and Gynaecology: A Medicolegal Handbook.* Edinburgh: Churchill Livingstone.

INDEX

Note – Page numbers in italic type indicate tables.